T0299502

TWOCHUBBYCUBS

FULL-ON FLAVOUR

TWOCHUBBYCUBS

FULL-ON FLAVOUR

100+ tasty, slimming meals under 500 calories

James and Paul Anderson

Photography by
Liz and Max Haarala Hamilton

yellow kite

CONTENTS

INTRODUCTION

Well, hello there! May we say, before we get started, how well you're looking! We love what you've done with your hair. We're already jealous, and we're only twenty-eight words in. If you're reading this, there's a very good chance you've either bought our book or are flicking through it in the shop trying to decide whether we're the right fit for you. Well, we're barely the right fit for a shipping container, but we try our best. Let's introduce ourselves and tell you why this book will work for you.

At this point in our adventure, regular readers will of course be familiar with our story, and we apologise for repeating ourselves, but we still have to get the formalities out of the way. We are James and Paul, the twochubbycubs – a married couple of ne'er-do-wells from Oop North who have inexplicably turned a sarcastic healthy food blog into a series of cookbooks. Paul is the chap who cooks and I'm the writer who strangles each and every metaphor he meets to within an inch of its life. Nice to meet you, or to see you again.

Twochubbycubs was born out of the sheer despair we felt at cooking 'healthy' recipes – they were nearly always tasteless, watery, joyless concoctions designed to fill you up with no real regard for the taste or appeal of the dish. We started cooking our own versions and discovered that taking a light-hearted approach (i.e. adding smut) seemed to resonate with folks who were tired of the same old slop. We used our recipes to lose weight, accelerated by a challenge for a TV show (how the sheer terror of appearing on ITV helps to focus the mind!), and managed to drop almost ten stone each. More importantly, we've kept it off, and we've never gone without our favourite foods or drink. Listen, I'm from Newcastle: if I gave up drinking I'd probably be asked to hand back my passport and be personally driven over the border by one of Ant or Dec.

As this book is based on the blogging style we are known for, you'll find each recipe is prefaced with either a few lines about the ingredients or some random puff-piece that seems entirely disconnected from the meal you see in front of you. That's our style and how we've kept ourselves entertained over the years . . . well, that and polyamory. That's our neighbour, she's a terror. As the writing is about us as a couple but written by me as a person, I sometimes slip into the wrong third person, but that's fine, I just apologise to Paul, promise never to do it again and take over the ironing duties for a few weeks as penance. We try our best to get it right, but also understand this may trouble the Grammar Buff. That's our other neighbour: she may be old, but she sure loves to show off her bits.

When it came to brainstorming ideas for the fourth book, we confess we were torn. We had already covered our classics in the first book (imaginatively titled *The Cookbook*), speedy and delicious meals in our second, *Fast and Filling*, and then for our third, we gave half the nation a reason to spit at us in the street by devoting a book entirely to *Dinner Time*, a selection of evening meals. You would not believe the venom some people have regarding whether the evening meal is called dinner or tea, I can tell you. So what for book four?

My initial suggestion of having a book of aubergine, cucumber and banana recipes and calling it *twochubbycubs: Hard to Swallow* was

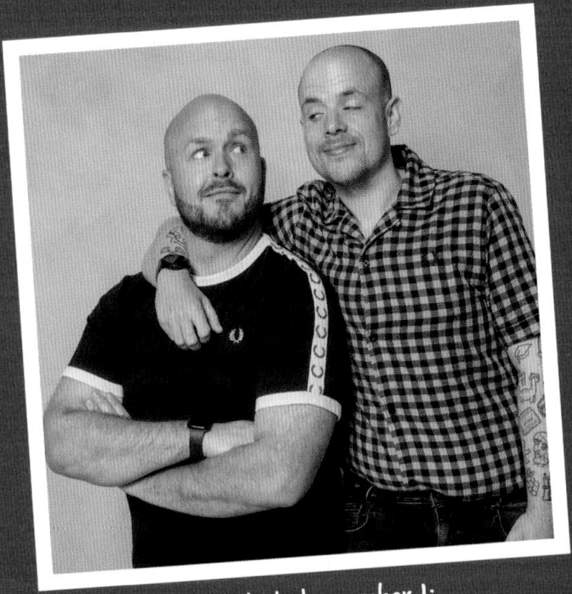

Rejected photo number 1:
Paul at wrong height, also looks like
James is breaking wind

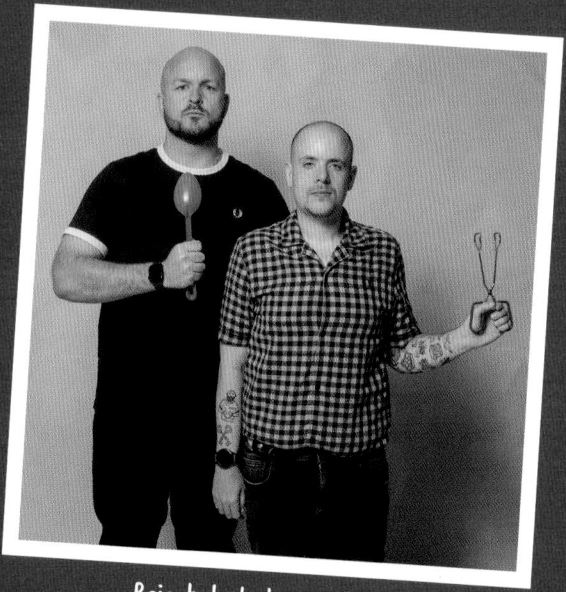

Rejected photo number 2:
Looks like we're about to give
someone a medical exam

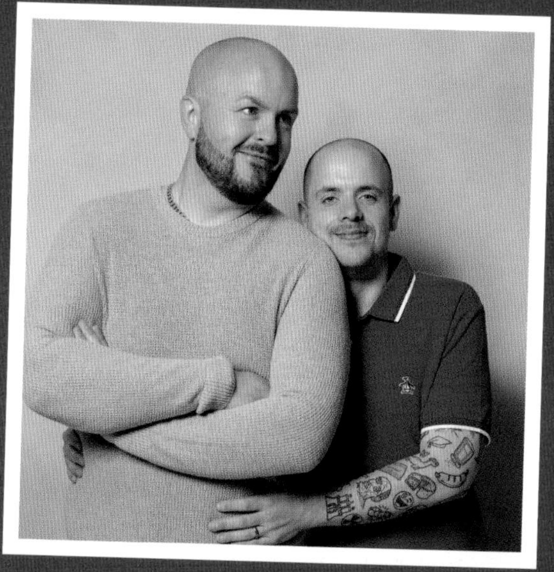

Rejected photo number 3:
Almost the winner, but James spotted
someone fit walking past the window
at the last second. Also looks like we're
announcing a pregnancy

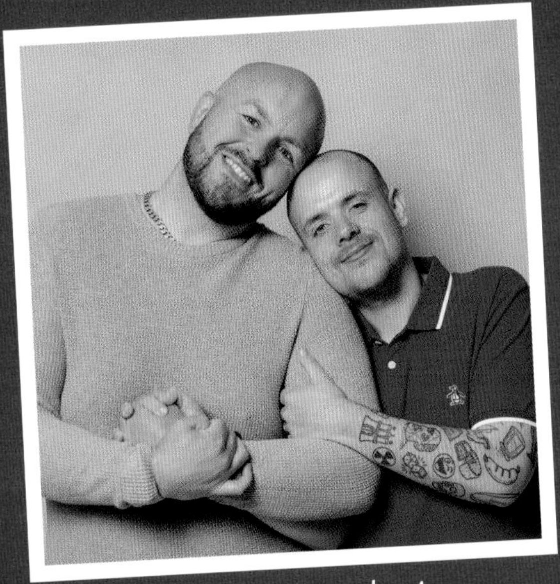

Rejected photo number 4:
Knew wearing superglue as hair
polish was a bad idea

deemed inappropriate. Fair enough, nobody needs more cucumber in their life. Paul suggested a pasta book, but we soon realised that I'd give myself an actual hernia trying to shoehorn even more pasta puns into print. Discussions went back and forth, usually consisting of me excitedly grabbing Paul's hand or shaking him awake and getting as far as 'How about we . . .' before being told absolutely not and the country isn't ready for a compilation of recipes made entirely in a blast furnace. Poor sport.

Two possible suggestions *were* seriously considered: a budget book and an air fryer book. We dismissed the air fryer book on the basis that, whisper it, if we're honest with one another, an air fryer is just a teensy-tiny oven. There, I said it, and it feels good to get that off my chest. They're wondrous little machines for saving energy, though, so we can't knock them – and it's always a treat to see the next 'big thing' in the home-cooking world: we've survived the slow-cooker era, the batch-cook times, the 'stick everything in a wrap' golden years . . . can't wait to see what's next!

We started writing a budget book instead, only to struggle with making our recipes even more budget-friendly than they are now. You must understand that Paul and I are both notoriously as tight as a tick's nipsy at the best of times, and as a consequence, our meals are always about creating delicious, healthy meals with cheap, easily sourced ingredients. We were *already* budget-friendly. There's a more serious side to this coin, too: what is considered budget for two chaps with pink pounds in their pockets might be well beyond the reach of others. I've always thought there was something slightly inappropriate about those more fortunate dishing out tips on how to eke out a roast dinner or what to do with leftover lamb, as though they know what it is to truly budget. I remember stealing potatoes out of nearby farmers' fields when I was young, Paul grew up on whatever microwave dinners were on special offer at the local shop, and when we got together we had barely a penny to rub together. Luckily, being in the first flush of romance, we found other things to rub to keep us busy.

So we ditched the budget idea, but instead incorporated a lot of those recipes into this book, which we believe is the most 'us' book we have done so far. We've concentrated on the three values that have kept us true throughout the decade we've been in this game, namely:

- **making healthy, full-of-flavour meals that don't taste like you're 'on a diet'**
- **using ingredients that are cheap, plentiful and easy to find**
- **cooking meals that everyone can enjoy together**

As a result, we promise that every single meal in this book – whether it's the **delicious breakfasts**, the **perfect brunches**, the **sumptuous snacks** or the **best-ever dinners** (or teas, don't send us letters!) – will leave you satisfied, full and more importantly, happy! They're all easy to cook, because as we have said before, we're not chefs – there's going to be no tricky cooking styles or fancy equipment needed. If you saw us in the kitchen, you would understand. It's like watching cats trying to parallel-park a burning car. If you've got a sharp knife, a good cooking pot and a can-do attitude, our delicious meals will be your reward. Each meal is designed to be enjoyed together: no cooking a special 'diet' meal while everyone else eats what they like. This is healthy eating done exactly as it ought to be and as we've always done it: fabulously.

Now, before we go, the plea we make in all our books: if you're picking up this book, there's a good chance you may be wanting to lose some weight. That's great, but make sure you're doing that for the right reason. If you're losing weight so you feel fitter, healthier and happier, then superb – but do it for yourself, and no one else. Cheesy as it is, it was only when we learned what worked for us personally, as opposed to being told by someone else the weight we should be, that it finally stuck with us. For the first time in our books we're including sections on calorie counting and exercise, purely so we can discuss how we've managed to keep the weight off, but please know that we're not insisting you do either of these. In words that I may as well get tattooed on my forehead (and believe me, there's enough space on there for two copies of this book and a list of why Paul is wrong in any given situation) – **whatever works for you, works for you**.

Anyway, look at the time, we've got cooking to do! Enjoy every mouthful, we certainly did!

James and Paul x

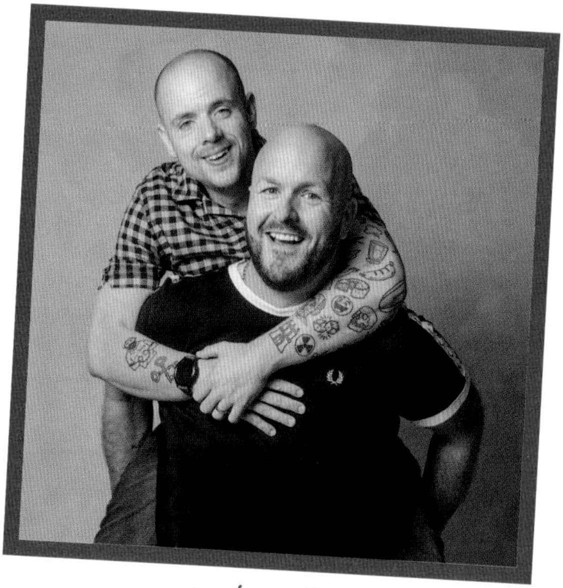

our favourite!!

KEEP IN TOUCH AND TAG US WITH YOUR FLAVOURSOME MEALS!

twochubbycubs

@twochubbycubs

@twochubbycubs

SOME HANDY SYMBOLS ON HOW TO USE THE BOOK:

Like our previous bestselling books, we've marked each recipe with our handy set of symbols to streamline your cooking needs.

Over 30 mins	30 mins or under	Freezes well
Easy to scale	Under 10 ingredients	Blog recipe
V Vegetarian	GF Gluten free	DF Dairy free

Don't forget, the calories given on each recipe are per portion!

CALORIE COUNTING

The eagle-eyed among you, and those with glasses that could set your neck on fire if you look into bright sunlight, will have spotted over the last few books that we are all about the calories these days. Although we have written in exhaustive depth across the blog and social media about why we made the switch, it seems we never committed our reasons to actual print. I know, a shocking lapse in attention, but then you are talking to someone who's had a pair of scratty white briefs stuck on the corner of his roof for over a year. Storm Antoni blew them off the washing line, and it would take a matter of moments to hook them down, but that's a lot of effort. Plus, I like to think the neighbours imagine we hurled them out of the window in a frisson of passion ... give them something to mull over.

Forever conscious of the fact that we don't want to look as though we're suggesting one type of weight loss is any better than another, let us say straight off that if whatever you're currently doing works for you, then you simply must carry on with it. Unless it's hard drugs and sleazy living: we can't really be seen to endorse that. When we ask if anyone 'has any numbers', we're only after the calorific value of a packet of microwave rice, thank you. No, the paean to calorie counting that follows is entirely our own experience, and we include it purely to offer up a different view.

Paul and I loved our weekly slimming club visit. Admittedly, I say loved in the sense one might love the relief following the removal of an ingrowing toenail, but even so. It's all we knew for a good decade or so – where other young couples were out partying and living it up, we were sitting in a church hall listening to someone extol the virtues of yoghurt while we played last-person-to-clap. There was always a great sense of camaraderie, which we enjoyed; we had (mainly) great leaders and, hand on heart, I can see why people keep going there because everyone having a common purpose (mainly being first to the chip shop afterwards) is helpful.

The weekly weigh-in also helped focus the mind and keep us from 'straying' – the fear of getting on those scales and seeing the numbers blink upwards rather than downwards was generally enough to stop us reaching for the biscuit tin. We would all troop in, pay our dues, queue up while Sandra plugged in the machine, reset the scales, found her pen, held a forty-minute conversation with the first person in the queue ...

We would take our seats, make polite small-talk about what we'd eaten that week and how uncomfortable the chairs were, get the latest on Andrew's troubling bowel movements, then a hush would descend and we would undergo an hour-long creative thinking class where everyone desperately tried to come up with ever more elaborate reasons for why they hadn't lost weight that week. A particular highlight for me was when a member took great pains to explain that she had gained four pounds as her neighbour was having their roof done that week. Now forgive me, but unless her air fryer and müllerlight stash was kept in her neighbour's loft, I couldn't see the link. Still, at least we all got our Silver Exercise sticker that week, thanks in no small part to the mental gymnastics we went through.

Actually, thinking about it now, as someone who had a full deck of roofers and scaffolders at his house for a few weeks after the house had burned down, I can see why eating healthily was the last thing on her mind. I walked around with such a lickerish leer for those six weeks that I'm surprised my glasses stayed on my ears.

Occasionally we would triumph and one of us would win the prize for losing the most weight that week, usually a fruit basket that you would have to sieve in order to find the one apple that wasn't halfway to being cider. Good times. Then out the door we would go (if the leader had decided to go through the group alphabetically, you best believe that us Andersons were already in the car backing out of the car park by the time she got to 'Anderton'), to celebrate our weight loss with some horrifically greasy food, and the cycle would continue. Lose some weight, hit a mini-target, reward ourselves with 'bad' food. Sometimes that reward would become a full week off, then we'd put off going back to class, then rejoin a few weeks later ever so slightly heavier.

And that's the issue, at least for us. We weren't losing weight, we were simply cycling through the same one or two stone over and over. Occasionally we'd scrape to three stone, but then fatigue would set in and we'd pile it all back on, eating what we liked, telling ourselves we could have the chocolate and the chips and the crisps and the booze because we would be able to rejoin and shift it 'for good' the next time. After all, it works, doesn't it?

Nope. When we managed to be good and swerve the above trap, we'd fall into an entirely different one. Our initial big weight losses would slow down, despite us sticking to what we'd been eating before. What used to be a 5lb or 4lb loss would become 2lb, 1lb, an inexplicable stay the same. Looking back now, with the endless benefit of hindsight, this slowdown in weight loss is inevitable as you lose weight for the reason I touch upon next, but what ticks me off something chronic is how much we used to beat ourselves up over it, or worse, be encouraged to lose big amounts each week without changing what we were doing. It was never really addressed, only ever put down to 'not following the plan correctly' or blamed on exercise. Bloody exercise! I kid you not: we once had a temporary leader tell us with barely concealed contempt that we shouldn't walk to work because too much exercise can affect losses. I responded by upping my walking immediately, namely across the hall and out of the door.

Speaking of which, the epiphany that it wasn't a good fit for us came when we started exercising properly as part of our big weight loss for television, and, newly conscious of the number of calories we were burning via the cheery displays on our smartwatch, began looking at exactly how many we were eating in our 'free' meals. Let me give you an example: one of the main meals Paul and I used to enjoy was a big plate of air-fried chips (done in oil, with a beef stock cube crumbled over at the start – try it, it's lovely) with a packet (each) of those instant pasta 'n' sauce meals on top, with our allowance of cheese scattered on top of that. My wrist used to ache carrying the plates through to the living room. A quick fag-packet calculation puts that dinner at 560 calories for the potatoes, 430 calories for the pasta and 130 calories for the cheese. 1,120 calories for a simple evening meal which was 'free'. Factor in a 500-calorie 'free' breakfast, a 750-calorie 'free' lunch and then the calories of all the snacks we had because 'we could use our points', and we would easily be topping out over 3,000 calories a day.

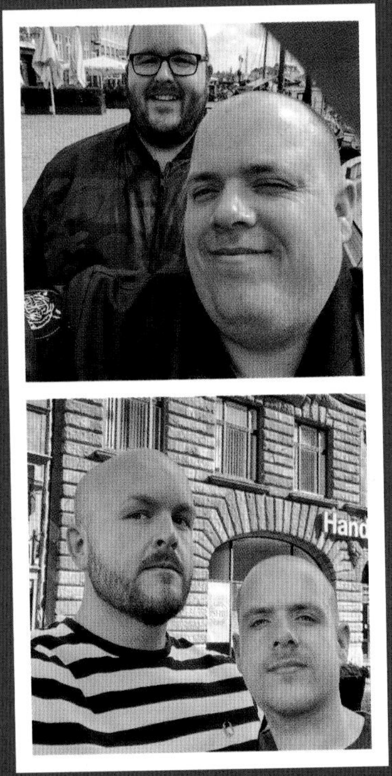

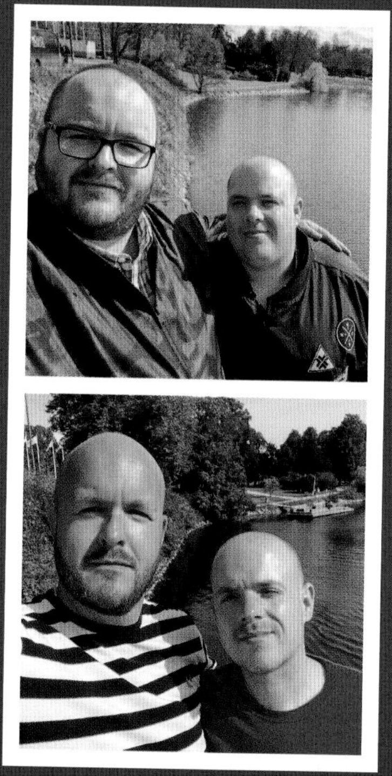

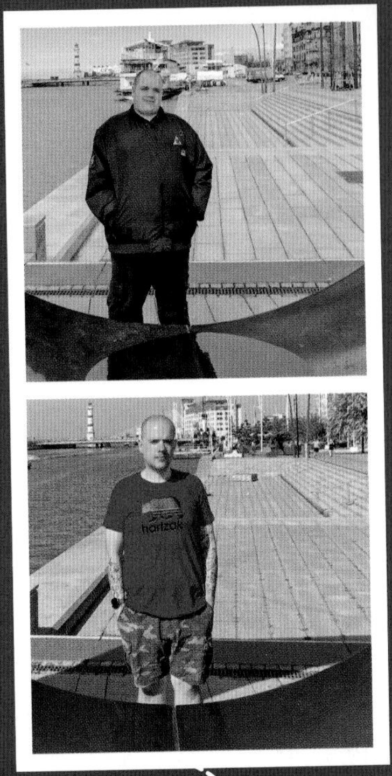

These photos were taken almost exactly five years apart in Copenhagen – from when we were at our heaviest (2018) to now (2023).

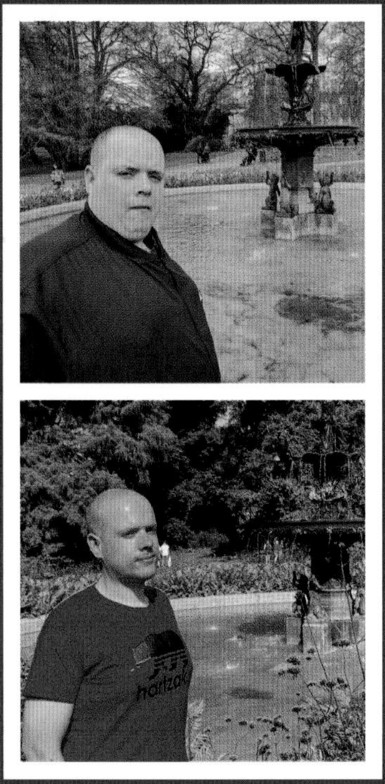

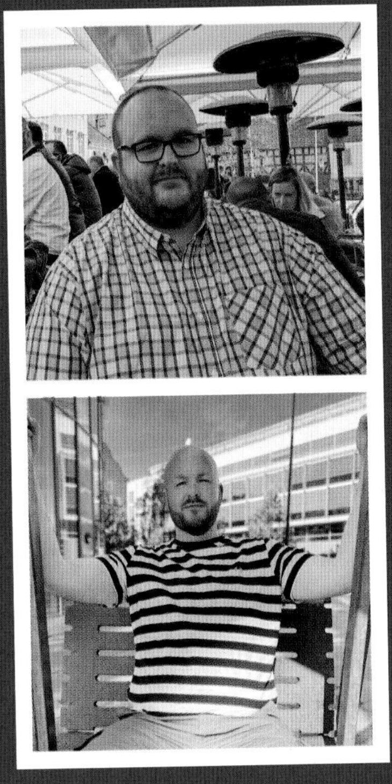

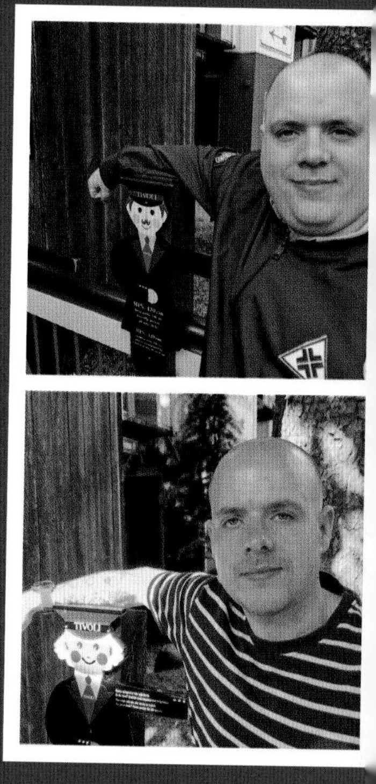

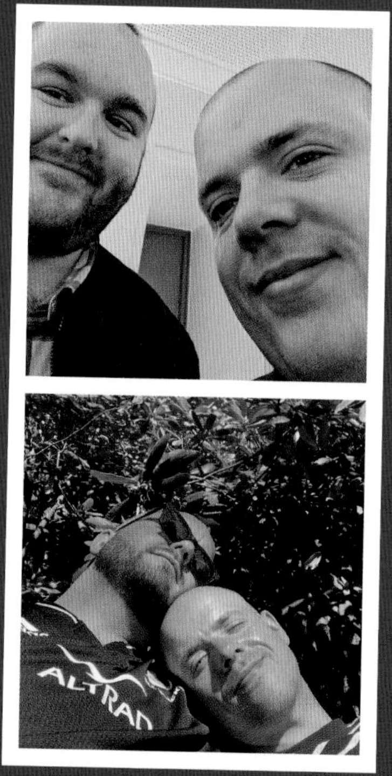

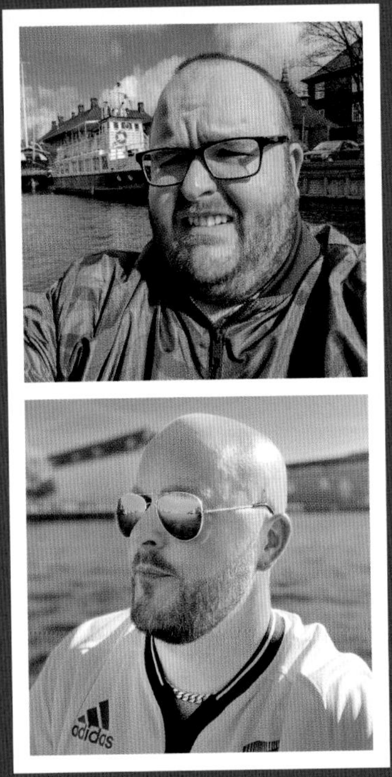

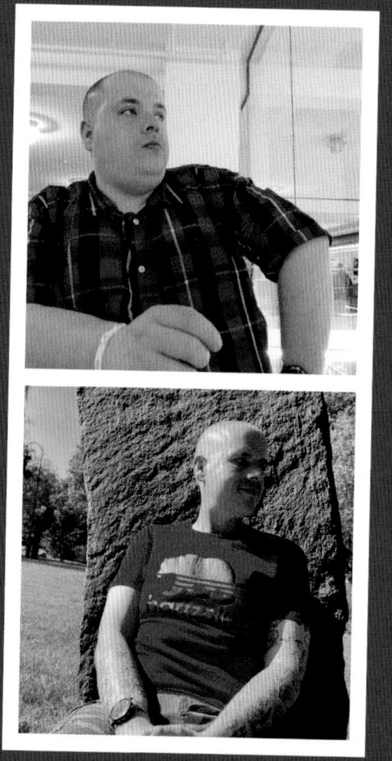

We tend not to 'see' our weight loss until we compare like this – still got those Freeman's catalogue poses down though!

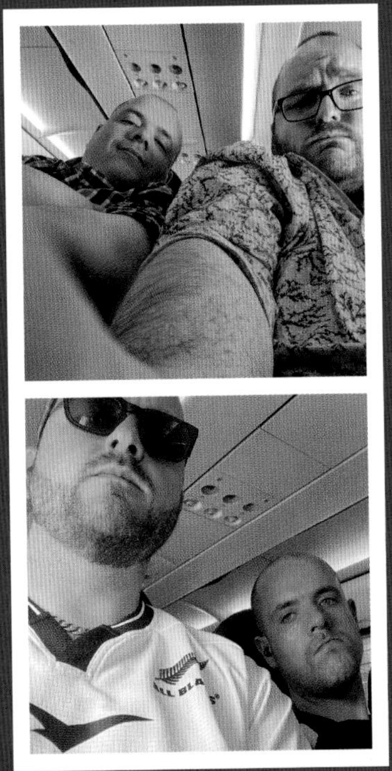

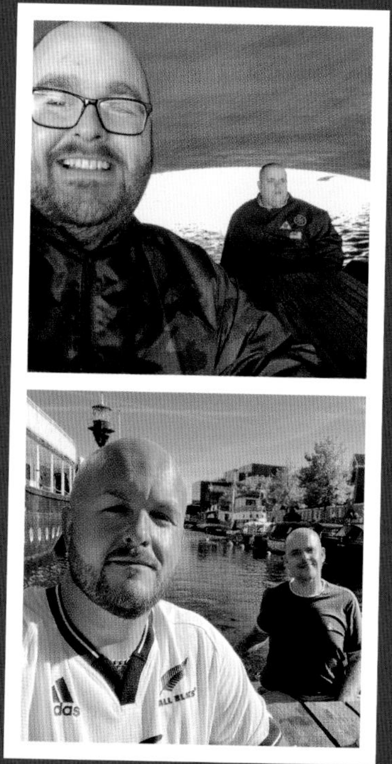

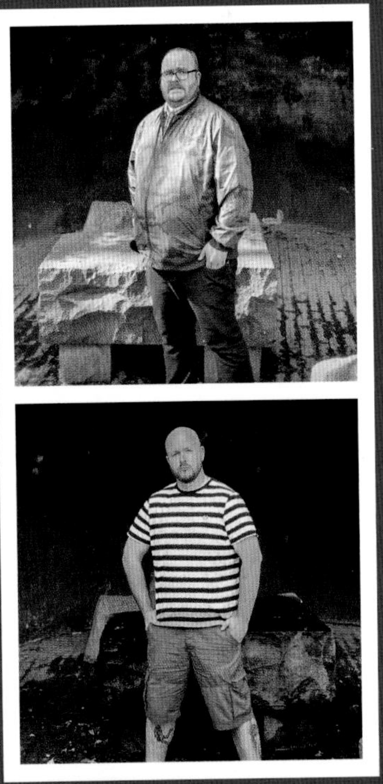

When you are as overweight as we were, your body burns more calories just through existence alone – everything from keeping your heart going to making sure you have enough energy to get out and about. It's why, as you lose weight, you need to lower your calorie intake as you go to compensate. A minibus needs less fuel than a coach, after all. This explained why we would lose the weight initially, but it would stall and slow down. It wasn't because we weren't trying, it was because we were ignoring the simple scientific fact that to lose weight, you need to reduce the amount going in. Plus, eating 3,000 calories a day under the guise of 'it's free, it's fine' is absolutely stupid.

We decided at that point that the slimming club model wasn't for us, and, buoyed with how easy everything had become in terms of tracking apps and new technology, decided to give calorie counting a go. We worked out our total daily energy expenditure (TDEE) via Nutracheck (our favourite calorie-tracking app – not paid to endorse it, just happy to mention it because it works so ruddy well), shaved a little bit off and started tracking everything that passed our lips.

Not going to lie: for the first couple of weeks, it was a hard habit to form. Especially coming on the back of years and years of half-heartedly counting our points, and sneaking in all those little extras that you didn't 'count', but it doesn't take too long to bed in. If you're using an app, it's even quicker – mostly you scan the barcode of what you're consuming and away you go. You can see through the day how much you have left, and work to that accordingly. It's tempting to consistently come in under your target, but that way lies ruin, not least because your body needs a set amount of calories just to function.

The weight loss that followed, although a shade slower than what we had experienced before, was significant and, more importantly, consistent. We didn't hit a plateau, just lost a little each week and kept on going. Those of you who bought our previous book, *Dinner Time*, will have read my piece about focusing on losing 1lb a week, and it's something I keep repeating – chasing big numbers will only ever lead to disappointment.

The most liberating thing with calorie counting is the freedom it gives you. Now, that might sound paradoxical, given you are having to track and stay loosely within your limits, but hear me out. No food is 'bad', there's no stupid rules to adhere to (for example, it doesn't matter whether you chew, mash or inhale your ruddy banana), and there's no guilt involved. My calorie target, at my weight and activity level, is around 2,500 a day for a consistent, slow loss. You'd be amazed how much you can fit into 2,500 calories, I can tell you. Paul's daily target is lower, because he's the height of an upturned matchbox, but even his gives him enough freedom to have a lunchbox of various snacks during the day in lieu of a big lunch. He prefers that, because he's such an Action Jackson.

Speaking of Action Jackson, let's quickly mention exercise. The more exercise you do, the more calories you gain to play with. You'd be surprised how much 'extra' you gain by simply upping the exercise, although it's important to note that your TDEE value already takes into account what you've said you do – so if you suggested you ran marathons when you first worked it out, you can't then decide to have another 600 calories on top of your allowance if you're not doing anything extra. But if your calorie target was worked out on the basis that you have an office job and sit on your bum all day, and then you start building a bit of swimming and walking into that, your target should adjust accordingly. Think of it like this: if you ordinarily put £70 of petrol in the car and that covers you for your commute into work each week, then you suddenly decide to go via a different town forty miles away each day because you're having a steamy affair, you'll need to top that tank up with more fuel. Also, you dirty bugger, you should be ashamed. Though think of the extra calories you'll burn (around four calories a minute, fact fans – and you best believe I spend that extra two calories well).

Some people ask us to include macros in the book – that is, the nutritional breakdown of each meal. There's a reason we don't: approximating calories is one thing (and just for clarity, all calorie counts in this book are approximate!), but macros are different. Say we suggest using one chicken breast in a recipe – we might use a chicken breast that looks like a shotputter's arm, you might use one that looks like a skinned goldfish. Thus, the protein level we worked out would be considerably different to what you have, and if you're looking at your nutrition on a macro level, it's important that it is recorded correctly. If you're taking note of your macros – whether for medical reasons, weight loss or curiosity – we again recommend Nutracheck – it works everything out for you. Other apps are available, of course.

Now that we have been doing calorie counting for a few years, we find it is entirely second nature to us. We don't need to use the app all the time because we can keep track in our heads roughly how many calories we have spent, and because it isn't an exact science, as long as we aren't going too crazy, we don't need the app. That does take time and you'll find yourself occasionally having to double check calorie counts if you aren't sure. There are days when we know we will be well over our calorie limit, but who cares (not me, because it usually means I'm out on the pop) – we just lower our limit a little the next few days and balance it out. I think it speaks to the success of calorie counting that my weight, previously like my underwear (forever up and down), has stayed consistent.

Interestingly, neither of us weigh ourselves as a matter of course these days. I'm hovering around the weight bracket I'm happiest in (between 17.5 and 18.5 stone), and I can tell by my clothes and, more importantly, the volume of noise I make as I ease myself out of a chair, how my weight is doing. I can't begin to tell you how liberating this is, especially after years of being so focused on my weight week-in, week-out. I do this with the luxury of being around my own target, of course – and I find that if I stray a little too far in either direction, a few weeks of focus on the calories gets me back on track mentally. As I've recently started weightlifting, I use the app to check I'm getting enough protein and ensure I've got enough calories in me to safely lift, but that's it.

In an ideal world, we wouldn't track calories at all. There's an argument to be made that focusing too much on calories can cause disordered thoughts, and if this is something you think you might struggle with, it's extremely important you tread lightly. There is a lot of tracking and focusing involved, especially when you first get started, and that can be overwhelming. If you can get yourself to the state I mention above – that is, not checking, and tracking almost in your head – that's the ultimate goal. But for now, if calorie counting helps, give it a go. We put it off for years, and wish we had started sooner.

EXERCISE

Let's address the elephant in the room, which admittedly seems a slightly insensitive phrase to use in a weight-loss book. A good diet will do wonders for your weight loss, but exercise – whatever form that takes for you – will only ever accelerate it. Exercise, especially when you're perhaps a shade more padded than you would like, can be a very daunting thing. When writing this chapter it became apparent that Paul and I have had very different 'blocks' to exercising over the years: with me, it's a mental battle against my own inherent laziness, while for Paul, the sheer physicality of getting moving always stopped him in his tracks. With that in mind, rather than us telling you to get off the bus a stop early and take the stairs instead of the lift and all that hackneyed crap, we thought it might be more useful to talk about our different paths to exercise in the hope that one of them will resonate with you. Fair warning: Paul sure loves a heady word count …

We must stress, though – if you're planning a new course of exercise, it's always worth having a quick chat with your doctor to make sure you're in good nick. The last thing we want is for you to set off hillwalking only to need an air ambulance back to hospital. Got to think about future book sales …

JAMES – THE MENTAL BATTLE

For me, exercise – both the inclination to do it and the will to continue – has always been a battle not against the limits of my physicality but against my own brain. Regardless of my size, I've always been what I would describe as fairly fat-fit – for as long as I can remember, I've been one for walking and exploring, but actual structured exercise has never seemed to stick. I've had more brief reunions with my gym than Liz McDonald, so I have, though I'm far less of a *heeur*.

The biggest battle for me was not what it was for Paul – bending down to get his shoes on unassisted – but rather the worry about what others would think. Would the gym be full of people whispering and pointing as I galumphed my way around the treadmills or I split my knickers trying to get on the stationary bike? If I ran outside, would traffic crawl to a halt as each white van driver took his turn to hurl an insult as my boobs slapped around under my chins?

I would spend so much time before going to the gym worrying about what might happen that I would talk myself out of going – and then one day missed became one week, then a month, and then my fitness folly would be forgotten entirely. It's called catastrophising (always thinking the worst) and I've written about it at length on the blog: those who endure anxiety are especially prone to it. Of course we are, it's not as if we don't have enough imaginary terrors to be cracking on with.

But the reality, of course, is that no one truly gives a tinker's toss what we do in the gym or how we exercise. We all like to imagine they do, because there are none so important as ourselves, but it just isn't true. Well, so far as I've encountered, anyway. I've had exactly one negative experience when exercising and it was actually what I jokingly referenced above: someone called me a fact hunt (I think – it was said at speed, but that's what it sounded like) as I jogged along. I was devastated and it set me back for a good few months, until I realised that the mantra I tell people regarding wearing whatever clothes they want applied right there: those vanishingly rare idiots who may pass comment will make a remark regardless of what you're doing. It's who they are, not what you are. You could be walking down that footpath looking like a Parisian model during Fashion Week and they'd find a flaw to attack. To put it in a less flowery way: a bumhole will always fart, it's up to you whether you breathe it in.

With the Hallmark-esque mantra above floating in my head, and with the stark realisation I'm hurtling towards (generously) middle-age now, I decided this year to do two things I've been wanting to do for ages but put off because I was so bloody self-conscious. The first was joining our local inclusive rugby team (Go Ravens!), which, at the time of writing, I'm halfway through a boot-camp with. I'm terrible at it: it was week three before I realised you could actually run with the ball – but I adore it. There's a great sense of community already and, well, I never need an excuse to stick my head between a chunky pair of thighs.

The second is weight-lifting and strength-training. This one was particularly scary because, let's be honest, it attracts the sort of person who could theoretically hurl you over the gym roof if you give them the wrong look. I was expecting to be shouted at and mocked and pushed into the bins, but none of this, of course, occurred. If anything, people are even friendlier – because there's such a risk of injury if you lift wrong, people go out of their way to offer advice and correction. No judgement, just help. I love going, which is handy because I'm there six times a week. It helps that I also have the most magnificently terrific trainer (more on him later in the book).

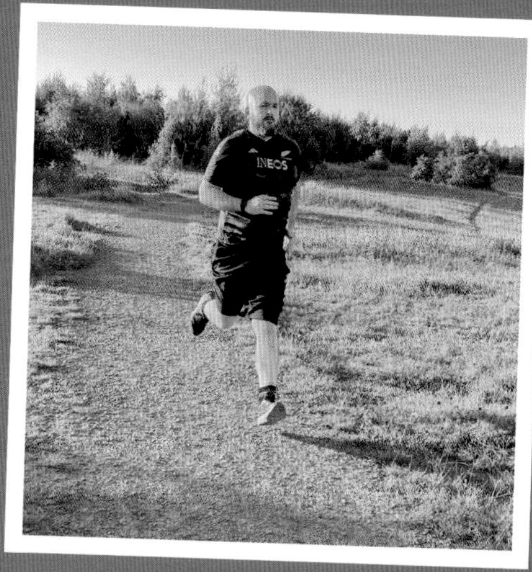

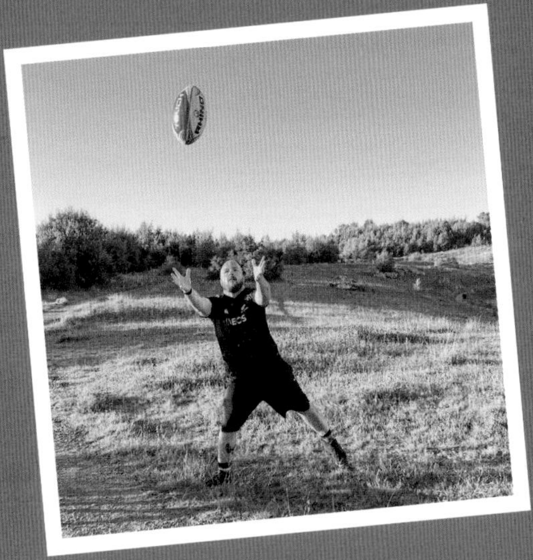

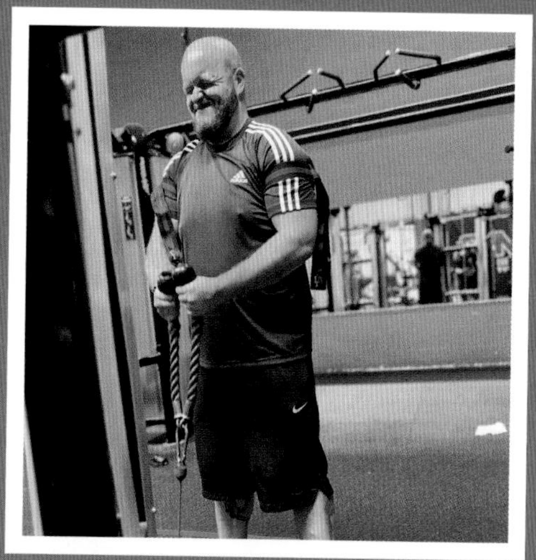

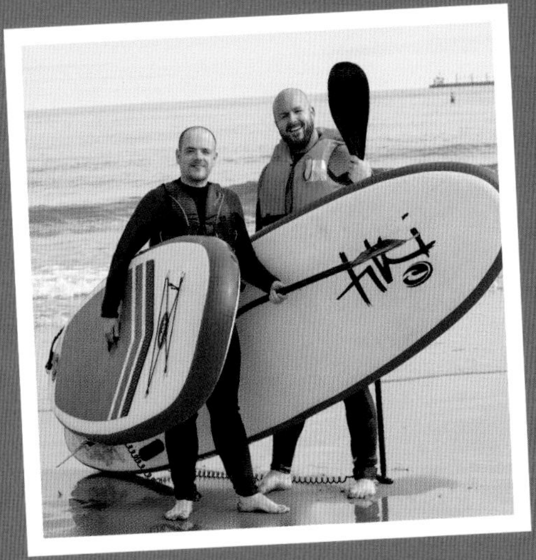

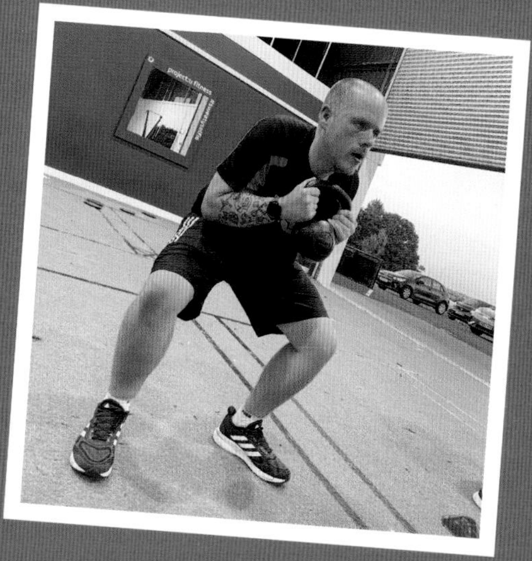

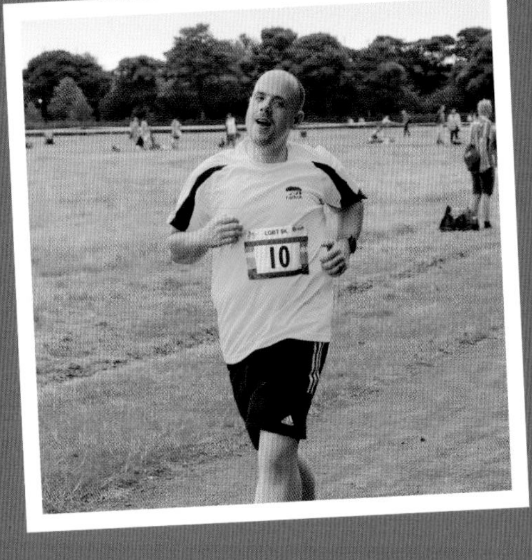

All of this brings me to my final point: if there's an exercise you've always wanted to try but have been put off by fear of judgement, or uncertainty, or just the sheer unknown quality of it – don't delay a second longer. I don't regret many things in my life, because lord knows we're not on this earth long enough for that level of angst and introspection, but I do regret not starting both my new activities sooner. For what? Some phantom comments that never materialised and judgement that never came? So frustrating, and all my own doing. So, fabulous as I am, don't be me. Get out there, get started, get on.

Oh, one final pro-tip if you're still struggling with mental attitude: it's not school PE. If you try it and hate it, you can leave and never see those people again. Actually, thank goodness it isn't school PE – my teacher was an absolute sadist who used to deliberately pick me to demonstrate various sports moves, knowing full well I couldn't do them. One of my favourite school memories (which I'm sure I've mentioned in a previous book but it's such a glorious image it bears repeating) was when myself and all the other PE rejects went on strike and refused to participate in his class. We went further than that, though: we all brought food and snacks and had ourselves a little picnic on the patch of grass we were sent to for misbehaving. The sight of his angry little face going pillar-box red as his renegades prepared a full high tea in response to his spittle and ire brings me great joy even now.

PAUL – THE PHYSICAL BARRIER

I'm sure I've mentioned this before but here I go anyway – my earliest memory is sneaking downstairs in the early hours, filling a little green plastic bowl with biscuits and chocolates, and eating them in front of the Open University on the telly. I would have been no older than three, four at the most, and that pretty much set the tone for the rest of my life until very recently. I was always the fat kid, and it was something I was acutely aware of. Whether it was something as simple as being called 'fatty' by schoolfriends, or not being able to play a Viking because I couldn't get into the costume, it was just something I was. PE was always a humiliating experience, seemingly egged on by the teachers (one particularly sadistic one made me do the 800m run on sports day – instead, I hid in a tree and smoked). Fortunately for me, I broke my arm around year 8 and somehow managed to wrangle never having to do PE again. Unfortunately for my waistline, though, this did absolutely nothing for my general size and I continued to grow.

Don't worry, the story cheers up soon, promise.

Looking back, I really would have appreciated and benefited from some education about nutrition and exercise. As I recall, it was almost non-existent and I'm not sure whether that has changed – I hope so. For all us fat kids a little bit of kindness back then could have done wonders, rather than just effectively bullying us into staying as we were.

But let's fast forward to modern day – as you've probably guessed, nothing changed. I continued to do very little exercise except for superficial 'bursts' that coincided with 'new starts' on a diet. For a while, I walked an hour into work and back, which was quite impressive for a dumpy little thing like me (nothing at all to do with me getting to shower with the binmen at the council when I got to work, nosiree), except I'd then reward myself with a load of snacks to say well done, so it made zero difference. We also joined a few gyms, which we'd go hell-for-leather at for a few weeks, but then that'd dwindle and it'd just be a line on my bank statement, reminding me to cancel after the year. The worst part? The pains and the aches after any exercise – I felt like a eighty-year-old.

I had resigned myself to two simple facts: I would always be overweight, and it would always be impossible to exercise because of it.

I got fatter and fatter, until – on my birthday, I might add – James *forced* me to start attending a local HIIT class. This was when we were in 'panic mode' during *This Time Next Year*, when we were roughly halfway through and had got barely anywhere. We knew that we had to really ratchet it up a gear, and this was it. I'll confess, I had no idea what HIIT was. It stands for High Intensity Interval Training – a method where you go full pelt for around 40 seconds, and then rest, and then go again. Some sort of *science* happens, resulting in weight loss. Don't ask me specifics because I haven't a clue, but it works! What was interesting was how the classes were scaled to fit everyone, including me at my heaviest and James with his inhaler, back-up inhaler and 999 already pressed on his phone. You were encouraged to do as much as you could, but weren't shouted at for what you physically couldn't. For the first time, I was exercising to my limits and enjoying it, and as the weight dropped off, those limits went through the roof. I went from being unable to do one 'burpee' to where I am now, fifty in a row. It still looks like someone's shot my knee-caps out as I collapse ungraciously to the floor, but I can do them.

This was the first time in my life I enjoyed exercise, and didn't feel as though my weight was stopping me from progressing. I could see the results, I could feel the improvement. It hit me then how much I enjoyed it! And for all that I'd complain about being sweaty and having sore knees and the initial dread of walking in, there really is nothing like the feeling of doing a good job, and I can hand on heart say there hasn't been a single session I haven't enjoyed. I might hate it at the time, but once it's over I know I had a good time. Plus, the weight loss is a nice little bonus.

I knew, however, being me, that I needed to branch out into other things. As I lost weight, more opportunities for exercise presented themselves. I studiously followed the Couch to 5K programme to completion and was able to run a solid 5km without stopping, which seems amazing given I used to get out of breath walking round the supermarket. I even joined parkrun, but soon knocked that on the head when I realised I'd have to get out of bed before 2pm on a Sunday. I never experienced a runner's high, though – I still think it's a myth. James reckons he sometimes gets one but he's probably sniffing the chalk from his weight-lifting gloves.

I love swimming and, having been a fat kid, was unsurprisingly good at it (superior buoyancy, see), but I found that there was a somewhat aggressive nature to a lot of the swimmers in our local baths, and I grew tired of being tutted at by people in crinkly-hats and goggles as they glided past. I gave badminton a go, but tittered like a child at the mention of a shuttlecock. James wants us to join the local wrestling team, but I fear he may have indecorous intentions.

But then I tried rugby! I joined a bootcamp for the local inclusive team up here and I bloody loved it. I started with Rugby Union but found it a bit full-on (I was concussed on my first real game), so switched to the Touch Rugby team and I'm still there now. I'll not pretend I'm anywhere near good at it, but it's a really fun game and the people are lovely. I have a brilliant time at training events and I've even played in a few games, and it's marvellous fun going round the country with your mates, having a laugh and a bit of a run-about. My confidence is growing, which again is that thing about self-perpetuating! James has just joined too, so having him to play with will make it even better!

For us, the key to weight loss has been the coming together of two elements – the right diet, and the right exercise. I think too many of us hope we can do the former without the latter, and many plans have come out saying it's easy to do. I'm sure many of us have our own traumas when it comes to exercise, whether it's getting picked on as a kid, being clumsy, or just not wanting to get out there, but I can't stress enough how much fun you can have. Finding the right exercise is important, but the process of finding it can be such a great experience! And – as I learnt – the perfect exercise for YOU might be the LAST thing on your list. If you'd told me to write an ordered list of exercises I wouldn't ever want to do, a HIIT class and rugby would have been top. But look at me now! Be prepared to move out of your comfort zone. Try something outrageous. Get a mate to go with you and just have a bloody good laugh! I played a game of rounders with some colleagues and it was one of the best days I've ever had. I don't think we hit the ball once. But it didn't matter. And I promise you – your worries about being laughed at, looking silly, feeling like a fool are all in your head. Don't listen to that voice, and just bloody go for it. It'll be worth it.

I'm still attending HIIT classes (I've actually moved to another place that's a bit more intense – and I'm loving it!) and touch rugby (I've recently won Player of the Match!), and my confidence is growing day by day. I'm always on the lookout for new things to try – next spring I'm going to do a watersports course (not letting James book that one) and I'm still going to try and get into running. I might make some silly mistakes with my diet, but because I'm exercising so much I'm really not that bothered. I've realised, now, that I'm a pig when it comes to food – always have been, always will be, but that's perfectly fine so long as I'm exercising to burn it off. I get to eat what I want, when I want, AND I get to have a load of fun in a warehouse, or running around a field with my mates.

I'll end on this: although I've talked about the physical restraints in getting going, the best part for me about exercising hasn't been the physical benefits, but the mental ones. It's helped my confidence and self-esteem massively, and it's also helped improve my sleep. It's helped loads with my stress – it's a great outlet. Whether I'm walking the dog around the lake, doing burpees or trying (probably failing) to catch a ball, it's brilliant for helping to melt away stress. Find what works for you, and, more importantly, what you enjoy, and go from there.

Back to us speaking to you as a pair now, like two elderly spinsters dishing out sage advice. Please don't take any of the above as a demand for you to exercise: if you don't want to, that's fine. We umm-ed and aah-ed about whether or not to include this section, because we know that for many of you, a lecture on moving will be the last thing you need. That's fair enough. We decided to add it because we both exercise more than before and it's become a big part of our weight management, and we thought it might be helpful for you to hear about two very different paths to consider. Much like choosing a diet plan, it's all about what works best for you.

Good luck and over to you with the recipes!

James and Paul x

If you fancy even more chat from us (and delicious recipes), check out our other *Sunday Times* bestselling cookbooks:

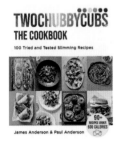

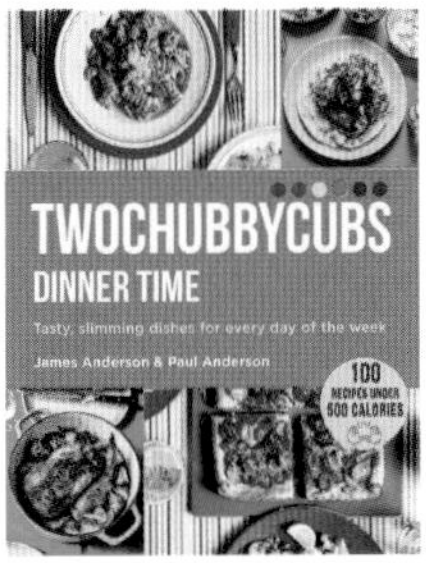

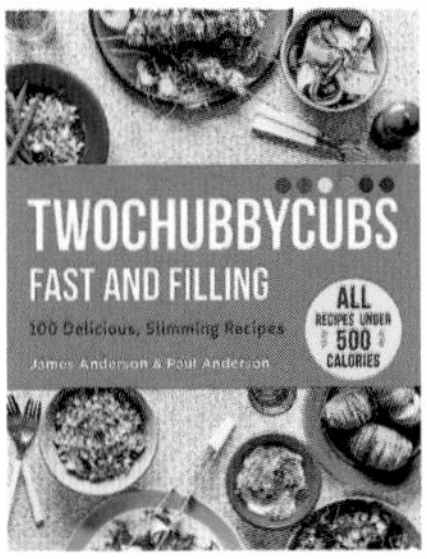

MO

MA

RNING

RVELS

SERVES: 1
PREP: 5 MINS
COOK: 5 MINS
CALORIES: 272

SMOKED SALMON & CREAM CHEESE TOAST

This recipe, egg and all, is one of the mainstays of 'Paul's lunchbox', which, for those who don't know, is a feature he sometimes remembers to post about on our social media. Paul realised a long time ago that having a big lunch at noon doesn't work for him, because he's hungry until then and sleepy after, which is far from ideal for someone who needs to be alert all day to spot when the chap comes to fill the vending machines. Instead, he packages up all sorts of little snacks (he calls them snackettes; I can't bring myself to do so without grimacing) and parcels them out during the day, meaning a nice sustained calorie intake. It works well for him, and he heartily recommends it for those looking for something different. Somewhat adorably, he carries them all into work in a little lunchbox in the shape of the Epcot monorail car. Along with his chocolate milk. Bless his heart! I do love him. Bet his coworkers don't though, what with the fish and egg in a small office . . .

- 1 medium egg
- 1 tablespoon reduced fat cream cheese
- 1 slice of toast
- 60g (2¼oz) smoked salmon trimmings
- 2 radishes, sliced
- 2 teaspoons chopped fresh dill (optional)

Bring a small saucepan of water to the boil. Add the egg and cook for 5 minutes (or to your liking), then remove from the pan, cool under running water and peel.

Spread the cream cheese over the toast and add the salmon, radishes and dill.

Slice the egg and arrange on top.

Notes: We use smoked salmon trimmings because they're much cheaper than the sliced stuff, and honestly, we can't tell any difference with taste, etc. Of course, though, slices will work just as well.

Have the radishes however you like – we love them chopped into matchsticks but it really doesn't matter. No radishes? Capers, sliced pickled onions and diced gherkins all work really well too.

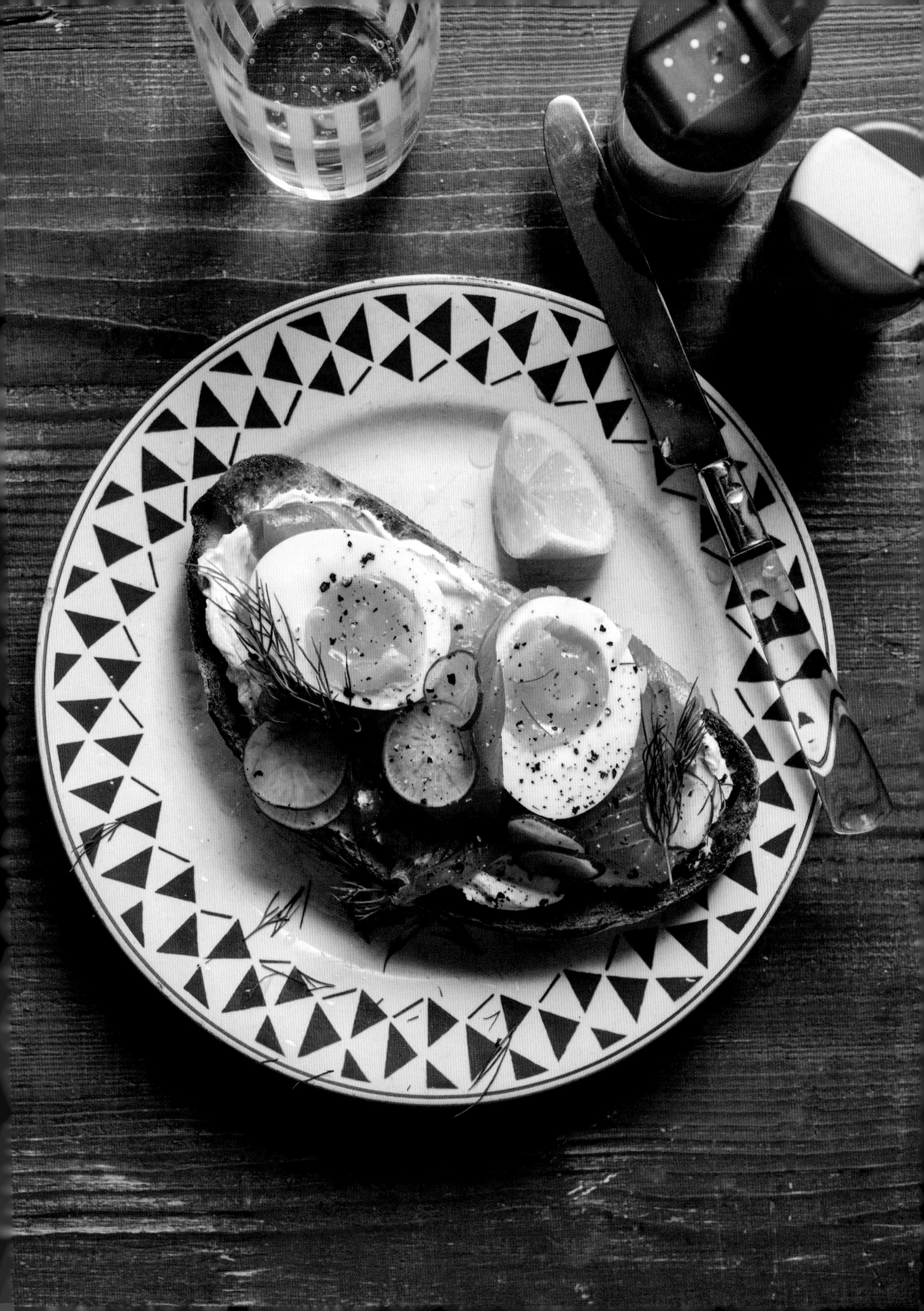

SERVES: 1
PREP: 10 MINS
COOK: 20 MINS
CALORIES: 491

BREAKFAST PIZZA

We're calling this a breakfast pizza despite the fact it's clearly a bagel. But what a bagel! Just so you're aware, the only acceptable way to eat this is to go all in, dislocating your jaw like a snake swallowing a sheep. But even so. A little recommendation – we both love a good bagel, and you'll find no better bagel for your buck than Brawsome Bagels in Partick, Glasgow. What those chaps manage to squeeze between bagel halves would make your eyes water, trust me. I had a Spicy Brat Bagel and thought I'd ascended. If you find yourself in Glasgow – and mind, lucky you, because it's my favourite city in the UK – give them a go. They're just a stop or two along on Glasgow's hilariously tiny and utterly cute subway system. That's worth a ride regardless of destination, because you will absolutely feel like a borrower as you board their tiny trains. They're on Instagram at @brawsomebagels. In the meantime, to keep you ticking over, here's ours.

- 1 reduced-fat pork sausage
- 2 bacon medallions
- 1 egg
- a splash of milk
- 1 tablespoon tomato purée
- 1 bagel, toasted and sliced
- 25g (1oz) reduced-fat Cheddar cheese, grated
- 4 fresh basil leaves, roughly chopped

Spray a large frying pan with a little oil and place over a medium-high heat. Cook the sausage for 12–15 minutes, until browned all over and cooked through. Add the bacon for the last 5 minutes or so and cook to your liking, then remove both to a plate.

Crack the egg into a bowl, add a splash of milk, and whisk well with a fork.

Pour the egg into the pan and stir continuously for just a minute or so, until nicely scrambled, then scoop on to a plate.

Slice the sausages and roughly chop the bacon.

Mix the tomato purée with 2 teaspoons of water and spread over the bagels halves.

Top with the sausages, bacon and egg, and sprinkle over the cheese.

Place under a hot grill for 2–3 minutes, until the cheese has browned, then remove from the grill and sprinkle over the basil.

Notes: A quick bit of research shows that snakes do not, in fact, dislocate their jaw in order to swallow their prey. Which is a pity, because I had questions. They probably don't eat sheep either, for that matter.

Also, you may be expecting me to make reference to the fact that the owners are terribly good-looking, tall and have that Scottish accent that pretty much pops my trousers off of their own accord. Of course, I won't be doing that.

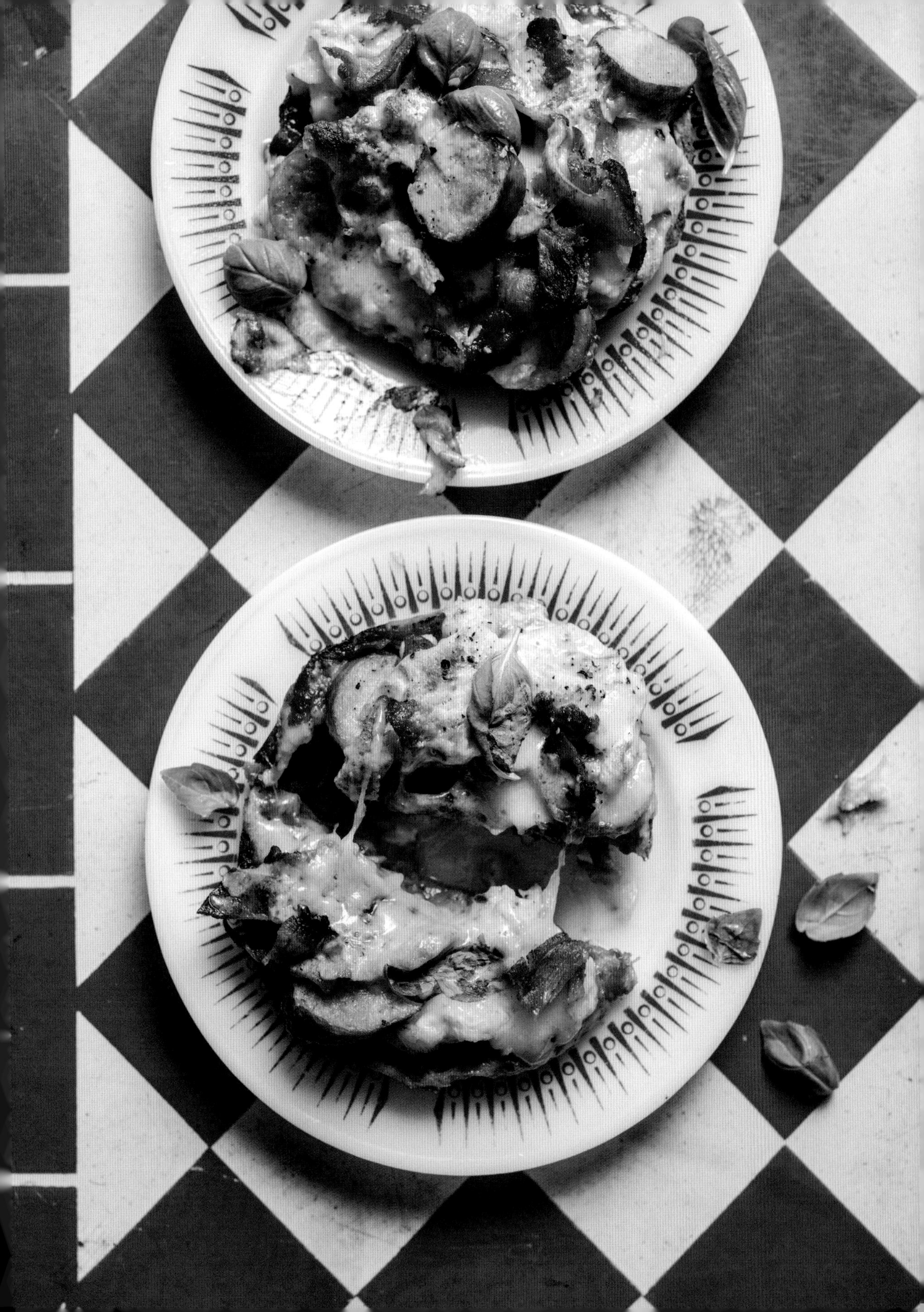

EGG FLORENTINE SANDWICH

SERVES: 1
PREP: 10 MINS
COOK: 30 MINS
CALORIES: 427

The elves at Google tell us that a true Florentine sandwich should be made with a bread known as schiacciata. But see, not only does schiacciata sound like something Paul shouts he's running off for the second he gets off an aeroplane, it is seemingly also difficult to find in the UK. You could make your own, of course, but you could also do as we do and swap it out for a ciabatta. Italy is top of our list of places to visit at the moment, mainly because I see myself in some fancy trattoria on the shores of Lake Garda, sipping a coffee as black as pitch from a cup that could fit on the head of a pin. So elegant. Naturally, the reality would be altogether more different – it would be the usual Anderson holiday: quarrels about public transport, drinking slightly too much and then eight hundred escape rooms compressed over two days. It's getting to the point where we can't relax on a holiday without someone in dungarees clapping their hands together, saying 'right guuuuuuys' in a sing-song voice and telling us we've got sixty minutes to solve a mystery / save the world / escape from a serial killer's lair. I know, I know, it's no life this. Here! Have a sandwich.

8 cherry tomatoes
1 tablespoon balsamic vinegar
1 ciabatta, sliced
whites of 3 eggs
1 tablespoon green pesto

Preheat the oven to 200°C fan/425°F/gas mark 7.

Place the tomatoes in an ovenproof dish and spray with a little oil, then pour over the balsamic vinegar.

Roast in the oven for 20–25 minutes, until the tomatoes are starting to blister and are tender.

Meanwhile, toast the ciabatta and set aside on a plate.

Whisk together the egg whites in a bowl until frothy.

Spray a small saucepan with a little oil and place over a medium heat. Add the egg whites to the pan and cook for a few minutes, stirring occasionally, until set to your liking.

Remove from the pan and place the egg whites on the ciabatta.

Top with the roasted tomatoes and drizzle over the pesto.

Notes: We have used just the whites for this one, but of course you can use the full egg if you like!

Can't be jiggered roasting tomatoes for a sandwich? Of course. Get good beefy tomatoes, slice them thick, add a touch of salt and leave for 10 minutes while you faff about with the rest. Rinse them off and bung them in your sandwich.

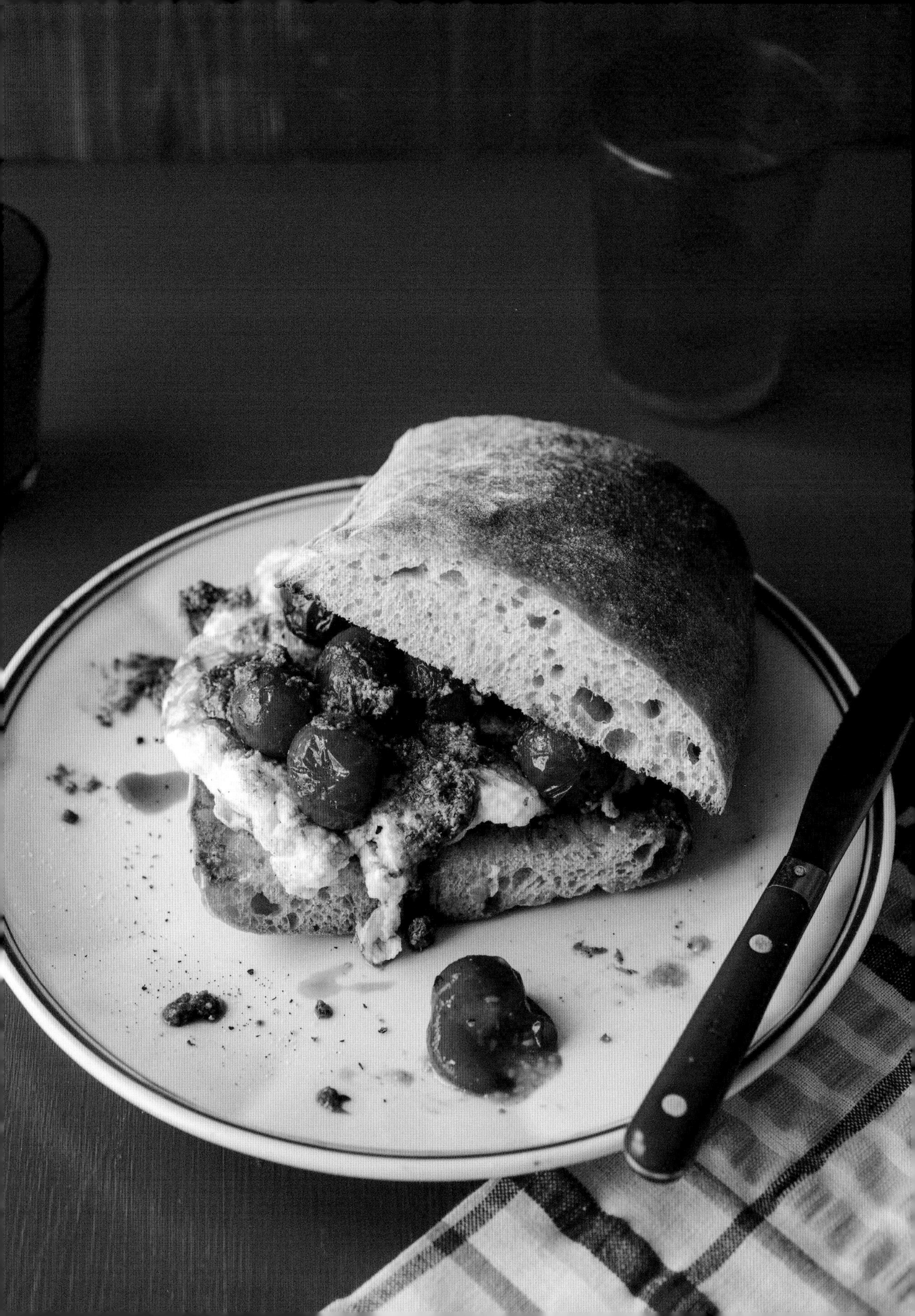

SERVES: 1
PREP: 15 MINS
COOK: 5 MINS
CALORIES: 333

THE FLUFFIEST OMELETTE YOU'LL EVER HAVE

Can you remember that craze for cloud bread not so long ago? Bloody awful, wasn't it – like eating a mist made from farts? Well, have no fear, this recipe is nothing like that, but just a slightly different way of making an omelette which yields, as Paul breathlessly says in the title, the fluffiest omelette you'll ever have. High praise indeed. We've kept the filling ever so simple, but if you want something a bit more substantial (and my personal favourite), add sliced sausage and Marmite. Perfect for putting hairs on your chest. Cast your eyes downwards past the recipe for an alternative serving suggestion for your ovo-wonder.

- 2 eggs
- 1 spring onion, sliced
- 1 green chilli, deseeded and finely chopped
- 1 tablespoon chopped fresh parsley (optional)
- 1 tomato, diced
- 40g (1½oz) Cheddar cheese, grated
- 1 teaspoon dried chilli flakes (optional)

Separate the egg yolks from the whites, and set them aside – try your best to keep them intact!

Whisk the egg whites (an electric whisk is best) until they reach soft peaks.

Spray a small frying pan with a little oil and place over a medium heat.

Add the egg whites to the pan and gently push out to the edges.

Add the egg yolks on top, one at each side, and cook for 2 minutes.

Sprinkle over the spring onion, chilli, parsley (if using) and tomato.

Flip the omelette over in the pan, and sprinkle the cheese over the browned base.

Use a spatula to roughly slice the omelette in half and fold it back over itself.

Sprinkle with the chilli flakes, and serve!

Notes: A good friend of mine, Martin (compact, aged), makes the second best omelette after this beauty: there's nothing especially different in the method, it's your standard affair, but he serves it betwixt two fat slices of white bread and enough bacon to warrant a Christmas bonus for the staff at the abattoir. He's a treasure.

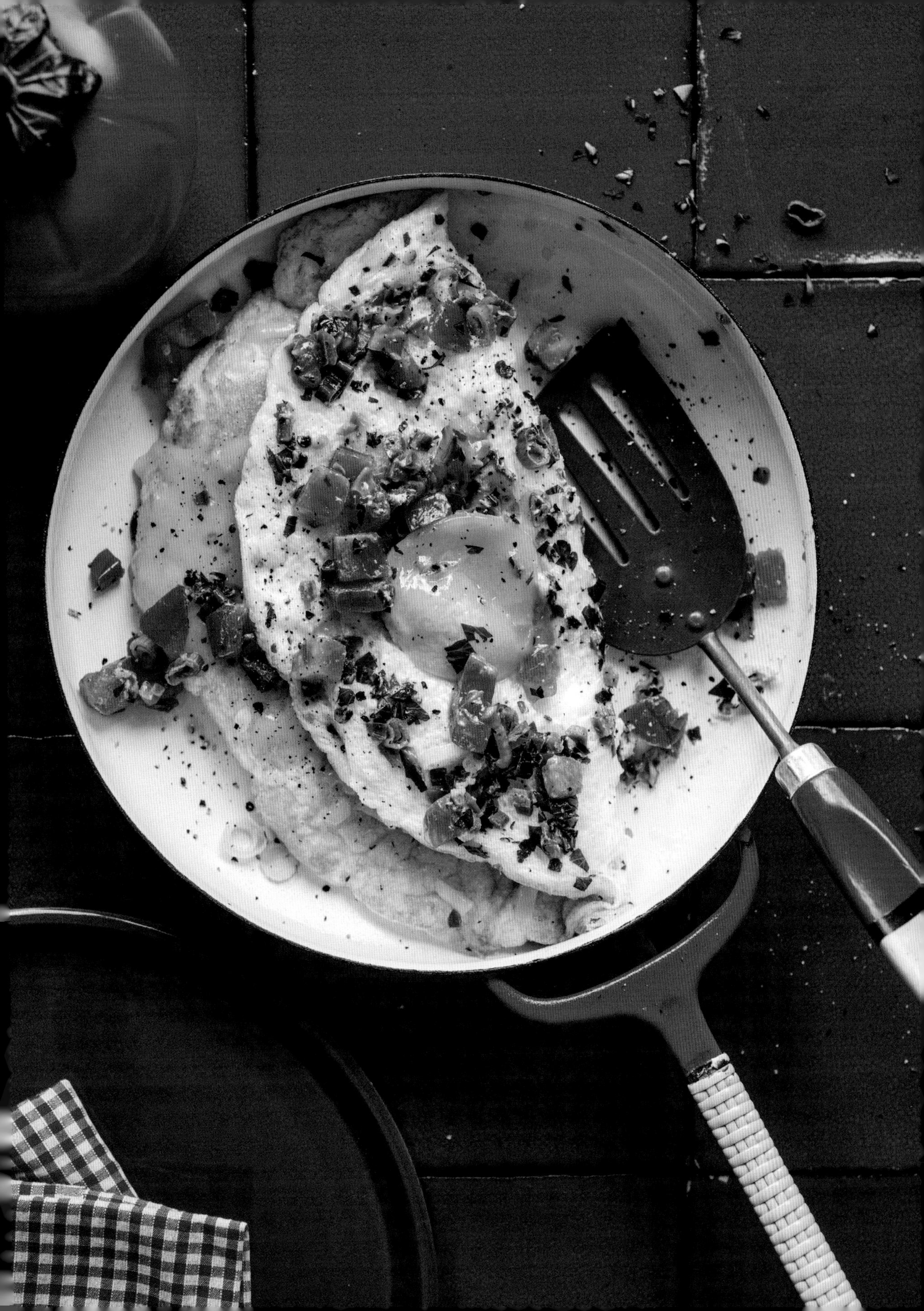

SERVES: 4
PREP: 10 MINS
COOK: 25 MINS
CALORIES: 471

JALAPENO POPPER CHEESE TOASTIE

One thing we try to stay cognisant of here at Chubby Towers is that, for all you try and make healthy, unprocessed food, for all you want to eat clean and smart and not allow stodge and slop into your temple of a body . . . sometimes you just need cheese on toast. So with that in mind, what you have here is a terrific version, souped up to add a little bit more taste to your day. If you're one of those sensible souls who still have a sandwich maker, you should absolutely be making this in that. For all the talk of air fryers and other fancy gadgets, it is the humble sandwich toaster that absolutely deserves a moment in the sun once more. When I was little I used to deliberately scatter cheese all over the machine so that once the sandwich was done, I'd have crunchy cheese to snack on after. Some might say it was genius, others may say it was a cry for help, but either way I was satisfied.

- 8 chilli peppers (see notes)
- 8 bacon medallions
- 150g (5½oz) reduced fat soft cheese
- 1 teaspoon garlic granules
- ½ teaspoon black pepper
- 8 slices of bread
- 4 tablespoons butter
- 200g (7oz) reduced fat Cheddar cheese, grated

Preheat the oven to 220°C fan/475°F/gas mark 9.

Slice the chillies in half lengthways, deseed, then spread out on a baking sheet, spray with a little oil and roast for about 15 minutes.

Add the bacon to the baking sheet after 5 minutes, then remove both from the oven, allow to cool, and roughly chop.

In a bowl mix together the chopped chillies, soft cheese, garlic granules and pepper.

Spread one side of each slice of bread with the butter.

Turn the slices over and spread half of them with the cream cheese mixture. Top each one with some of the chopped bacon and grated Cheddar, then place the remaining slices of bread on top, buttered side up.

Heat a large pan over a medium heat and add the sandwiches. Cook for about 4 minutes per side.

Notes: Jalapeños, obviously, work best for this, but if you can't find those easily any green chilli will do, as hot as you dare, but mild ones are probably best.

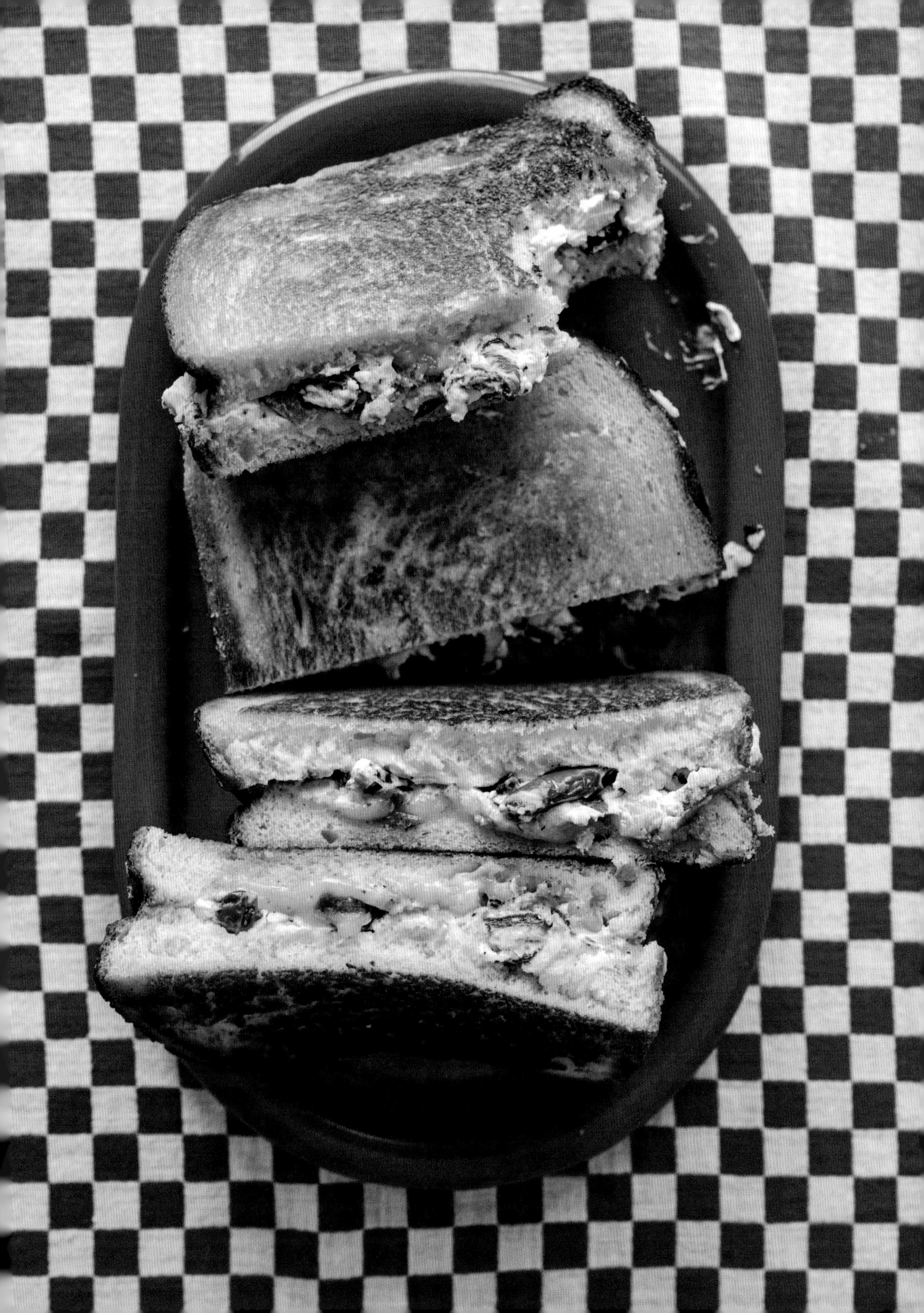

SERVES: 1
PREP: 10 MINS
COOK: 35 MINS
CALORIES: 487

- 1 small onion, peeled and thinly sliced
- 1 small courgette, trimmed and sliced lengthways into ¾cm (⅜ inch) slices
- 1 teaspoon wholegrain mustard
- 2 slices of white bread
- ¼ teaspoon dried thyme
- 40g (1½oz) reduced-fat Cheddar cheese, grated
- 2 slices of ham (optional)
- 1 tablespoon butter, softened
- 1 egg

CROQUE MADEMOISELLE

A little education for you here, which I only share with you because I had to double check whether we can get away with calling this a croque mademoiselle if it has ham in it. Technically, no: there should be no meat in a mademoiselle (poor cow), but we're including it here just in case you're the sort who can't get through the day without some slab of protein passing your lips. No, the education is this: a croque monsieur is, in essence, your traditional cheese and ham toastie. A croque madame is the monsieur but with an egg sat on top. The croque madame is thusly named because it looks like a lady's hat and not, as I had assumed in my infantile and uncultured manner, because the egg looks like a big old boob. The more you know! So, with all that in mind, whatever you want to call this, enjoy it! Also, traditionally, you would use cucumber, but Paul has decided on courgette. To his credit, it does work delightfully.

Spray a frying pan with a little oil and place over a medium-high heat.

Add the onion and cook for 20–25 minutes, until caramelised, then remove to a plate.

Add the courgette slices and cook for 4–5 minutes each side, then remove to the plate with the onions.

Spread the mustard over the bread and sprinkle over the thyme.

Top one slice of bread with the onion, courgette, cheese and ham (if using), and put the remaining slice of bread on top.

Spread the butter over the top and bottom of the sandwich and cook in the pan for 2–3 minutes each side, until browned. Then remove to a plate.

Crack the egg into the pan, fry to your liking, and serve on top of the sandwich.

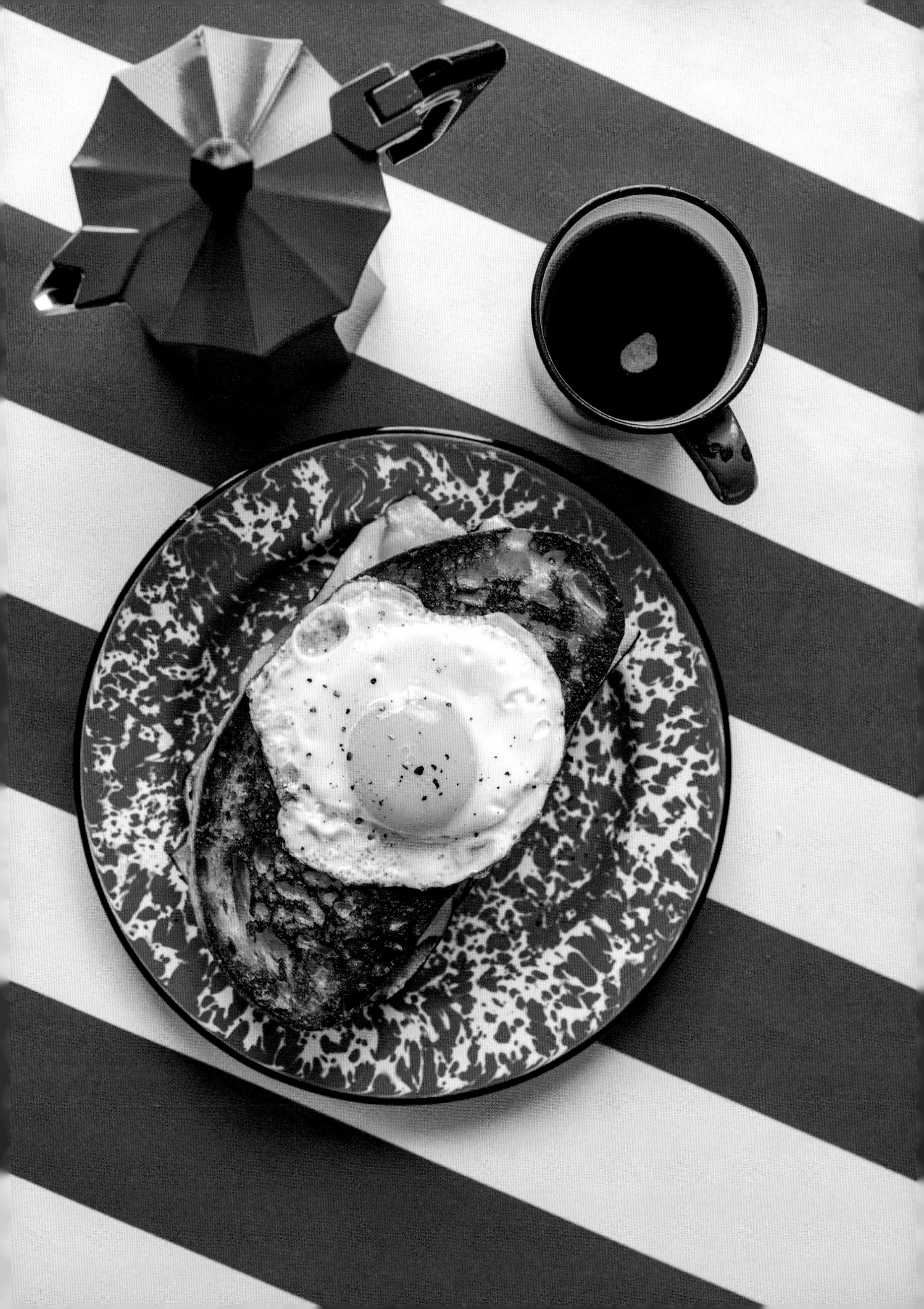

SERVES: 4
PREP: 10 MINS
COOK: 30 MINS
CALORIES: 498

DF

- 700g (1lb 8oz) potatoes, finely diced (no need to peel)
- 1 large brown onion, peeled and finely sliced
- 2 cloves of garlic, finely chopped
- 340g (12oz) corned beef, diced
- 100g (3½oz) bacon medallions, diced
- 125g (4½oz) black pudding, diced
- 4 eggs

GEORDIE HASH

We're calling this Geordie Hash for two simple reasons: we've found the best local supplier of black pudding up here in the North East (Geordie Banger Company, if you're interested), and we always try and get a little bit of Newcastle into our book. It was either this or have our photographers shoot us with paintballs so that we could recreate the famous 'blinding' scene from Byker Grove. We appreciate that black pudding is a contentious ingredient for a lot of people, given what it is. We recommend simply not thinking about it too deeply and getting it in there. If you can't get past the ick, though, some chopped sausages will also do the trick. If you're reading this book for the simple reason of wanting some delicious recipes and aren't too fussed, take a wee look at the notes. Those of us watching our waistlines, don't even peek.

Bring a large pan of water to the boil and add the potatoes. Boil for 2 minutes, then drain and return to the pan to steam dry.

Spray a large frying pan with a little oil and place over a medium heat.

Add the onion and garlic and cook for 3–4 minutes, until softened.

Add the potatoes and cook for 10–15 minutes, stirring occasionally, until crispy (add a bit more oil if needed).

Add the corned beef, bacon and black pudding and cook for another 10 minutes.

Crack the eggs on the top of the hash and cook for a few more minutes, until cooked to your liking.

Notes: Serving this with 2 fat slices of fried bread, for a total carb-bomb, is just magnificent. Remember the golden rule with fried bread, though: never use fresh slices. They'll soak up all the delicious fat and become a greasy chore to eat. Stale bread will give you perfectly fried, crunchy slices, and that's what you want.

Though of course, you don't, because this is a slimming recipe. Sssssh.

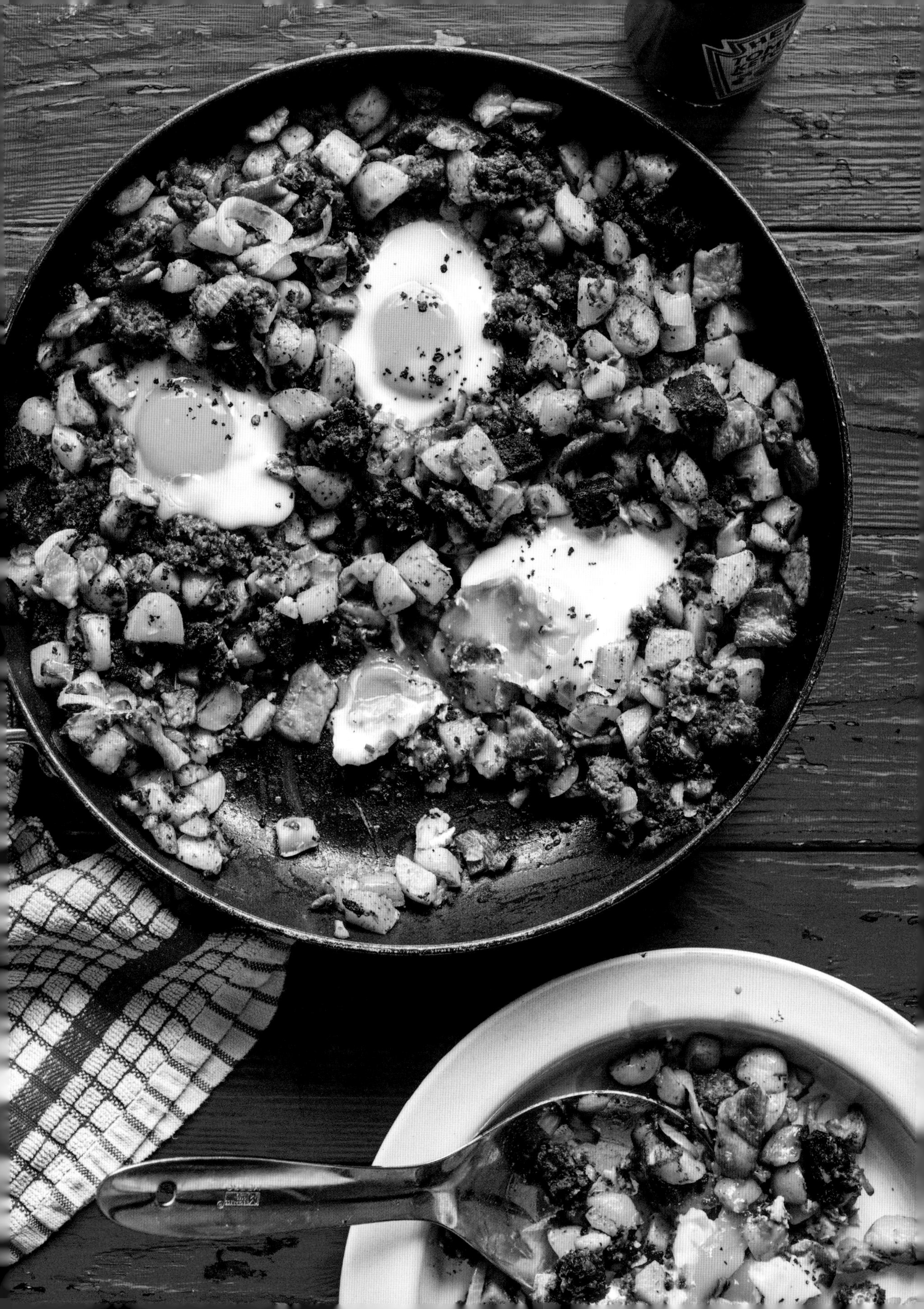

SERVES: 4
PREP: 5 MINS
COOK: 8 MINS
CALORIES: 373

CHEESE 'N' ONION FRENCH TOAST

As there isn't much I can say about this recipe, I'm going to use this moment to make a public apology. Imagine my delight when a few months ago I spotted someone else driving around our town in the exact same car I have: the same urine-yellow souped-up boy-racer model, no less. I had a CAR FRIEND. The law of motoring dictates two things: you must never let an Audi in unless it's pulling into a crematorium with at least four crying people inside, and if you see a matching car, you must wave. Since then, every time we've seen one another we've given a big elaborate gesture – finger-guns, hi-fives, jazz-hands, a Captain's Salute. I like to think it brightens his day as much as it does mine. However, today, in a mischievous mood, I held my nerve as he drove up to me, with his wife and kids in the back, giving me a double-handed wave and a cheery smile, and I locked eyes and scrunched my face as if to say 'Who the hell are you?' as I passed. You know that bit in The Simpsons where Lisa dates Ralph and Bart pauses the exact moment you see Ralph's heart break? Imagine that, but in a Golf going 40mph in a 30mph zone. I felt awful. Might move town. Anyway, where were we? Something about cheese on toast, right?

- 4 eggs
- 150ml (5fl oz) semi-skimmed milk
- ½ teaspoon ground turmeric
- 1 teaspoon paprika
- 8 thick slices of bread
- 100g (3½oz) reduced fat Cheddar cheese, grated
- ½ a brown onion, peeled and sliced
- 2 tablespoons chopped fresh chives

In a bowl, whisk together the eggs, milk, turmeric and paprika and pour into a shallow dish.

Spray a large pan with a little oil and place over a high heat.

Dip the bread into the egg mixture and allow to soak it up for 15–20 seconds on each side, then remove, shake off any excess and place on a chopping board.

Top 4 slices of bread with the grated cheese and sliced onion and put the other slices of bread on top.

Place in the hot pan and cook for 2–3 minutes on each side.

Serve on plates and sprinkle over the chopped chives.

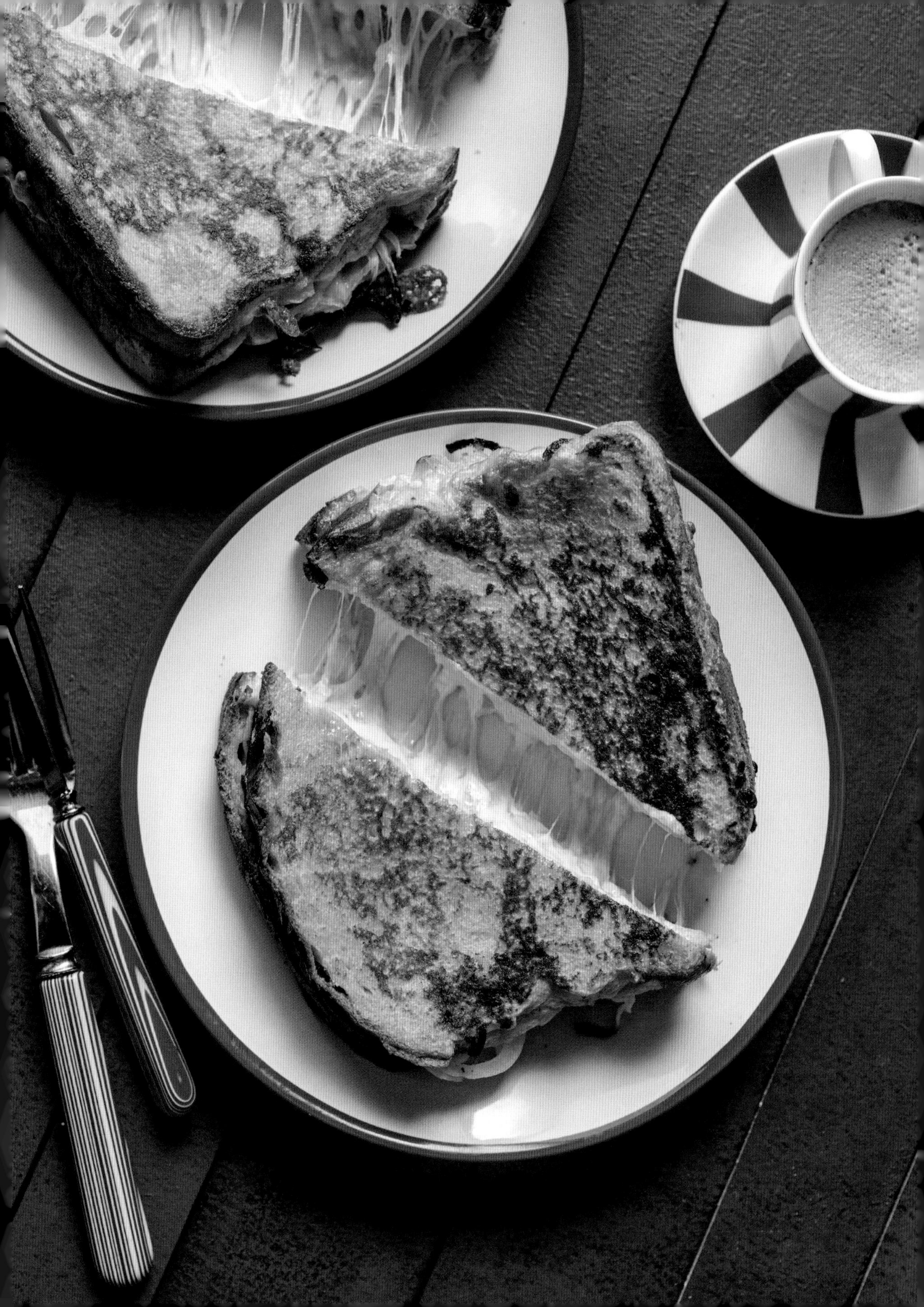

SERVES: 4
PREP: 10 MINS
COOK: 1 HR 20 MINS
CALORIES: 500

- 100g (3½oz) cherry tomatoes, halved
- 1 tablespoon mixed herbs
- 6 eggs
- 4 tablespoons semi-skimmed milk
- 1 onion, peeled and diced
- 1 green pepper, deseeded and sliced
- 150g (5½oz) button mushrooms, sliced
- 85g (3oz) goat's cheese
- 100g (3½oz) baby spinach
- 4 bagels
- a handful of salad leaves
- 4 tablespoons reduced-fat ranch dressing

EVERYTHING & EVERYTHING BAGEL

One hour and twenty minutes to make a bagel‽ I know, ridiculous, but if you take a moment to catch your breath, you'll see that most of that is letting the tomatoes roast in the oven. The world won't crack apart like a dry reservoir bed if you just slice some tomatoes and pop them in raw, but we do encourage you to go down the roasting route. If you're savvy, like we very much are not, you will roast a glut of tomatoes all in one go, and then blend any remainder into a good pasta sauce. If I'm entirely honest with you – and I like to think we have that sort of friendship now, given you've bought our book and judged our author photos – my incredulity at the start was entirely set up purely so I could copy and paste in my favourite punctuation mark: the interrobang. What could be more twochubbycubs than ending a sentence on a dramatic squeal?

Preheat the oven to 140°C fan/325°F/gas mark 3. Roast the tomatoes with a little olive oil, salt, pepper and mixed herbs for 45 minutes, until softened, then set aside. Increase the oven to 180°C fan/400°F/gas mark 6.

Meanwhile, beat the eggs with the milk and a pinch of salt and pepper, and set aside.

Spray a saucepan with a little oil and place over a medium-high heat. Add a quarter of the onions and fry until golden brown and crispy, then scoop on to a plate and set aside. Reduce the heat to medium, then return the pan to the heat with another spray of oil. Add the green peppers and the rest of the onions to the pan and cook for 4–5 minutes, until the peppers are soft, then reduce the heat to very low and stir occasionally.

Next, spray an oven-safe frying pan with a little oil and place over a medium heat. Add the mushrooms and cook for 4–5 minutes, stirring occasionally. Add the roasted tomatoes, goat's cheese and spinach and stir well, then spread out in the bottom of the pan. Give the eggs a final whisk and pour into the pan. Cook for about 5 minutes, until the edges have browned, then transfer to the oven and bake for 5 minutes.

Tip the frittata out on to a chopping board and cut into quarters.

Toast the bagels. Top them with the green pepper and onion mixture and add the frittata and the salad leaves. Drizzle over the ranch dressing and sprinkle over the fried onions.

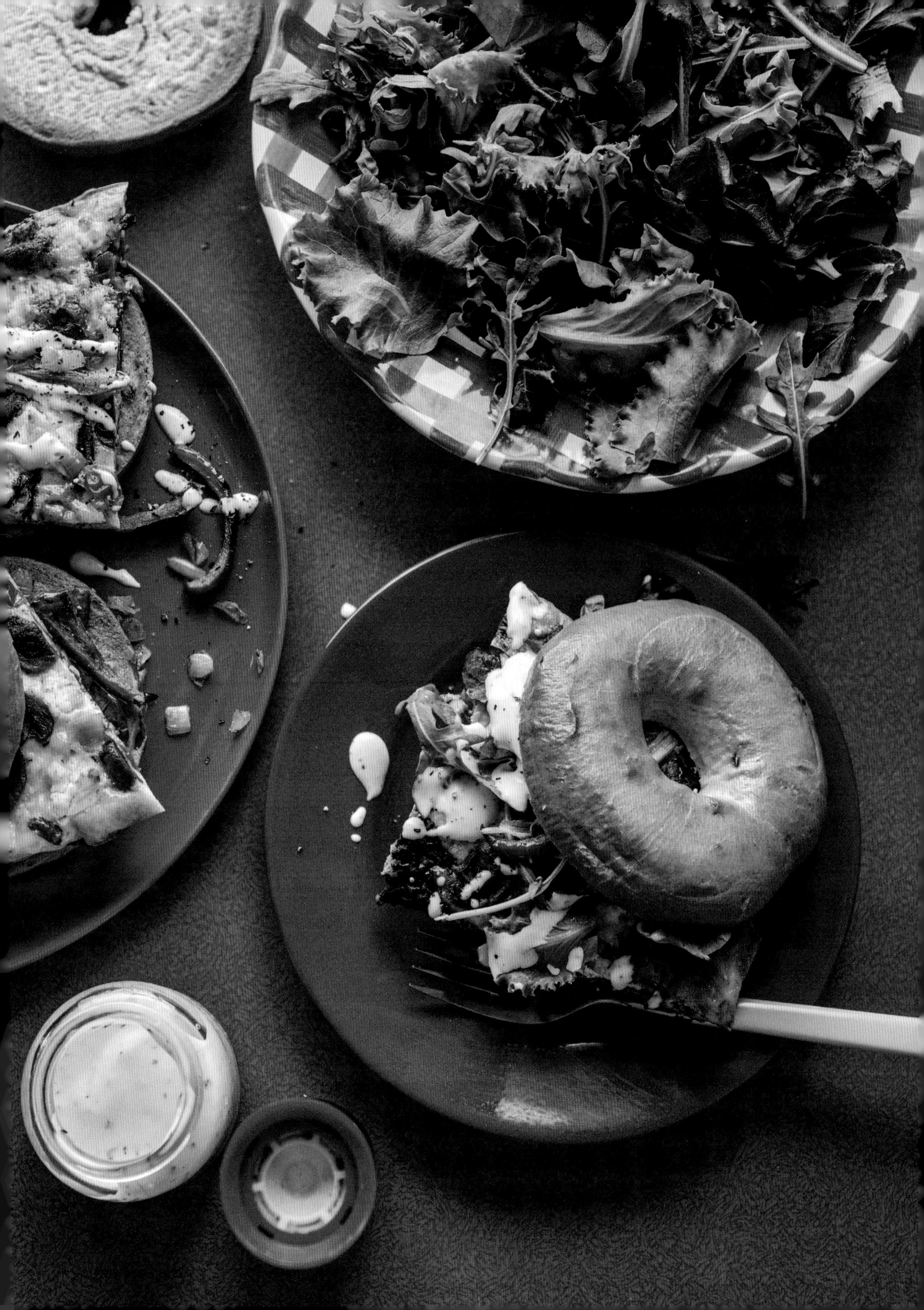

LI
LU

GHTER

NCHES

SERVES: 4
PREP: 5 MINS
COOK: 55 MINS
CALORIES: 472

30 mins | DF

- 2 red onions, sliced
- 2 teaspoons sugar
- 1 tablespoon balsamic vinegar
- 2 cloves of garlic
- 3 skinless boneless chicken thighs
- 4 eggs
- 950ml (32fl oz) chicken stock
- 250g (9oz) dried medium noodles
- 3 spring onions, sliced
- 2 pak choi, sliced
- 2 tablespoons dark soy sauce
- 2 tablespoons light soy sauce
- 2 tablespoons hoisin sauce
- 1 teaspoon black mustard seeds

WHAT CAME FIRST SOUP

Over the years we have posted a few recipes that use both chicken and egg, and they never fail to elicit the same responses from a fractured few: you can't, you mustn't, you monsters! We hear you, we are terrible people, but nevertheless we recommend you swallow your horror and give this soup a go. It's one of those dishes you can customise to your liking, and is perfect for what I call the 'fridge door sweep'. You know: that moment of guilty panic you have when you gaze into the fridge in search of cheese and note all those vegetables you bought at the start of the week to 'start again', currently all sat slightly on the turn as monument to your indecisiveness. Chop them up and throw them in. Of course, with us being such fine specimens of health, you will not find such a vegetable graveyard in the bottom of our fridge. Oh no. Because that's where we keep all the cheese.

Spray a saucepan with a generous amount of oil and place over a low heat.

Add the red onions, along with the sugar and a pinch of salt, and cook for 35 minutes, stirring occasionally. Add the balsamic vinegar and cook for a further 5 minutes.

Peel and grate the garlic, put it into a bowl with the chicken thighs and a good spray of oil, and mix well.

Spray a frying pan with a little oil and place over a medium-high heat.

Add the chicken thighs to the pan and cook for 5 minutes on each side, then set aside and roughly chop.

Meanwhile, bring a pan of water to the boil. Add the eggs and cook for 7 minutes, then cool in a bowl of cold water. When cold, peel and cut in half.

While the eggs are boiling, pour the chicken stock into a pan and bring to the boil.

Add the noodles, spring onions, pak choi, soy and hoisin sauces to the pan, stir, and simmer for 5–6 minutes.

Serve the noodle soup in bowls, with the chicken, caramelised onions and egg on top, and the mustard seeds sprinkled over.

Note: No pak choi? Celery or even spring greens work just as well.

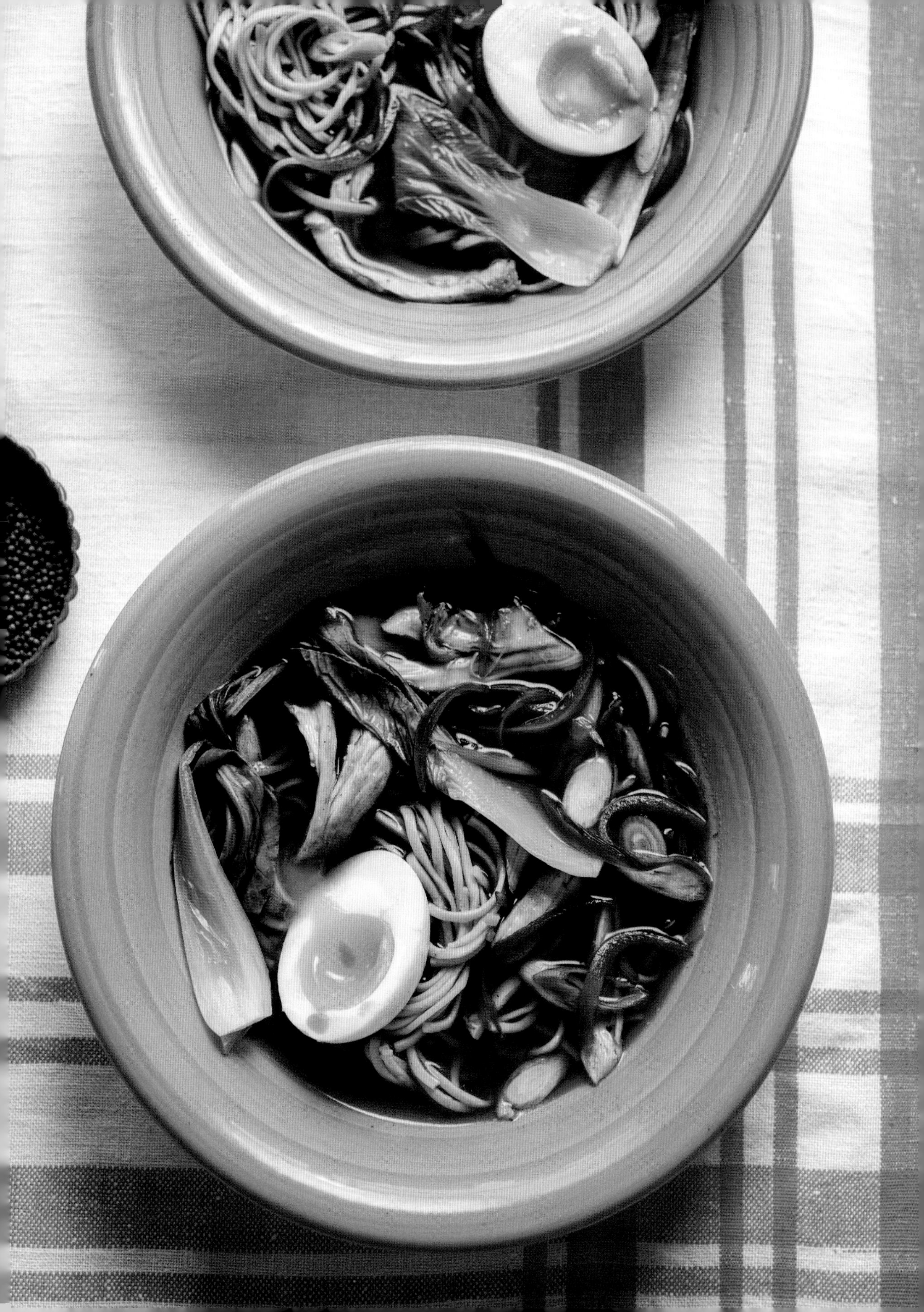

SERVES: 4
PREP: 5 MINS
COOK: 30 MINS
CALORIES: 254

30 mins, Freezable, Family, V, DF

- 650ml (23fl oz) whole milk
- 3 tablespoons oil
- 200g (7oz) concentrated tomato purée
- ½ teaspoon garlic granules
- ¼ teaspoon mixed herbs
- ¼ teaspoon black pepper
- 4 tablespoons balsamic vinegar
- ½ teaspoon lemon juice
- 1 teaspoon sugar
- 1 tablespoon cornflour
- 2 teaspoons reduced-fat vegetarian green pesto
- a handful of fresh basil leaves (optional)

CUPBOARD TOMATO & BASIL SOUP

The seven people who bought our diet planner might recognise this soup from there, although we have tinkered with it to make it more filling. Forgive us our duplicity, but this recipe deserves the love. Whole milk? In a slimming recipe? My goodness – but you simply cannot use anything else here. The creaminess of the milk is what makes this recipe sing like a boiling kettle. We tried skimmed milk, but it was like drinking a salmon-coloured glass of water. No, embrace the slight hike in calories and stick to whole milk: your stomach will thank you. If you're a fan of the 57-variety tomato soup that we all used to slop down our fronts when we were poorly children, this is the best take on that, although we've added a bit of pesto because we're so bougie these days.

First step is to set aside 150ml (5fl oz) of the milk to use later on. Pour the rest into a jug.

Put the oil into a saucepan and place over a medium-high heat. Add all the tomato purée and stir continuously, but gently, for 3–4 minutes.

Reduce the heat to medium-low and stir in the garlic granules, mixed herbs and pepper.

Pour in 100ml (3½fl oz) of the milk in the jug and stir until well mixed, then keep repeating this until all the milk from the initial 500ml (18fl oz) is gone (don't forget to keep that 150ml (5fl oz) you reserved earlier).

Once all the milk has been added, leave to cook for another minute or so, then add the balsamic vinegar, lemon juice and sugar. Stir and cook for another 10 minutes.

Stir the cornflour into the reserved milk, pour into the soup, and whisk until smooth. Increase the heat to medium and simmer gently for 7–8 minutes.

Serve in bowls, stir in the pesto and top with fresh basil leaves (if using).

Notes: You can use fresh basil leaves instead of pesto if you prefer! If you want to really gussy this up, serve garlicky-cheesy-toast with it. Slice a ciabatta in half, brush with garlic and butter, toast, then add a conservative three inches of extra mature cheese on top. Grill and serve by dunking it in the soup like a big cheesy finger.

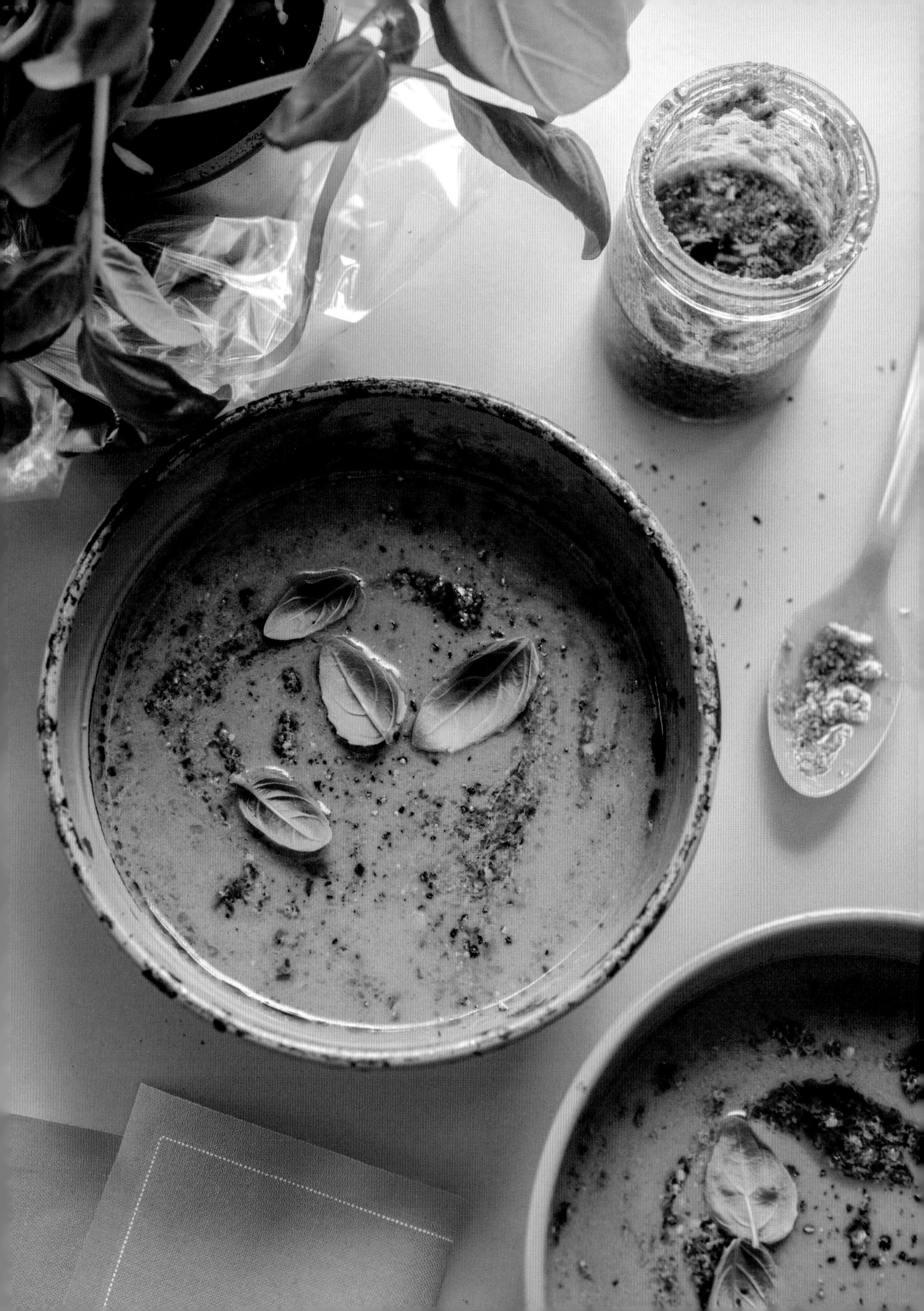

CRISPY BUTTER BEAN SALAD WITH CREAMY FETA DRESSING

SERVES: 4
PREP: 15 MINS
COOK: 30 MINS
CALORIES: 266

30 mins · V · GF

- 2 × 400g (14oz) tins of butter beans, drained and patted dry with kitchen paper
- 1 teaspoon smoked paprika
- 1 teaspoon dried mixed herbs
- 1 teaspoon garlic granules
- 2 eggs
- 1 romaine lettuce, chopped
- 100g (3½oz) cherry tomatoes, halved
- ½ cucumber, chopped
- ½ red onion, thinly sliced
- 3 roasted red peppers from a jar, drained and sliced

For the dressing

- 100g (3½oz) fat-free Greek yoghurt
- 75g (2¾oz) reduced-fat feta cheese, crumbled
- 1 clove of garlic, crushed
- zest and juice of 1 lemon
- 30g (1oz) chopped fresh dill

Butter beans, like my trainers and my husband, deserve far more love than they get. Perhaps you're of a generation like us for whom they were used as a vegetable of last resort, first put on to boil eighteen months before they were due to be served. If that's the case, then we understand your distrust: they're very much like broccoli and sprouts in that if they're overcooked they're ruddy awful, whereas cooked simply (and in this case, roasted) they're just wonderful. Quick side recipe: a tin of butter beans, a good pinch of garlic salt, some olive oil and a tiny bit of paprika blended together makes a really good fake houmous. Don't call it bummus though.

Preheat the oven to 220°C fan/475°F/gas mark 9. Spread the butter beans over a lined baking tray and spray with a little oil. Sprinkle over the smoked paprika, mixed herbs and garlic powder and season with salt and pepper. Cook for 25–30 minutes, turning once. Leave to cool.

Meanwhile, cook the eggs in a small pan of boiling water for 7 minutes. Drain, then cool under cold water and peel.

Mix the yoghurt, three-quarters of the crumbled feta, the garlic, lemon zest and juice and most of the dill with 1 or 2 tablespoons of cold water to make a creamy dressing. Set aside.

Divide the lettuce, tomatoes, cucumber, red onion and sliced peppers between serving plates and drizzle over the dressing. Top with the spiced crunchy butter beans, then halve the eggs and put one half on each plate. Add the rest of the feta and dill, and serve.

Notes: This is good with toasted pitta bread. If you don't like dill, then use parsley instead.

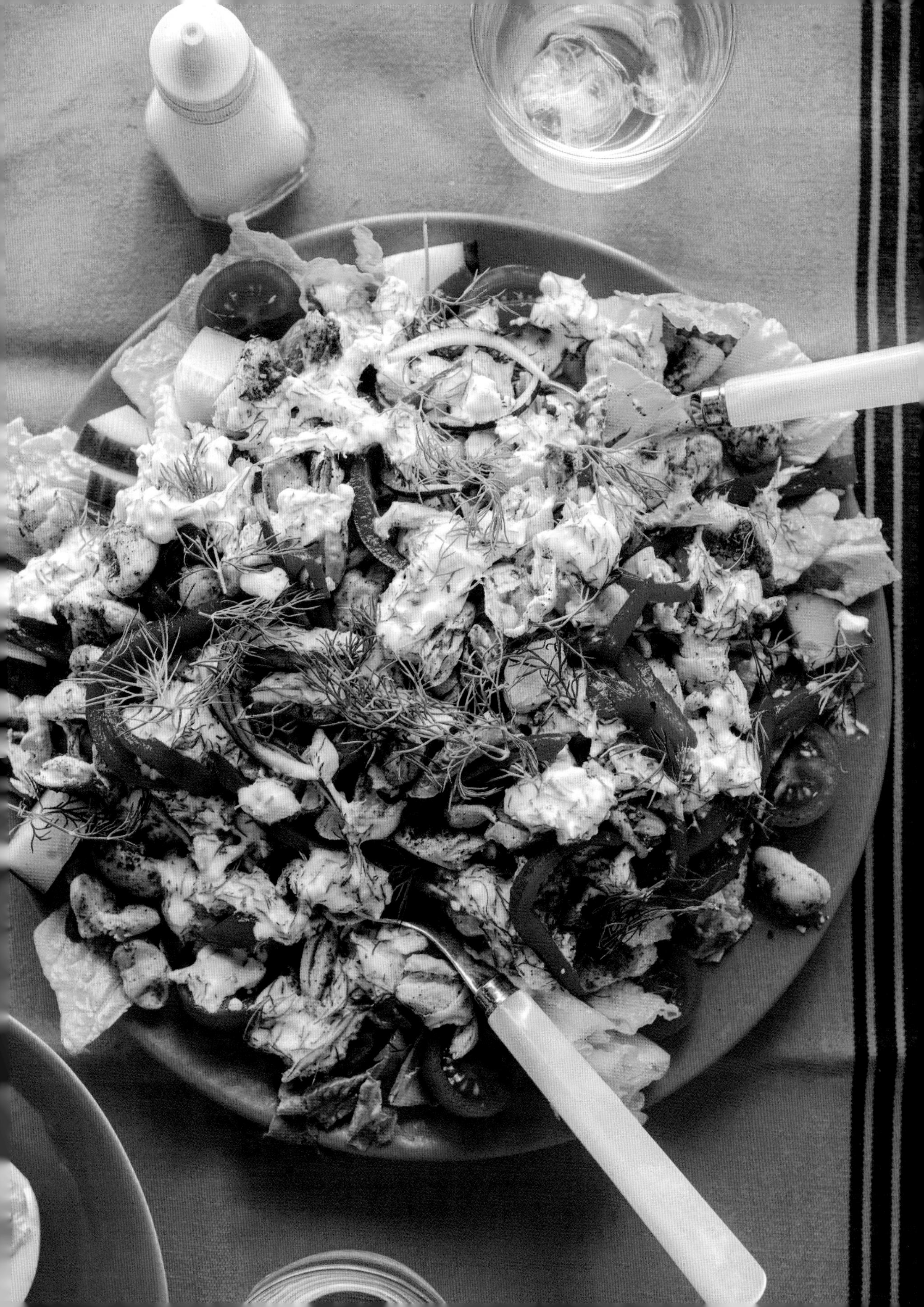

SERVES: 4
PREP: 10 MINS
COOK: 25 MINS
CALORIES: 195

EASY MUSHROOM SOUP

There is simply no getting away from the fact that this soup is a hard one to love, based on looks alone. We wanted to call it sink-trap soup, but apparently that wouldn't sell. It's a mushroom soup – it'll never set the world alight. Paul has added cashew nuts in a fit of fancy, and they really do add another note of flavour, but you're fine to leave them out if you're not a fan. While we talk about grey, a moment of reflection. Earlier in the year I was peering at my face in a mirror when I spotted, much to my chagrin, several grey hairs poking out of my beard. After checking they were indeed mine, I spent a further ten minutes examining my chest hair. Sure enough, I'm now officially 'salt and pepper' at the grand old age of thirty-eight. Each morning glance in the mirror reveals more lines, more sags, more grey, and it's all happened so fast. In my mind I still feel eighteen, but I know deep down I'm only one cold winter away from a tartan blanket over my legs and a subscription to *Puzzler* magazine. Still, at least I won't need to pop my teeth in for this lovely soup!

- 2 cloves of garlic, crushed
- 2 brown onions, chopped
- 750g (1lb 10oz) button mushrooms, chopped
- a handful of cashew nuts
- 500ml (18fl oz) milk
- 500ml (18fl oz) vegetable stock
- a handful of fresh dill (optional)

Spray a saucepan with a little oil and place over a medium heat.

Add the garlic and onions and cook for about 8–10 minutes, until golden.

Add the mushrooms and cashews and cook for a further 4–5 minutes, then remove from the heat.

Put the mixture into a blender, add the milk, and blend until smooth.

Put the mix back into the pan and cook over a low heat until it begins to simmer.

Add the vegetable stock, stir well and cook for 2–3 minutes.

Serve in bowls topped with fresh dill (if using).

Note: Swap the milk for a plant-based milk to make this vegan.

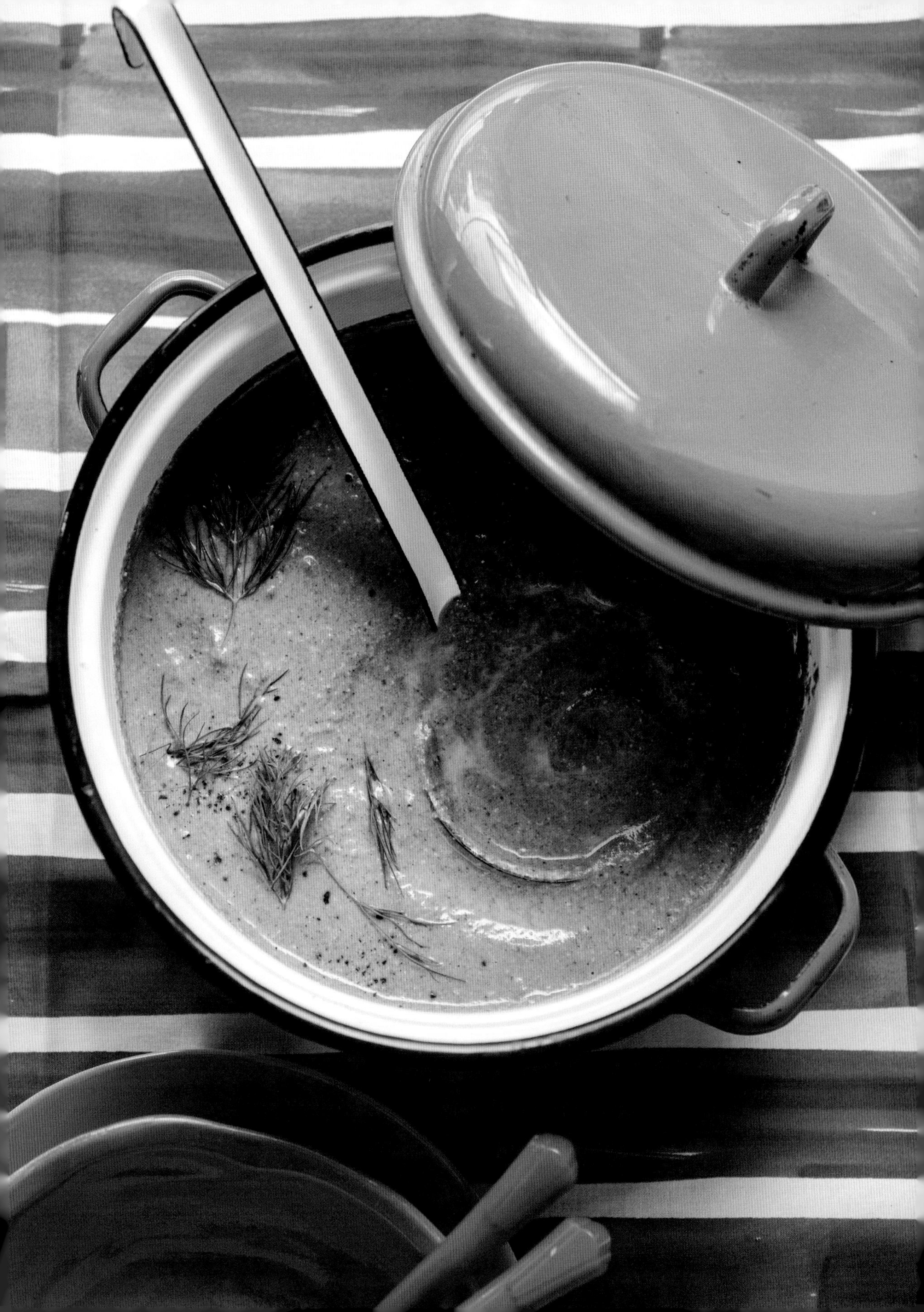

SERVES: 4
PREP: 10 MINS
COOK: 25 MINS
CALORIES: 155

30 mins · V · GF · DF

- 1 large onion, chopped
- 1 red chilli, deseeded and chopped
- 1 jar of roasted red peppers, drained and roughly chopped
- 2 × 400g (14oz) tins of chopped tomatoes
- 1 vegetable stock cube
- 3 tablespoons dried red lentils
- 1 tablespoon sugar
- 1 teaspoon dried basil

NANA BOB'S TOMATO, RED PEPPER & LENTIL SOUP

This recipe is the first in our BATTLE OF THE NANAS! I've certainly given my nana a good airing over the last three books, so we thought it might be neat to ask two other nanas for their full-on flavour recipes. We'll leave you to pick the winner, of course, and we won't try to influence you except to say . . . check the back pages. Nana Bob, as we all know him, has picked this entirely simple and very filling tomato and lentil soup recipe. If times are tight, you can absolutely whack more lentils in to bulk it out, though please do adjust the stock accordingly if it is looking a little thick.

Boil a kettle.

Spray a large pan with a little oil and place over a medium-high heat. Add the onion and chilli and cook for a few minutes, until softened (but not browned!).

Add the peppers and tomatoes and mix well.

Crumble the stock cube into 800ml (27fl oz) of boiled water in a jug and stir well to combine, then pour into the empty tomato tins. Then pour that into the pan, to get as much of the tomatoey goodness as possible.

Add the lentils, sugar, basil and a pinch of salt and pepper, mix well and bring to a simmer.

Cook for about 20 minutes, until the lentils have softened, then use a stick blender to blitz to your desired consistency.

Notes: If you're not serving this with a wedge of buttered bread that you could prop a fire door open with, then are you even living? Also, this freezes ever so well.

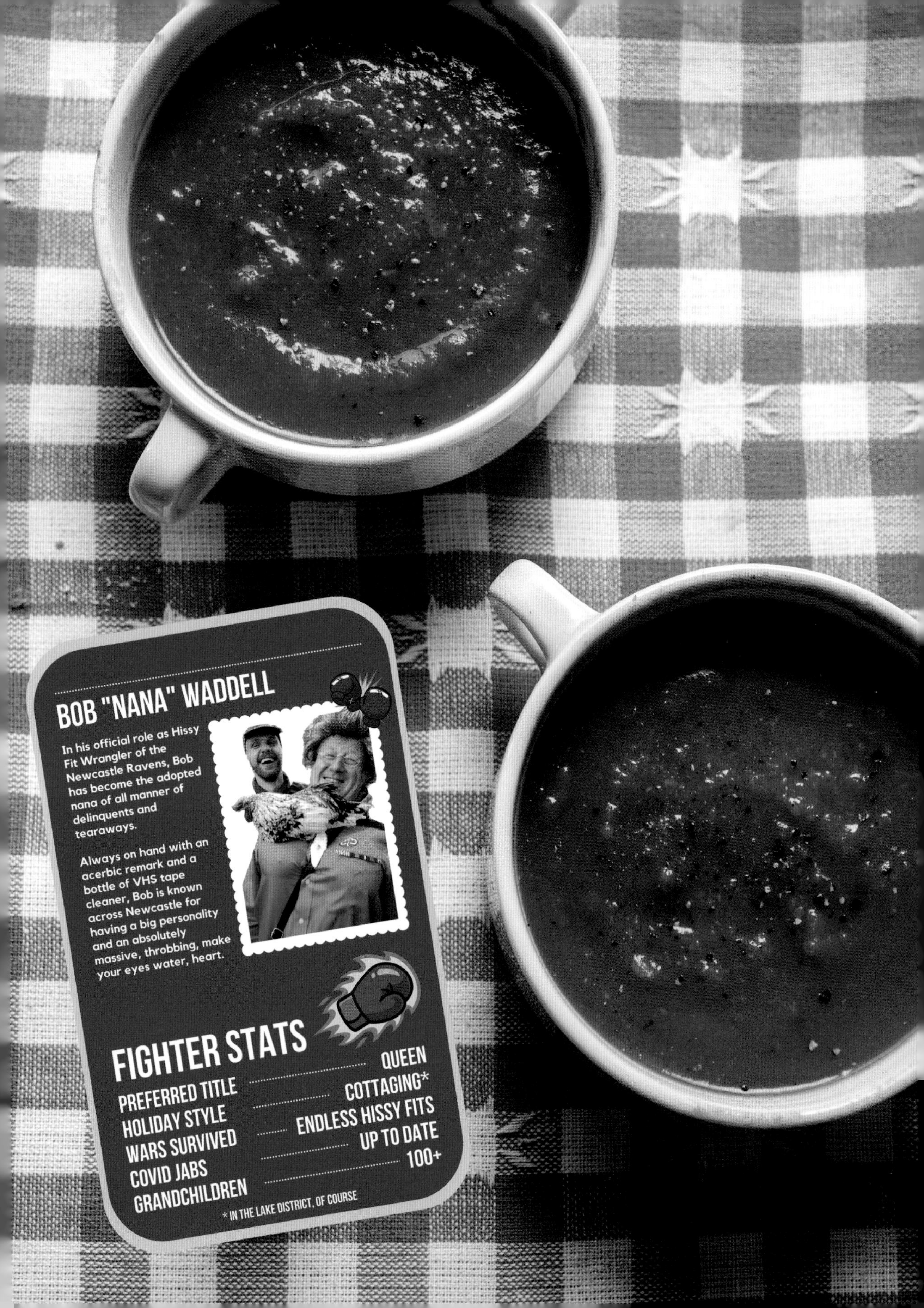

BOB "NANA" WADDELL

In his official role as Hissy Fit Wrangler of the Newcastle Ravens, Bob has become the adopted nana of all manner of delinquents and tearaways.

Always on hand with an acerbic remark and a bottle of VHS tape cleaner, Bob is known across Newcastle for having a big personality and an absolutely massive, throbbing, make your eyes water, heart.

FIGHTER STATS

PREFERRED TITLE	QUEEN
HOLIDAY STYLE	COTTAGING*
WARS SURVIVED	ENDLESS HISSY FITS
COVID JABS	UP TO DATE
GRANDCHILDREN	100+

* IN THE LAKE DISTRICT, OF COURSE

SERVES: 4
PREP: 10 MINS
COOK: 25 MINS
CALORIES: 363

WHITE BEAN SOUP

The addition of fennel and peanut butter may seem a touch froufrou for a bean soup, but as ever, you need to trust us. Fennel gets a bad reputation and certainly, if you're really not a fan of that slightly liquorice, slightly aniseed taste, by all means swap it out for sliced leeks. But if you have never tried it, this is the recipe to ease yourself in. Just cut off what we colourfully refer to as the fennel pubic hair, get rid of the hard root at the bottom, then slice thinly, like you would an onion. You can actually cook the chopped fennel fronds in the soup, if you really want to walk on the mild side.

- 2 thick slices of bread
- 2 tablespoons smooth peanut butter
- 2 teaspoons sesame oil
- juice of 1 lemon
- 1 brown onion, diced
- 1 fennel bulb, trimmed and sliced
- 3 cloves of garlic, crushed
- ½ teaspoon dried thyme
- 3 × 400g (14oz) tins of cannellini beans, drained
- 4 teaspoons dried dill
- 750ml (1½ pints) vegetable stock

Preheat the oven to 190°C fan/400°F/gas mark 6.

Slice the bread into cubes and spray them with a little oil, then spread them on a baking sheet and toast in the oven for 15–20 minutes, turning halfway. Remove from the oven and set aside.

In a small bowl, mix together the peanut butter, sesame oil and lemon juice until smooth, and set aside.

Spray a large pan with a little oil and place over a medium-high heat.

Add the onion and fennel along with a pinch of salt and cook for about 6–8 minutes, until the onion is starting to brown. Add the garlic and thyme and cook for another minute.

Add the cannellini beans, dill and vegetable stock and bring to the boil over a high heat, then reduce the heat to medium and simmer for 15 minutes, stirring occasionally.

Reduce the heat to low and stir in the peanut butter mixture.

Serve in bowls and top with the croutons.

Note: For the green-fingered among you, fennel is surprisingly easy to grow. I know this, because the few plants I stuck into our vegetable patch a few years ago keep popping back up. They even survived the shed fire – hardy indeed!

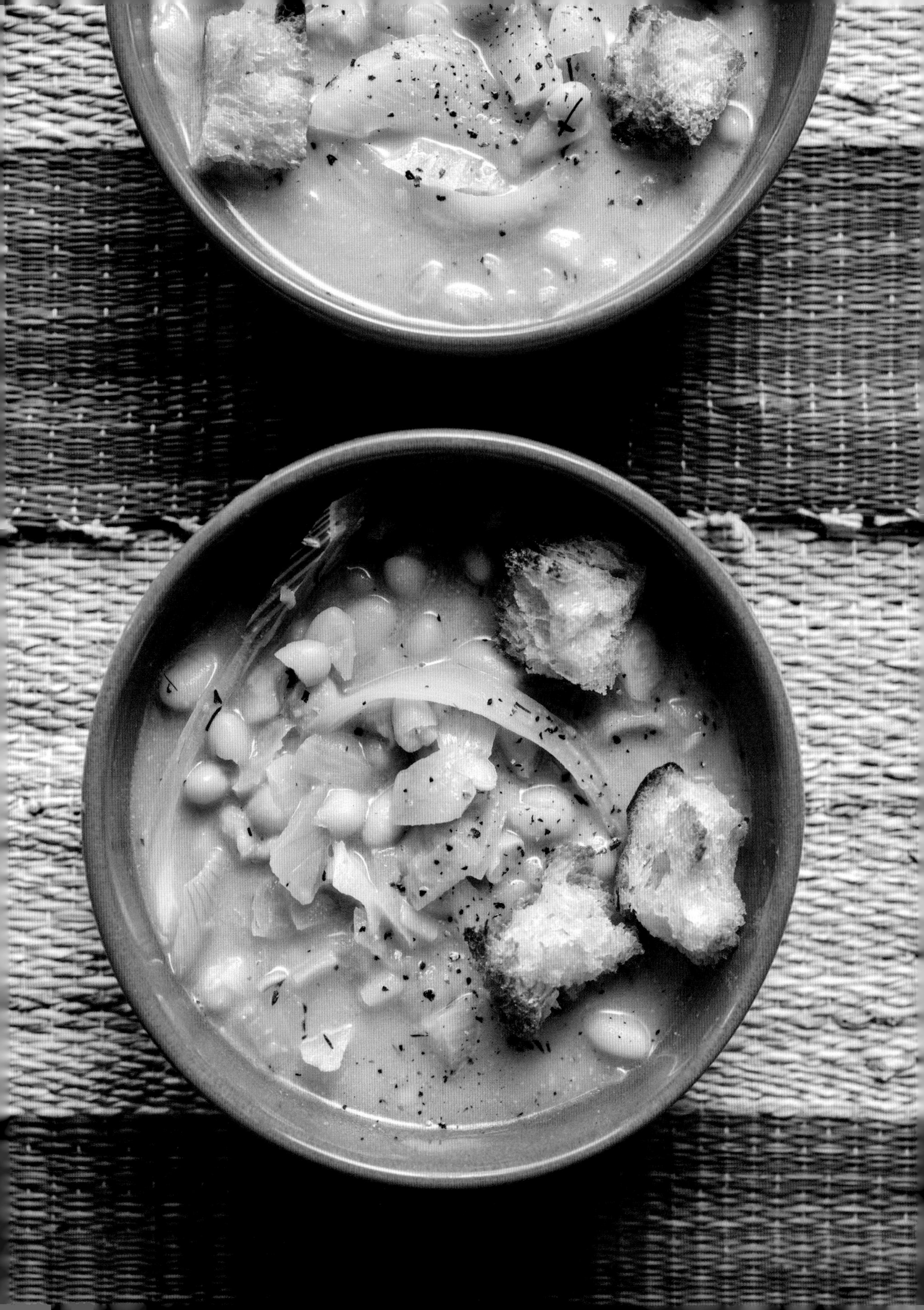

SERVES: 4
PREP: 10 MINS
COOK: 25 MINS
CALORIES: 496

- 4 chicken breasts
- 4 bacon medallions
- 4 tablespoons low-fat mayonnaise
- 3 tablespoons fat-free natural yoghurt
- 1 teaspoon English mustard
- juice of ½ lemon
- 1 clove of garlic, crushed
- 8 slices of wholemeal bread
- 2 hard-boiled eggs, sliced
- 1 avocado, sliced
- 150g (5½oz) cherry tomatoes, halved
- ¼ iceberg lettuce, sliced
- 30g (1oz) blue cheese, crumbled

CHICKEN COBB SALAD SANDWICH

A Cobb salad is perhaps one of my favourite dishes to have when we've managed to drag our carcasses over to the US – just a salad with chopped cheese, egg, bacon and other bits, but utterly delicious. You could cheerfully forgo the bread (we've added it purely because we're gluttons) and just have it as a salad – either way works well. We were lucky enough to revisit Florida and experience this salad anew. I needed something to calm me down: Paul had rashly decided to jump on the world's tallest swing ride – one of those giant structures where you're buckled into a little seat, taken 450 feet into the air, and spun around. I'd sooner walk into a burning house wearing a coat made out of petrol than trust my life to someone who looked as though they'd struggle to blink without prompting, but Paul has no such fear. So it was that I watched my husband disappear upwards into the night, supported only by two little chains, shrieking and screaming. He looked like an especially camp shooting star. Once he returned to the ground – thankfully not in freefall – he told me it wasn't frightening at all, but that's Paul all over: the queen of understated emotion.

Spray a frying pan with a little oil and place over a medium-high heat.

Add the chicken and cook for 6–8 minutes each side, then remove to a plate and slice.

Return the pan to the heat and add the bacon. Cook for 6–8 minutes, until crispy, then remove to the plate with the chicken.

In a bowl, mix together the mayonnaise, yoghurt, mustard, lemon juice and garlic, and season with salt and pepper.

Toast the bread, and spread half the slices with the mayonnaise mixture.

Top with the lettuce, avocado, sliced chicken, bacon, eggs, crumbled cheese and tomatoes and finish with the remaining slices of bread.

Notes: As we said, feel free to skip the bread. All we ask is that you present your salad in lovely uniform chopped-up lines. We like it that way.

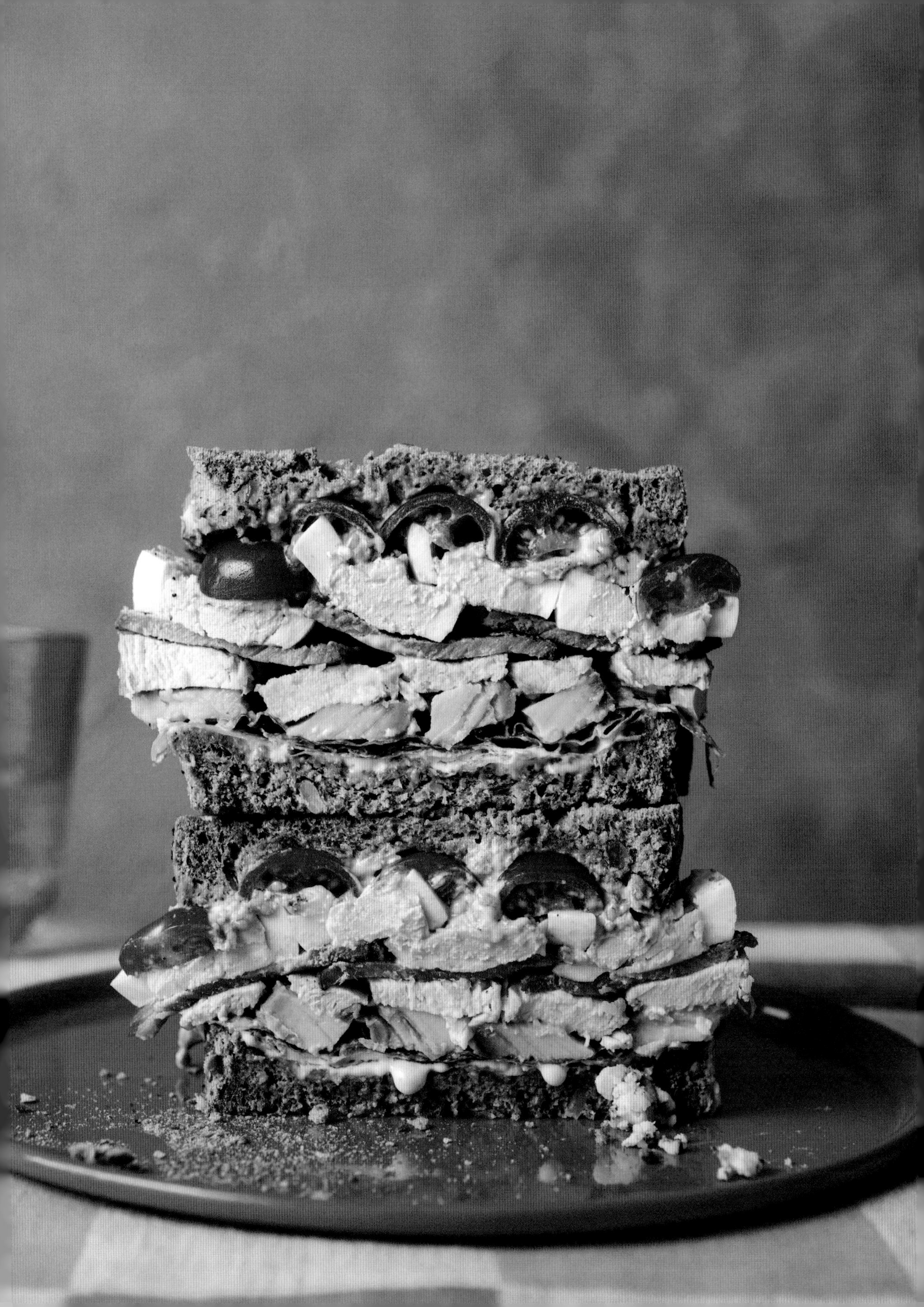

SERVES: 4
PREP: 10 MINS
COOK: 2 HRS 5 MINS
CALORIES: 165

30 mins, GF, DF

- 2 tablespoons olive oil
- 1 brown onion, chopped
- 2 garlic cloves, crushed
- 1 large cabbage, chopped
- 1 × 400g (14oz) tin of chopped tomatoes
- 1 carrot, peeled and chopped
- ½ green pepper, deseeded and diced
- 1 litre (1¾ pints) chicken stock
- 1 teaspoon paprika
- 1 teaspoon ground cumin
- 1 teaspoon hot chilli powder
- ½ teaspoon salt
- ¼ teaspoon black pepper

SPICY CABBAGE SOUP

A big, thick, spicy cabbage soup which is utterly delicious, but let's be honest, a sprinkling of hot chilli powder does not a spicy dish make. It's all so objective though: we've created recipes on the blog before that could reignite a dying sun and ne'ry a word of objection from folks, but dish out the most milquetoast of madras and you can guarantee we'll receive comments from people suggesting we've turned their dirty-basket to molten lava. So add the spice, leave it out, doesn't matter: the soup will absolutely stand on its own without it. Now the question you must consider before you turn to the recipe: did I engineer the whole paragraph above just for a reason to slip the word milquetoast into the narrative? I mean, it is one of my favourite words and you know me, why use a standard descriptive word when I can barrel something out covered in cobwebs? Well the answer is no, I didn't, but the publishers nixed a recipe for Not Milquetoast Milky Toast, so this is a compromise. Look carefully at the very end of this book though . . .

Put the oil into a large pan and place over a medium-high heat.

Add the onion and garlic and cook for about 5 minutes, until softened.

Add everything else to the pan and bring to the boil, then reduce the heat to low and simmer for 1½–2 hours.

Serve in bowls.

Notes: Stop buying your spices in those little jars – have a wander down your 'World Foods' aisle and you'll find far bigger containers and bags for considerably cheaper. Keep those spices in an airtight container in a cupboard and they'll last for ages. That said, do check your spices every now and then – they lose their potency over time.

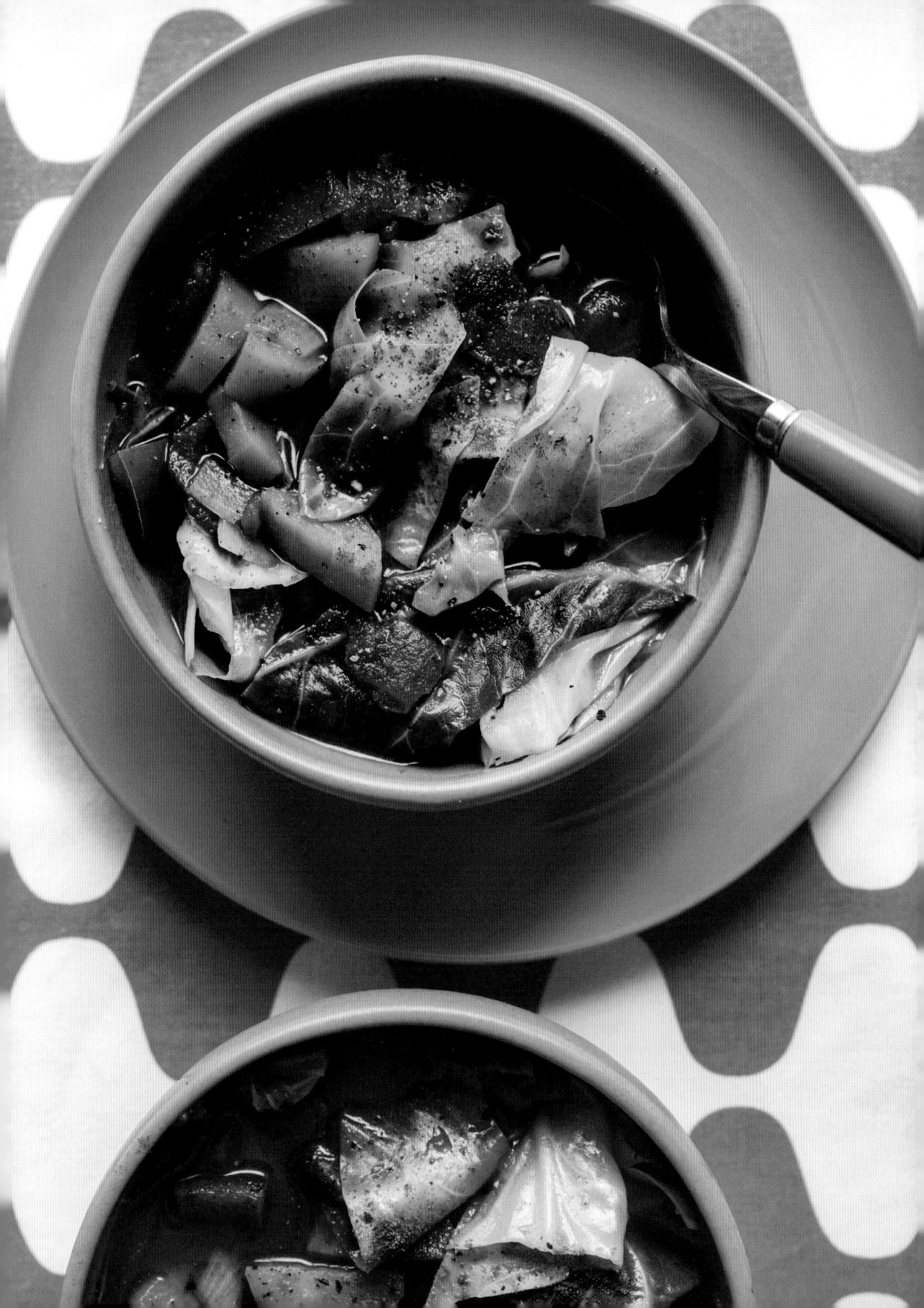

SERVES: 4
PREP: 15 MINS
COOK: 25 MINS
CALORIES: 251

30 mins · GF

CHICKEN IN THE GARDEN SALAD

As Lisa Simpson was told via the medium of song, you don't win friends with salad. And that's true: if you turn up to a barbecue with a wilted bowl of lettuce and some tomatoes that are two months away from flavour, you'll be rightly turned away. It's just common decency. That said, turn up with a bowl of this and you'll be warmly welcomed – we're talking fond pats on the back, the good liquor coming out of the cupboard and someone throwing their keys into the bread-bowl and fixing you with a libidinous leer. All this is to say that this salad isn't your typical boring salad, and frankly, if you're looking for a meal to delight and excite, this is the one. Trust your Cubs!

- 5 medium potatoes, peeled and diced
- 3 carrots, peeled and diced
- 1 × 290g (10oz) tin of garden peas, drained
- 2 skinless boneless chicken thighs
- 70g (2½oz) gherkins, diced
- 2 spring onions, sliced
- a handful of fresh parsley, chopped
- 25g (1oz) reduced-fat mayonnaise
- 25g (1oz) natural yoghurt
- 1 tablespoon mustard
- 1 tablespoon cider vinegar

Put the potatoes and carrots into a large pan and cover with cold water, then bring to the boil and simmer for 10–15 minutes. Add the peas for the last 2–3 minutes, then drain and allow to cool.

Meanwhile, spray a pan with a little oil and place over a medium-high heat. Open out the chicken thighs, add them to the pan, and cook for 5 minutes on each side. Check that they are cooked through, then remove them to a chopping board. Allow to cool, then cut them into cubes.

Put the chicken, gherkins, spring onions and parsley into a bowl, then add the cooled veg and stir gently.

In a separate bowl, mix together the mayonnaise, yoghurt, mustard and cider vinegar. Season with salt and pepper, then pour over the salad, mix well and serve.

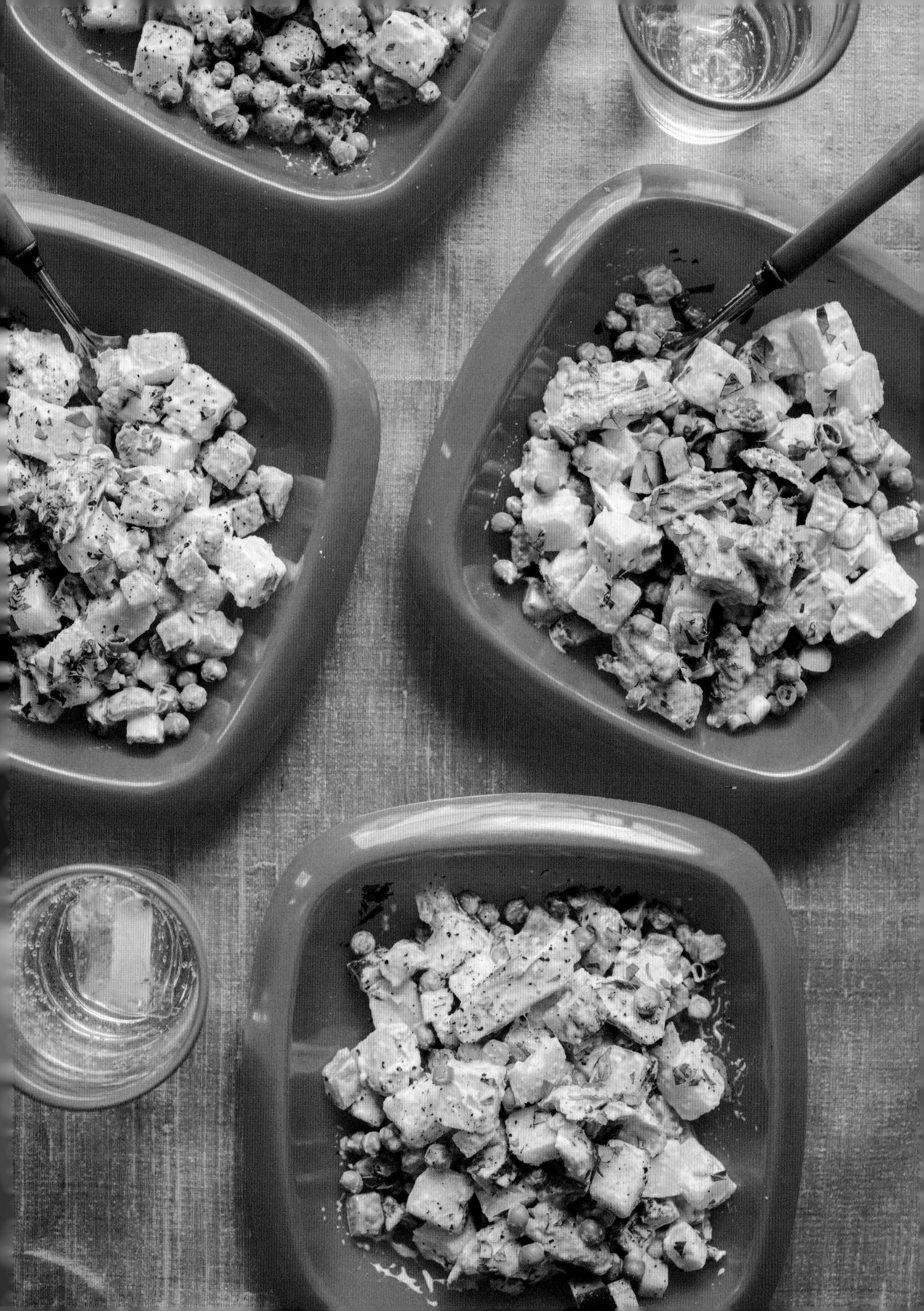

SERVES: 4
PREP: 10 MINS
COOK: 1 HR 15 MINS
CALORIES: 228

BACON & POTATO SOUP

Another one from our childhood, although I have to confess the soft cheese addition isn't part of the original recipe but simply my fervent need to add it to everything. If cheese doesn't sit right on your tummy, feel free to leave it out. I do wonder whether these older, simpler recipes are on the way out: I hope not. Most of the recipes from our childhood seem to be those with just a few ingredients, cooked simply, served without fuss or fanfare. More so in Paul's family, admittedly, although that hardly counts because the hob on the gas cooker was only ever clicked on when his mam couldn't find a lighter for her cigarette. But there's a lot to be said for stodgy simplicity, and we're sure this soup proves that right. As another aside, we often make jokes about Paul's mum's laissez-faire approach to parenting, and perhaps it's a little unbalanced. After all, it was my parents who left me in a carpet shop for an hour after I disappeared (after several increasingly thin-lipped warnings) between the giant rolls of carpet.

- 6 bacon medallions
- 1 brown onion, diced
- 3 cloves of garlic, crushed
- 2 large potatoes, diced
- 1 litre (1¾ pints) chicken stock
- 1 teaspoon dried thyme
- 200g (7oz) reduced-fat soft cheese

Spray a large saucepan with a little oil and place over a medium-high heat.

Add the bacon and cook until crispy, then remove from the pan and set aside to cool. Once cool, chop finely.

Add the onion and garlic to the pan and cook for 4–5 minutes, stirring frequently.

Add the potatoes, chicken stock and thyme and bring to the boil, then reduce to low and simmer for 1 hour.

Remove from the heat and use a stick blender to blend until smooth (or to your liking), then stir through the soft cheese.

Serve in bowls, topped with the chopped bacon.

Notes: We think keeping the skins on the potatoes is best, but you do you babe.

If freezing, add the cheese and bacon once you've reheated the soup.

Oh, not to mention the time they left me and my sister on a service station slip-road on the A20. Still, we did have a lovely summer touring with Eddie Stobart.

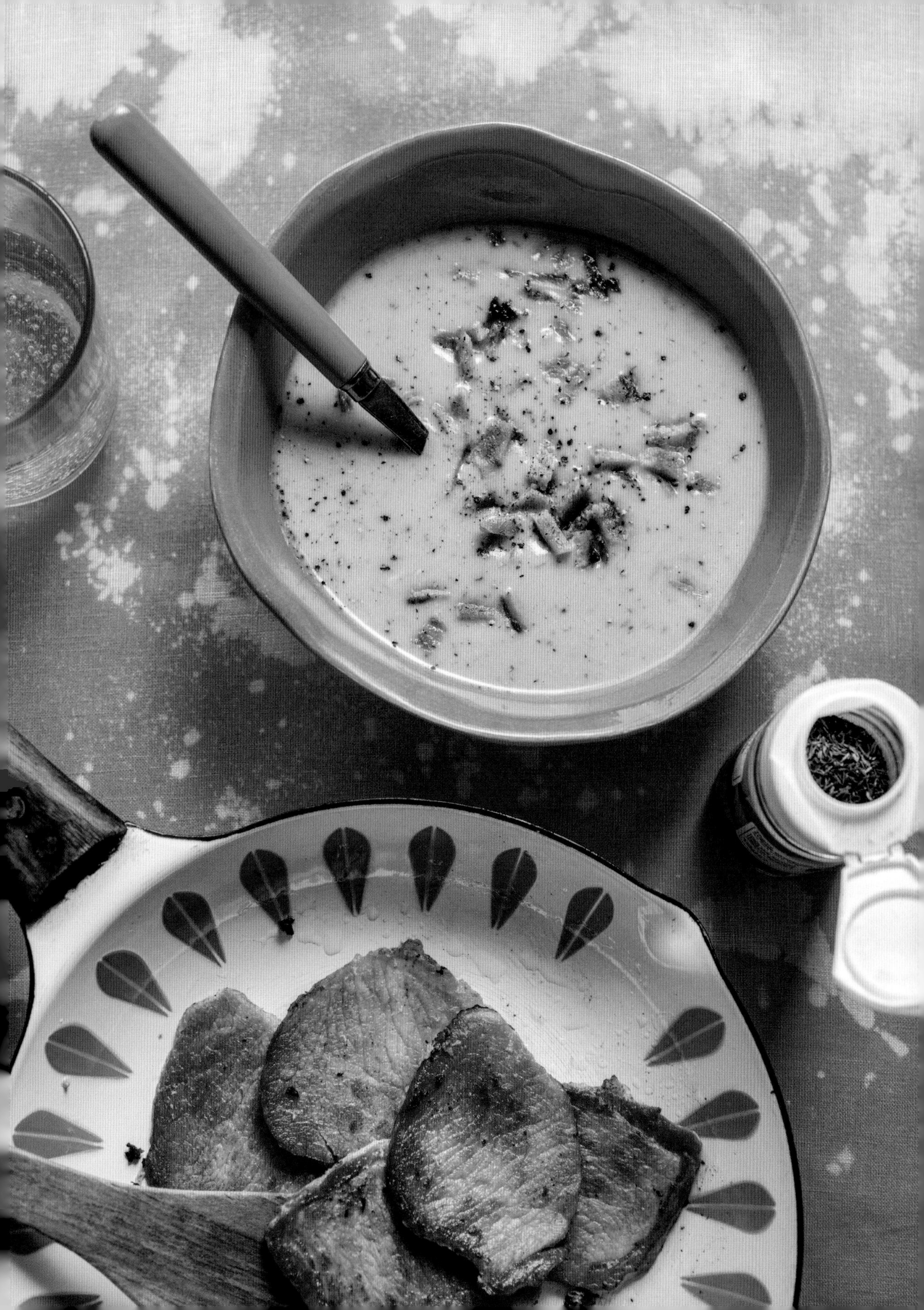

SERVES: 4
PREP: 15 MINS
COOK: 15 MINS
CALORIES: 150

30 mins · V · GF · DF

- 1 large broccoli, chopped into florets
- 500g (1lb 2oz) asparagus stalks, chopped
- 1 large leek, chopped
- 1 brown onion, chopped
- 3 cloves of garlic, crushed
- 1.5 litres (2½ pints) vegetable stock
- zest and juice of 1 lemon
- ½ teaspoon fennel seeds
- ½ teaspoon salt
- ¼ teaspoon black pepper
- 125ml (4fl oz) almond milk
- fresh dill
- 2 teaspoons olive oil (optional)

GREEN GOBBLIN' SOUP

As a lover of the colour green, this is one of my favourite-looking recipes in the book – and that's a high bar indeed, given that our designers seem to have poured a rainbow across the pages at the best of times. It always amazes me that I can say to our utterly wonderful team that we want a 'colourful' book and they come back with the most glorious designs. Of course, we know all about colour here: why, we're official colour experts. See, we went to the Museum of Colour at the start of the year. You would think a museum devoted to colour would be boring, but we learned so much, not least that the official colours to match our personalities are 'acidic lime' (James) and 'chilli red' (Paul). I assume that's why they called me a bitter old tart as I left, but who can say? Anyway, they also say red and green should never be seen, so Paul and I will be getting a divorce just as soon as we can. Enjoy your colourful dinner: an electric sapphire such as yourself will surely be delighted.

Put the broccoli, asparagus, leek, onion, garlic and stock into a large pan and bring to the boil, then reduce the heat and simmer for 10–12 minutes, until the vegetables are tender.

Remove the pan from the heat and add the lemon zest and juice, the fennel seeds, salt and pepper. Mix well, then blend with a stick blender until smooth.

Ladle the soup into bowls and swirl the almond milk over the top. Sprinkle over the dill and drizzle over the olive oil (if using).

Note: No almond milk? Use 80g (2¾oz) of soft cheese instead.

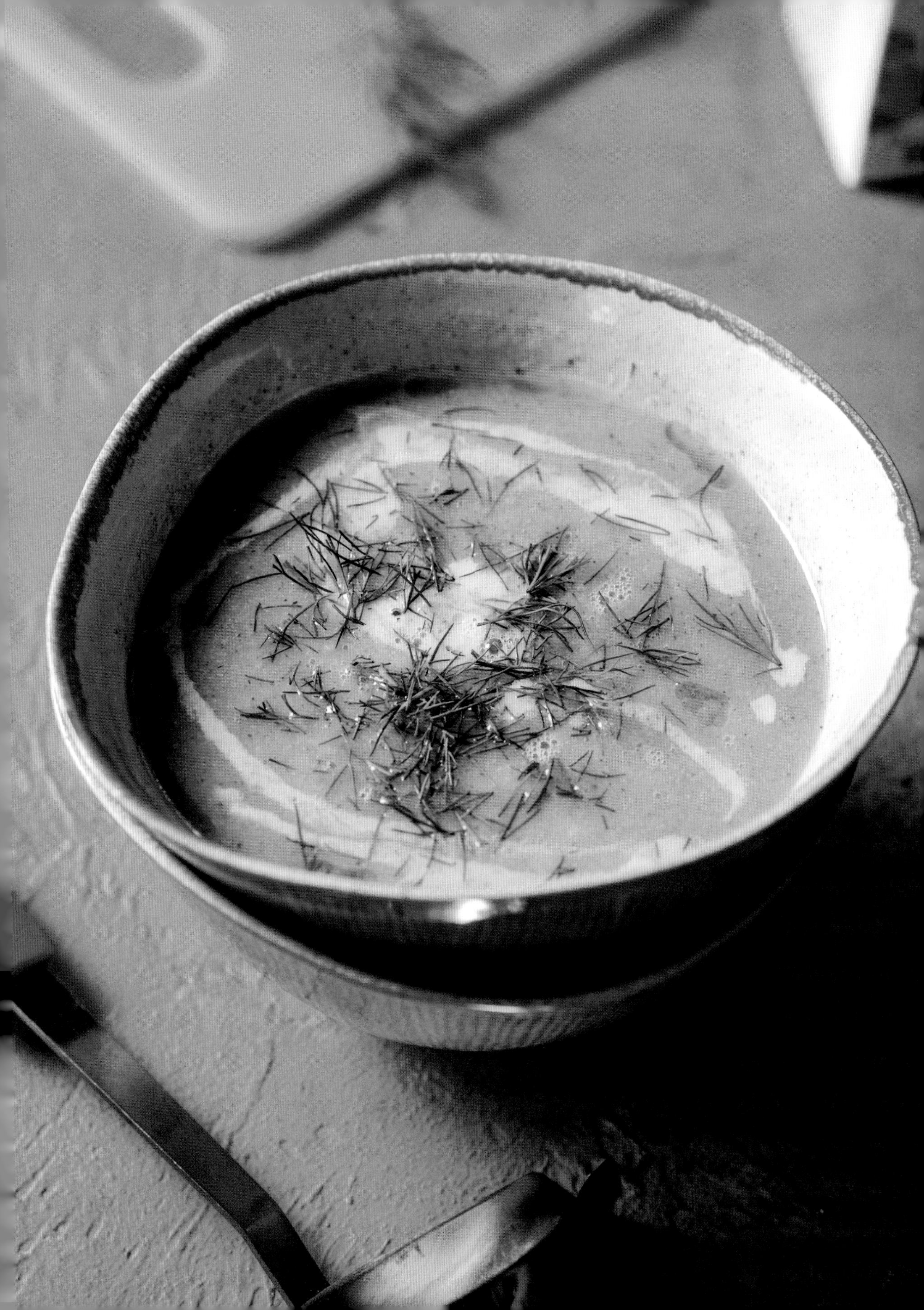

SERVES: 4
PREP: 20 MINS
COOK: 10 MINS
CALORIES: 279

30 mins · V · DF

SPICY PEANUT TEMPEH WITH CRUNCHY SALAD

New ingredient alert: tempeh! Ever mindful of the fact that people might view tofu with the same wrinkled-nosed expression you might adopt if you saw a spider scuttling into your shoe, we're switching to its sort-of-cousin. Tempeh is still soy, but using the whole bean – it's harder, it's fitter, it's got so much protein in it you'll be punching your way through a wall in no time at all. It does look rather like those bars of soap your mum used to make from all the smaller offcuts of leftover soap, mind. Or was that just my mother, so tight the people on her ten pound notes used to blink when they were brought from her purse? If you can't find tempeh, firm tofu will see you right. Mind, you find you've opened a box and 'Written in the Stars' starts playing, you've accidentally bought Tinie Tempah, and I assume he'll be very vexed.

- 200g (7oz) tempeh, cut into small pieces
- 1 tablespoon sriracha
- 2 tablespoons smooth peanut butter
- 100ml (3½fl oz) reduced-fat coconut milk
- juice of 1 lime
- 2 tablespoons soy sauce

For the crunchy salad

- ½ red cabbage, finely sliced
- juice of 1 lime
- 1 teaspoon honey
- 1 red pepper, finely sliced
- 2 carrots, grated
- ½ cucumber, halved lengthways and sliced
- 4 spring onions, sliced on the diagonal
- a handful of roasted salted peanuts, crushed

First, put the red cabbage into a bowl with the lime juice, honey and a good pinch of salt. Leave to stand for about 10 minutes – this will just soften the cabbage a little.

Heat a non-stick frying pan over a high heat and spray with a little oil. Add the tempeh to the pan and cook until crisp, then toss with half the sriracha.

Mix the peanut butter and coconut milk together and heat in a small pan until just warm (don't let it boil or it will split). Remove from the heat, add the soy sauce and the rest of the sriracha, and season with salt and pepper.

Divide the cabbage between plates. Top with the red pepper, carrot, cucumber, spring onions and crisp tempeh, then drizzle over the warm spicy peanut sauce and sprinkle the crushed peanuts over the top.

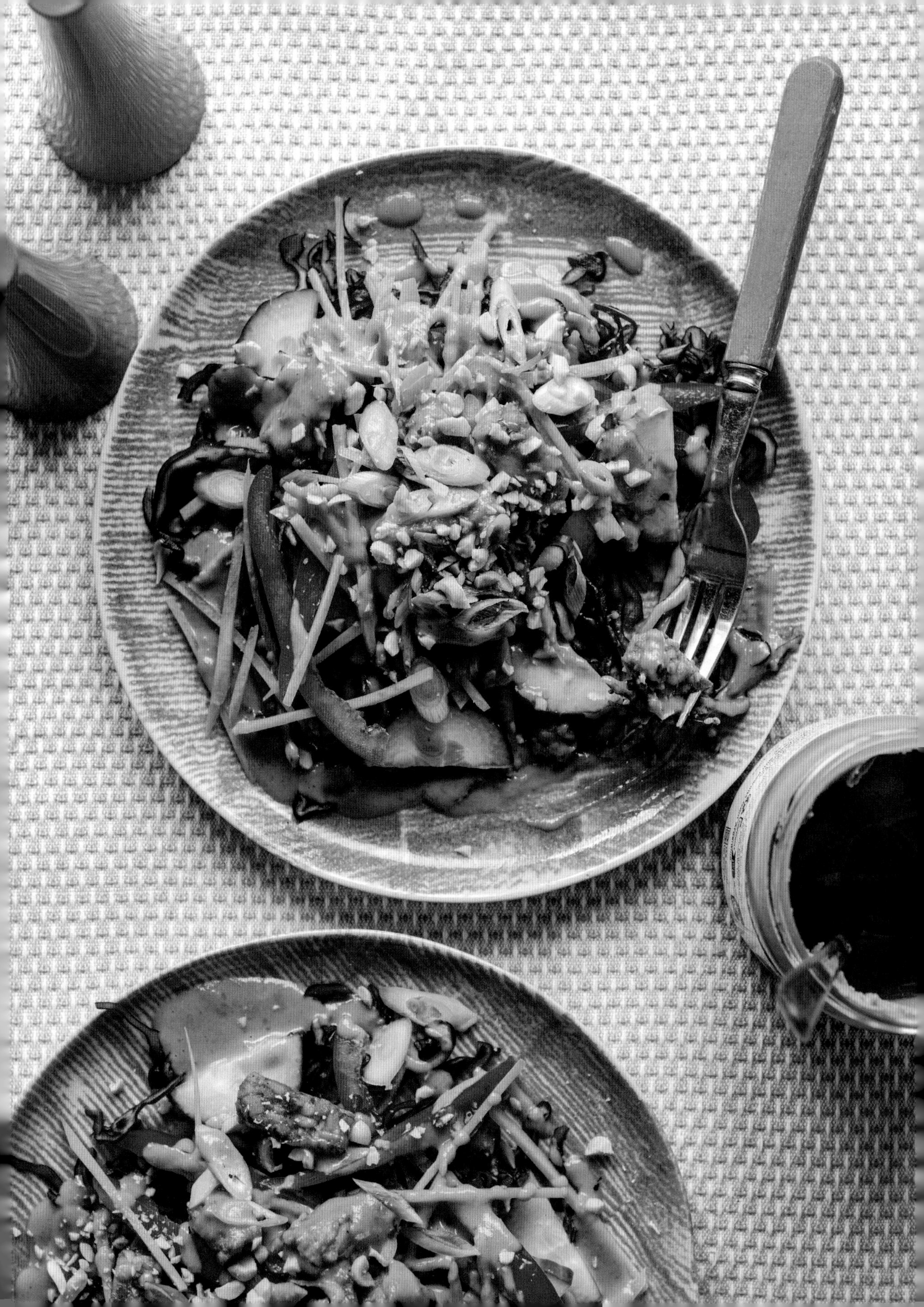

SERVES: 4
PREP: 15 MINS
COOK: 50 MINS
CALORIES: 319

1 brown onion, quartered
3 cloves of garlic, crushed
2 tablespoons curry powder
1 teaspoon ground cumin
1 teaspoon ground coriander
1 teaspoon ground turmeric
1 teaspoon paprika
1 teaspoon salt
1 teaspoon black pepper
1kg (2lb 4oz) cauliflower florets (frozen or fresh)
400ml (14fl oz) coconut milk
1 litre (1¾ pints) vegetable stock

CURRIED CAULIFLOWER SOUP

I must impress on those with delicate sensibilities that you may do well to skip straight to the recipe, as a rather windy conversation is about to take place. In all our books, we submit a recipe that, although suitably sapid, will leave you with the incredible ability to clear a room with a simple trouser-cough. This curried cauliflower soup is one such recipe: delicious, but deadly. I mean, to be fair, you stand no chance: cauliflower smells dreadful right from the get-go – it announces its intentions before you've even had a chance to mellow it with coconut milk. It follows the example of those slabs of wafer-thin ham you can buy where it must be someone's sole job to break wind in the packet immediately before it's hermetically sealed. That said, if you're happy to live with the blowy repercussions of a cauliflower soup, you'll be richly rewarded here: this is a soup to put hairs on your chest and a warmth in your tummy, let alone your keks.

Spray a large pan with a little oil and place over a medium-high heat.

Add the onion and garlic and cook for 3–4 minutes, stirring frequently.

Add the curry powder, cumin, coriander, turmeric, paprika, salt and pepper and cook for 1–2 minutes, stirring often.

Add the cauliflower, coconut milk and stock, bring to the boil, then reduce the heat and simmer for 30–40 minutes, until the cauliflower is tender.

Remove the pan from the heat, allow to cool for a few minutes, then blend with a stick blender.

Serve in bowls.

Notes: We find at Chubby Towers, cultured little sods that we are, that a fart is immeasurably improved with a rejoinder such as '. . .a little more choke and she would have started', '. . .hold tight Mr Brown, we'll send someone immediately', or, a personal favourite, '. . .that's gonna itch when it dries'. As I say, we're not a classy household.

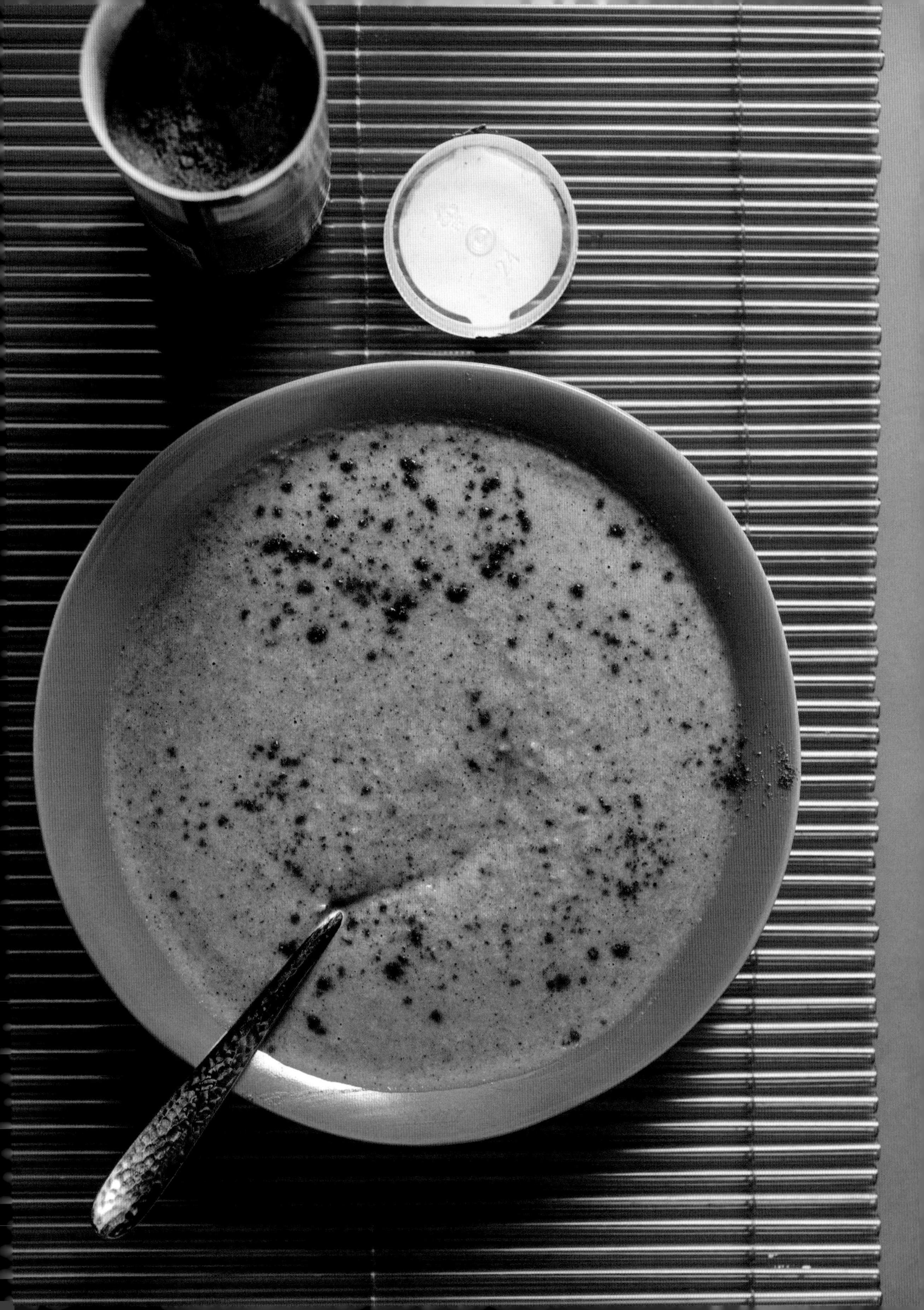

GREEK SUMMER SALAD

SERVES: 4
PREP: 15 MINS
CALORIES: 230

30 mins · V · GF

This is exactly the type of salad my parents would throw together with bits from the garden when I was young, though perhaps not with such a florid dressing: we were very much a Sarson's vinegar on your salad household. But it was just the thing coming back starving from a morning throwing pebbles down wells and building dens, which I hope is still very much a thing among the youth (good lord, I'm old). For the record, the best den we ever built as a group of village ruffians was one that still stands to this day. We stole several large pallets from a building site, tramped them into the woods and put together what can only be described as a ramshackle hut. It was terrific: our own place to hide from Pennywise. We once had the bright idea of having a small campfire inside this poorly ventilated wooden den, and to make things even more risky, we used a spare tyre we found to keep the fire contained. Clearly we survived, although it goes some way to explaining why I can taste colours. So yes, kids: do build dens, don't build danger-huts. Your parents will thank you, and may make you this delicious salad as a reward.

- juice of 1 lemon
- 1 tablespoon honey
- 1 clove of garlic, crushed
- 1 tablespoon olive oil
- 1 × 400g (14oz) tin of chickpeas, drained and rinsed
- 325g (11½oz) cherry tomatoes (about 15 or so), halved
- 70g (2½oz) feta cheese, crumbled
- 1 cucumber, diced
- 1 red onion, sliced
- 1 yellow pepper, deseeded and chopped
- a handful of fresh parsley, chopped
- 100g (3½oz) baby spinach

Whisk together the lemon juice, honey, garlic and olive oil to make a dressing, and set aside.

In a bowl, mix together the remaining ingredients and top with the dressing.

Notes: We used a yellow pepper to add a bit more colour, but any colour will do! No cherry tomatoes? A normal chopped tomato will work fine!

There's also an entire tent strung up in a tree just outside of Horsley, Northumberland. It's still there because I spotted it only a few months back. Probably charge £400 a night on Airbnb for it now . . .

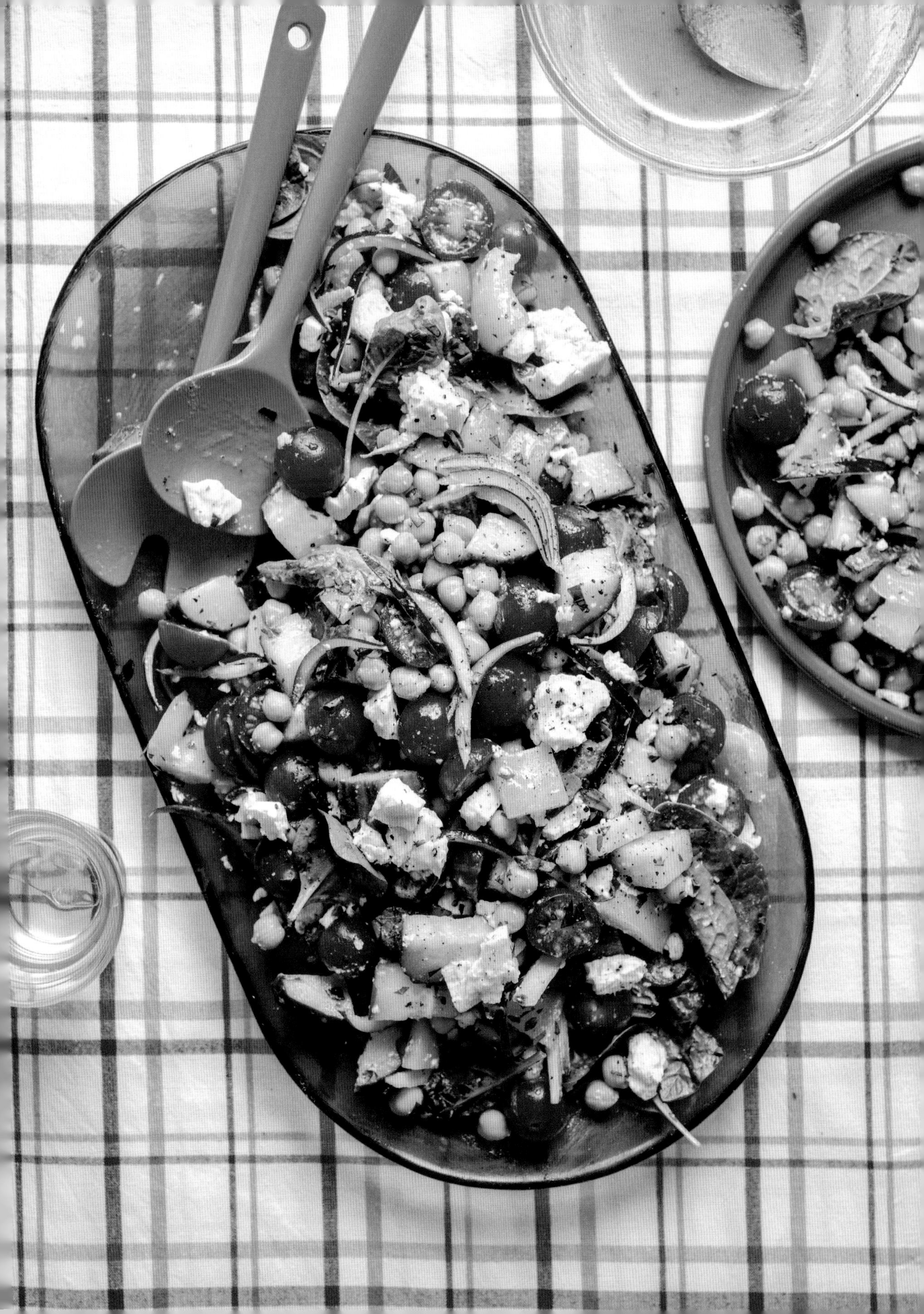

SERVES: 4
PREP: 10 MINS
COOK: 1 HR 20 MINS
CALORIES: 269

CHORIZO BARLEY SOUP

Now on first glance at the ingredients you may think we've taken leave of our senses including orange juice in a soup, but it really works to cut through what is quite a heavy, rib-sticking soup. Pearl barley is one of those ingredients that acts as a little flavour sponge, and that's why it's the star of the show here. We bought a big bag of pearl barley a few months ago as we started our little health kick, to up our protein, not realising that it isn't the best grain for that purpose. It's full of fibre, though, which keeps you regular, so there's always that. This push for 'protein-high' products can be such a swiz, and we recommend caution – we've often bought the 'protein' editions of regular products only to find just the slightest uptick on the protein macro, usually accompanied by a non-insignificant price increase. But we digress, as ever and always. This soup might not fill out your macro charts the way stuffing a chicken breast with mushy peas might do, but it will leave you satisfied and smiling. Isn't that all we can ask in this work-a-day world?

- 100g (3½oz) pearl barley
- 1 medium leek, sliced
- 150g (5½oz) broccoli florets
- 1 red pepper, deseeded and diced
- 120g (4oz) chorizo, diced
- 700ml (1¼ pints) chicken stock
- juice of 1 orange
- 2 teaspoons balsamic vinegar
- ½ teaspoon dried thyme
- ½ teaspoon sriracha
- a handful of fresh basil leaves

Put the pearl barley into a large saucepan with 500ml (18fl oz) of water and bring to the boil over a high heat. Boil for 10 minutes, then reduce the heat to low and simmer, covered, for 50 minutes, topping up the pan with extra water while cooking, if needed. Drain and set aside.

Spray a large pan with a little oil, add the leek, and cook for 5–6 minutes, stirring occasionally.

Add the broccoli, pepper and chorizo and cook for another 5 minutes.

Add the pearl barley to the pan along with the stock, orange juice, balsamic vinegar and thyme, stir well, then bring to a gentle boil.

Remove from the heat and serve in bowls, drizzled with the sriracha and sprinkled with the basil.

Notes: Couscous, quinoa, orzo and even rice are good alternatives for pearl barley, if you prefer. Just be sure to cook them according to the instructions on the packet.

I don't know about you, folks, but I'm glad Paul felt it necessary to add 'cook according to the instructions' in the note regarding possible barley swaps. We'd hate for anyone to start cooking their quinoa by hurling it into the sun or staring at it angrily until it yields of its own accord.

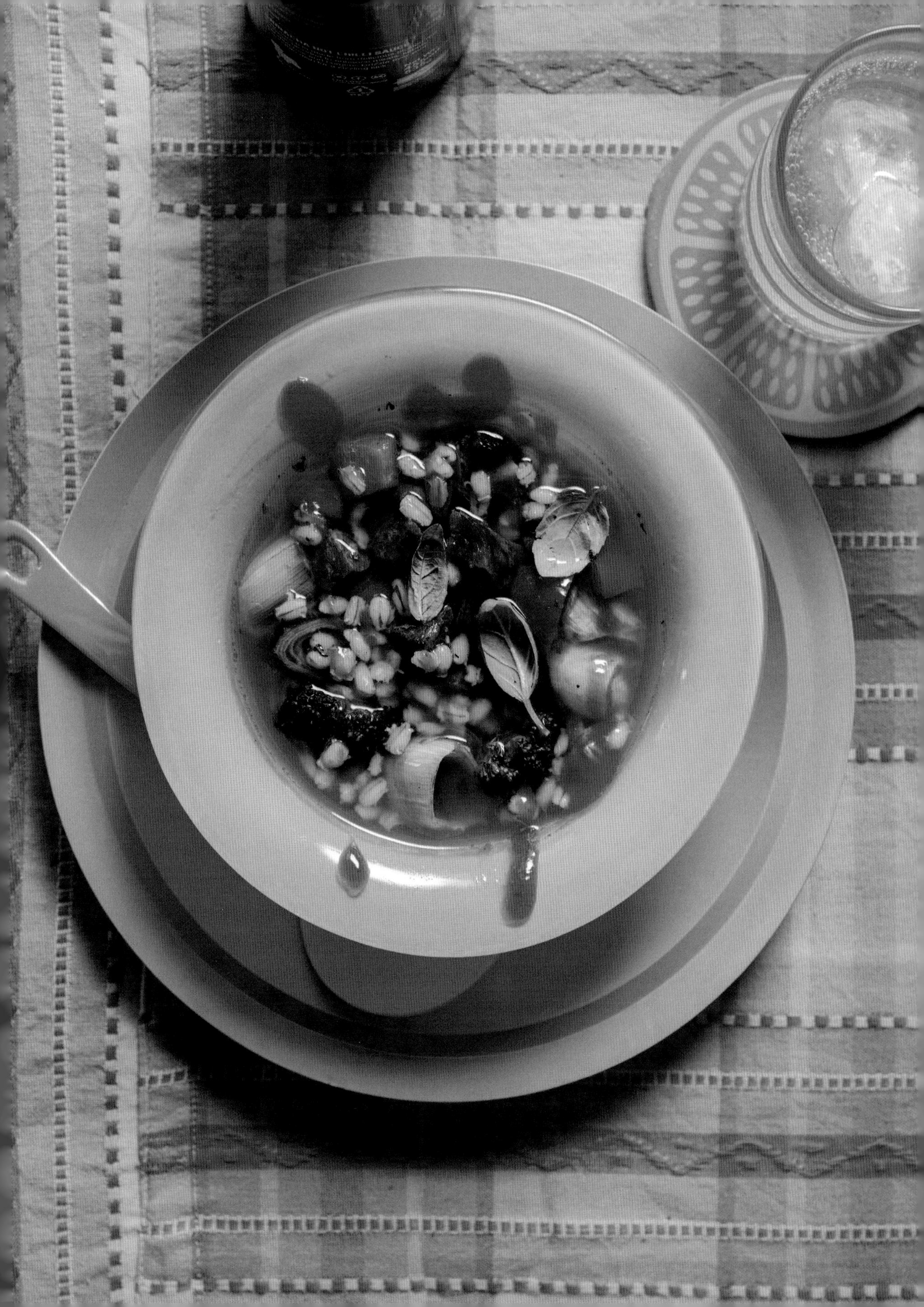

SERVES: 4
PREP: 10 MINS
COOK: 40 MINS
CALORIES: 236

2 brown onions, diced
600g (1lb 5oz) parsnips, peeled and roughly diced (reserve some of the peelings – see notes)
600g (1lb 5oz) Bramley apples, peeled, cored, and diced
2 cloves of garlic, crushed
1 litre (1¾ pints) vegetable stock
150ml (5fl oz) semi-skimmed milk

CREAMY PARSNIP & APPLE SOUP

It's been over two years since we brought Goomba, our popcorn-scented Springer Spaniel, into Chubby Towers, and over that time so many plus points have made themselves known. For example, the absolute joy of watching him take offence at an entirely random new object and spend a good twenty minutes barking furiously at it: his latest target is a lamp we have rotated ninety degrees. There's also the matter of him deciding when we're taking a little too long to rise of a morning – he's learned that our living-room door doesn't close properly, so he can nose it open and then spend ten minutes knocking his head on our bedroom door until one of us bursts forth in a vision of fat to get his breakfast sorted. But perhaps the most rewarding benefit is to be found via all the walks we have to take him on. I mention this purely because it's where we get the apples for this warming, autumnal soup. See, around September, we find ourselves mysteriously walking through an entirely different neighbourhood, simply because there's a house overlooking the path whose garden is full of apple trees, the fruits of which will often be stuck in a basket for people to help themselves.

Spray a large pan with a little oil and place over a medium heat.

Add the onions and parsnips and gently fry for about 15 minutes.

Add the apples and garlic and cook for another 3–4 minutes, then pour in the stock and bring to the boil. Reduce the heat to a simmer and cook for another 20 minutes.

Remove from the heat and blend with a stick blender until smooth.

Pour in the milk, stir, and serve.

Note: For extra fanciness, we like to toss the parsnip peelings in a little curry powder, spray them with a little oil, and roast them in a hot oven for a few minutes to crisp them up. We then use them to top the soup. It's well worth it. This is all completely optional, though.

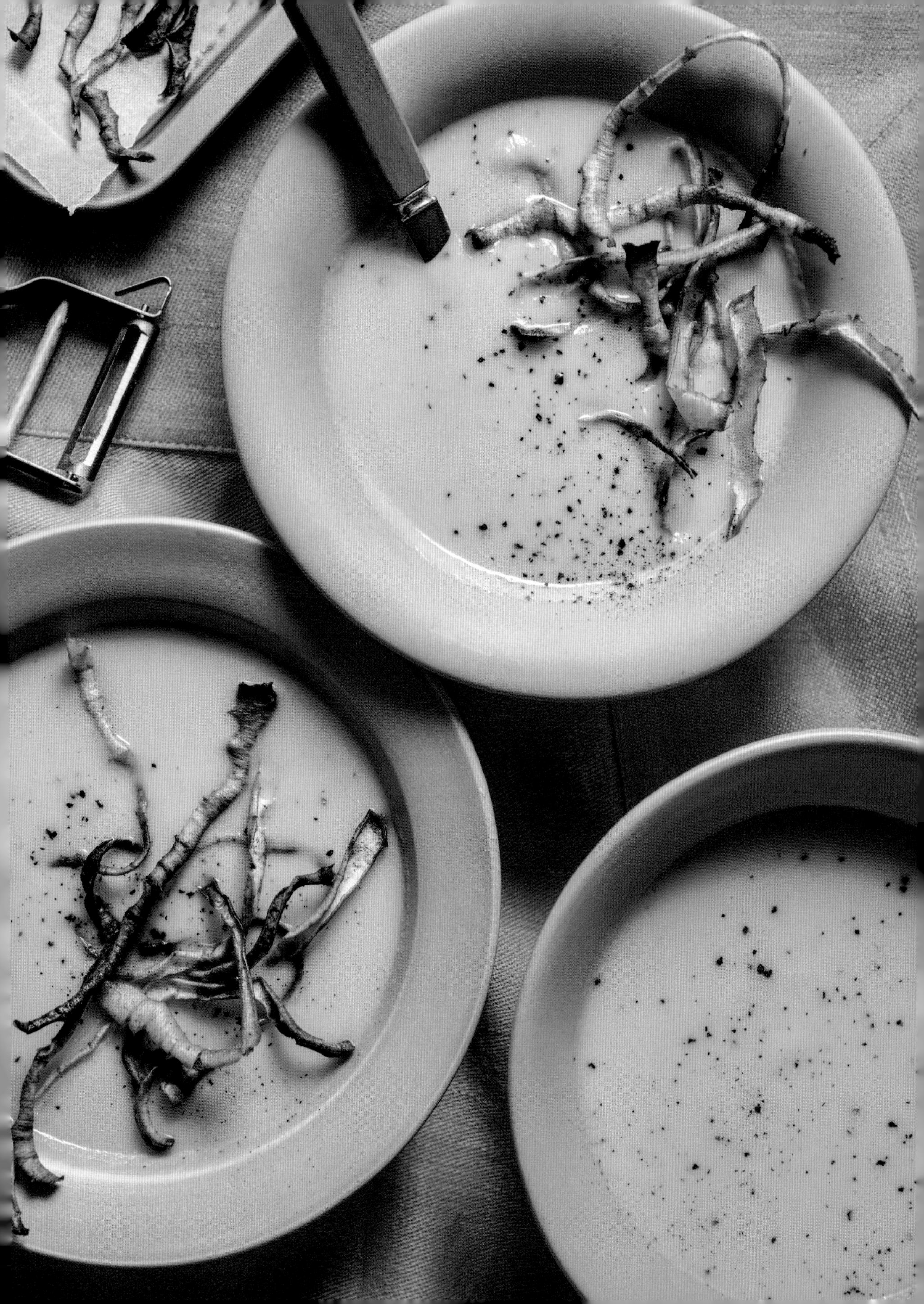

MAKES: 4–6
PREP: 20 MINS
COOK: 20 MINS
CALORIES: 234

SPINACH & FETA MUFFINS

Although we are sliding these little muffins over to you as a suggestion for a full meal, they also serve as the most delicious 'grab and go' breakfast. Cook them, freeze them, then grab one as you leave in the morning. By the time you arrive at work, assuming you don't schlep to work across the Siberian tundras, it'll be defrosted and ready for action. While we're on the topic of breakfast, a quick hooray for the return of full buffet breakfasts at those Inns who are Premier, after their COVID-demanded exile. I've never been one for a breakfast that extends beyond a black coffee and some form of nicotine delivery, but when I'm on holiday I want more. I want a rotary toaster that gives me slightly heated toast on the first rotation and pure carbon on the second. I want a trough of sausages to build a fort on my plate. Most importantly, though, I want to eat slightly more than I decently should, discreetly burp into my sleeve and then proclaim that 'I am as full as a bull's bum.' Paul expects it of me. But as we aren't on holiday, you should turn your attention to these muffins, and I'll go back to daydreaming of bacon and indiscreet acts under purple mood lighting.

- 250g (9oz) frozen spinach
- 200g (7oz) self-raising flour
- 1 teaspoon onion granules
- ½ teaspoon paprika
- 1 teaspoon salt
- 2 eggs
- 300ml (10fl oz) semi-skimmed milk
- 150g (5½oz) reduced-fat feta cheese, crumbled
- 50g (1¾oz) reduced-fat cottage cheese

Preheat the oven to 180°C fan/400°F/gas mark 6.

Put the frozen spinach into a bowl, pour over boiling water and leave for a few minutes to thaw. Once thawed, drain in a colander and leave until cool, then squeeze the spinach to remove as much water as possible.

In a bowl, mix together the flour, onion granules, paprika and salt and set aside.

In another bowl, beat the eggs, then add the spinach and milk, and mix.

Add the egg mixture to the flour mixture, along with the feta and cottage cheese, and stir gently, being careful not to overdo it.

Spoon the mixture into muffin cases into a Yorkshire pudding tin and bake for 20 minutes.

Notes: You could, of course, use fresh spinach here, but we all know how that dance goes: you put a quarter tonne of fresh spinach into a pan, wilt it down and then look aghast at the pan as you lift out half a teaspoon of green mush. It's no life, is it?

If you make teeny-tiny versions of these, you could use them as cheesy little dumplings to pad out meals. I know this, because my own cheesy little dumpling told me so.

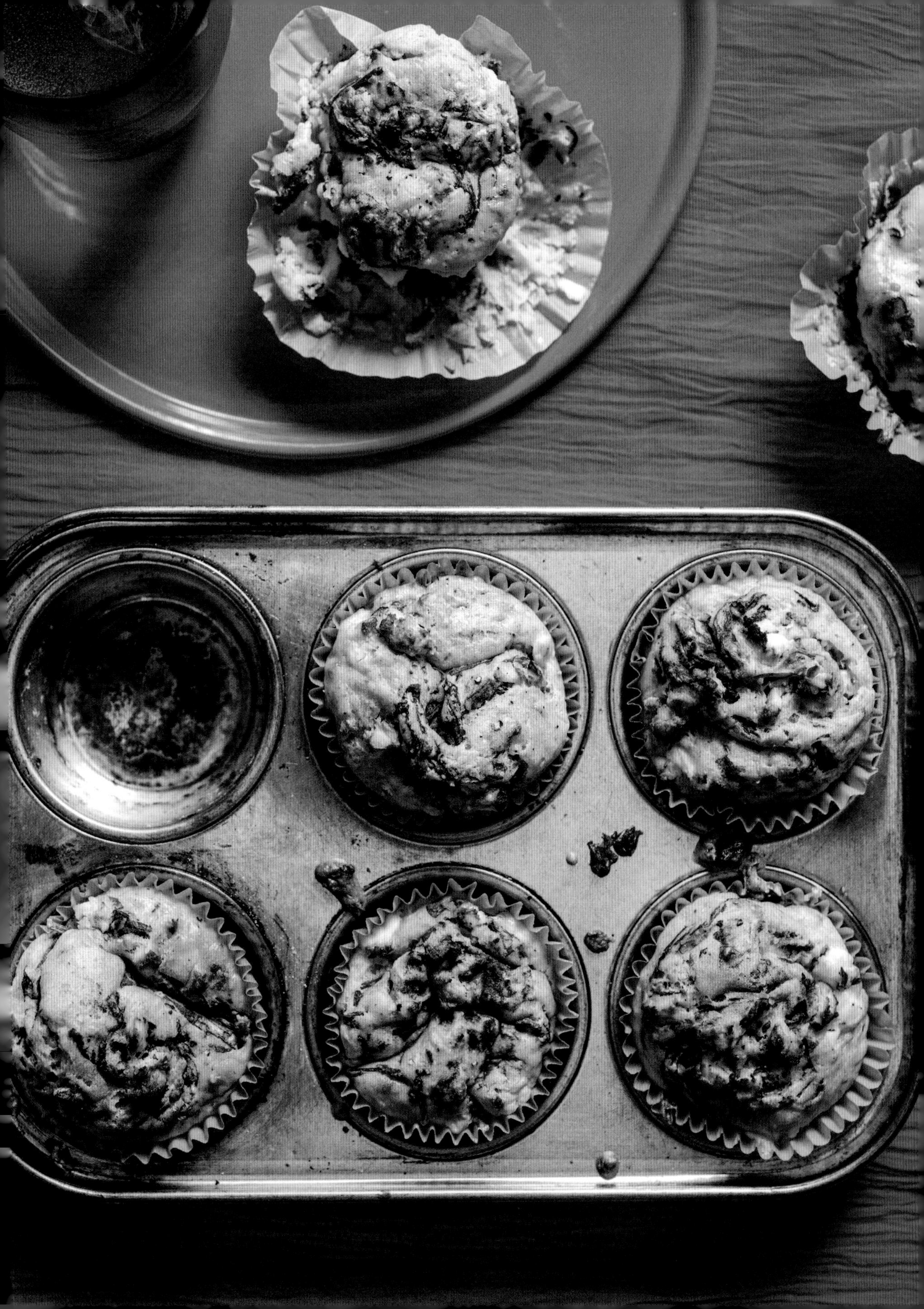

FUSS

FAKE

-FREE

AWAYS

SERVES: 4
PREP: 1 HR 10 MINS
COOK: 20 MINS
CALORIES: 78

GF

- 1 teaspoon lemon juice
- 12 jumbo king prawns, peeled
- 200g (7oz) low-fat natural yoghurt
- 1 teaspoon garlic and ginger paste
- 1 teaspoon paprika
- 1 teaspoon garam masala
- 1 teaspoon hot chilli powder
- ½ teaspoon ground fenugreek

TANDOORI PRAWNS

Folks who have been with us over the previous three books will know that we've been on quite a journey with prawns. At first I described them as 'icky pink fish commas', which remains true of those tiny pots you get slathered in pink mayo at the seaside, but over time, we've grown to love the 'big' versions. Proper prawns, that is. Don't get me wrong, they still freak me out and if I look too closely at them I can't quite process their alien faces, but done in this lovely tandoori style, they're delicious. This recipe is perfect for a barbecue should you be so inclined, and indeed, the 'paste' can be used for any other meat you fancy.

Sprinkle the lemon juice over the prawns and set aside.

In another bowl, mix together the yoghurt, garlic and ginger paste, paprika, garam masala, chilli powder and fenugreek.

Add the prawns to the marinade and leave in the fridge for about an hour.

Preheat the oven to 230°C fan/475°F/gas mark 9, or its highest temperature, and push the prawns on to skewers (3 per skewer). Place the skewers in the oven and cook for 10 minutes, then turn and cook for another 10 minutes.

Serve!

Notes: I have no notes to add here, so I'll leave you with my favourite seafood joke – what do you call a seafood restaurant that powers itself? A fission-chip shop.

I'll get my coat.

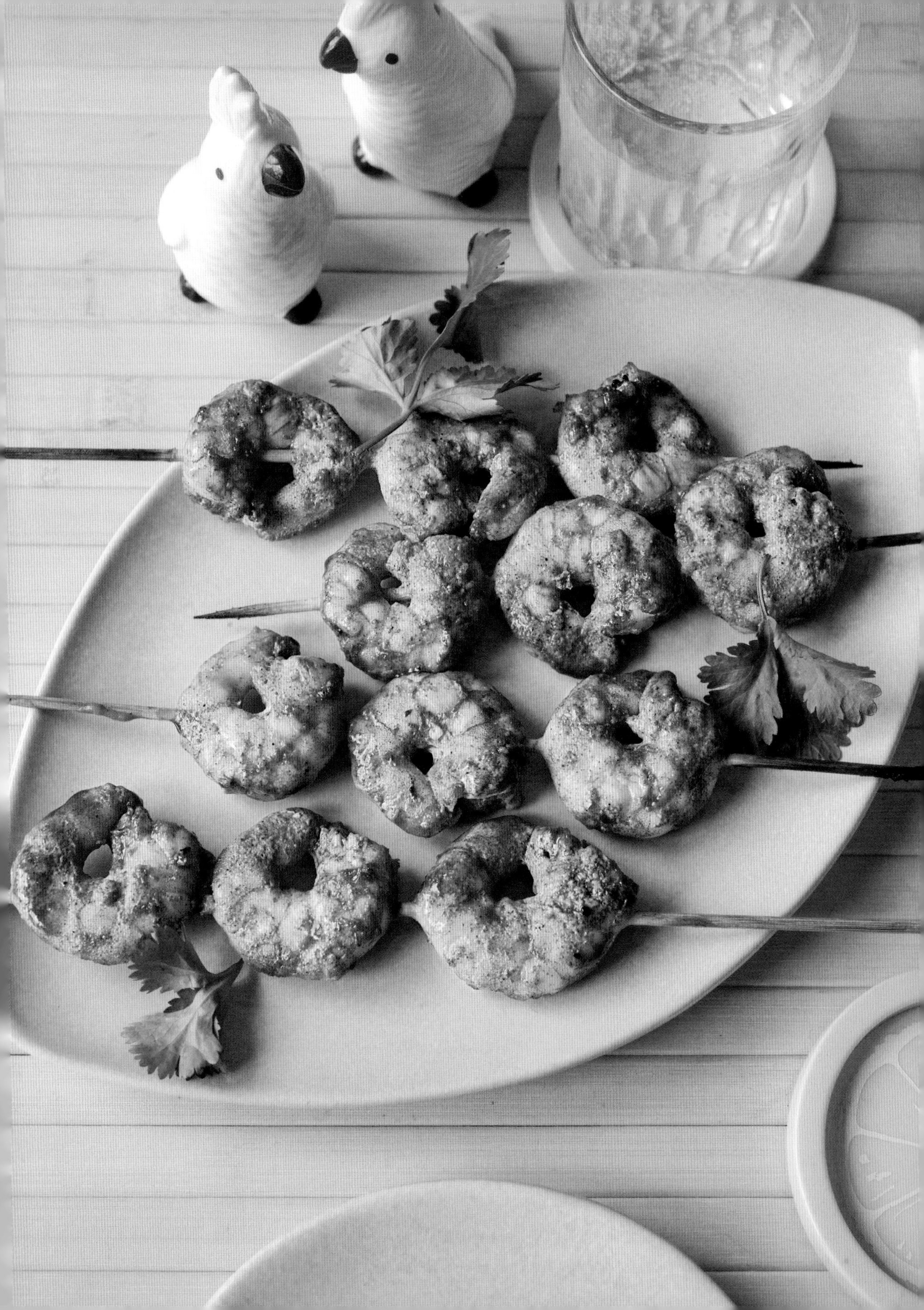

SERVES: 4
PREP: 10 MINS
COOK: 20 MINS
CALORIES: 483

30 mins, family, 10 basket, GF, DF

SPAM MASALA

Spam! We're huge fans of the stuff here at Chubby Towers, to the point where we are throwing caution to the wind and not replacing it with a non-branded equivalent. Over in America there's all manner of Spam flavours (including the frankly outrageously delicious teriyaki flavour), but here in Blighty, you're stuck with the classic. That's just fine though, because it sings in this recipe. Spam reminds me entirely of a Saturday night dinner singeing my buttocks in front of a coal fire eating Spam, egg and chips, and that's a very precious memory. Doubly so if there was an episode of *Bugs* on the telly, and triply so if my sister had been sent to her room for being a precocious little brat. If you're entirely averse to the idea of a brick of spiced ham then, of course, feel free to swap it out for chicken for a quick alternative. But if you're on the fence, I beg you to give it another go.

- 1 brown onion, sliced
- 2 cloves of garlic, crushed
- 2.5cm (1 inch) piece of ginger, grated
- 1 green chilli, deseeded and finely diced
- 1 tomato, diced
- 1 × 340g (12oz) tin of Spam, cubed
- 2 teaspoons curry powder
- 1 teaspoon hot chilli powder
- ½ teaspoon garam masala
- 250g (9oz) basmati rice, cooked

Spray a large pan with a little oil and place over a medium-high heat. Add the onion and fry for about 5 minutes, then add the garlic and ginger and cook for a further 30 seconds.

Add the diced chilli and tomato and cook for 2–3 minutes, then lower the heat to medium, add the cubed Spam and stir well to combine.

Add the curry powder, chilli powder and garam masala and stir, then add a splash of water.

Cook for 10 minutes, stirring frequently, then serve with basmati rice.

Notes: You could use the other staple from my childhood here: bacon grill. It's utterly awful yet somehow delicious stuff – hissing and spitting under the grill, always one moment away from setting the kitchen on fire – but it'll do the job.

Check the flavours before seasoning with salt: Spam is as salty as a scorned lover. There's low-sodium versions out there, but life can't be devoid of all joy, can it?

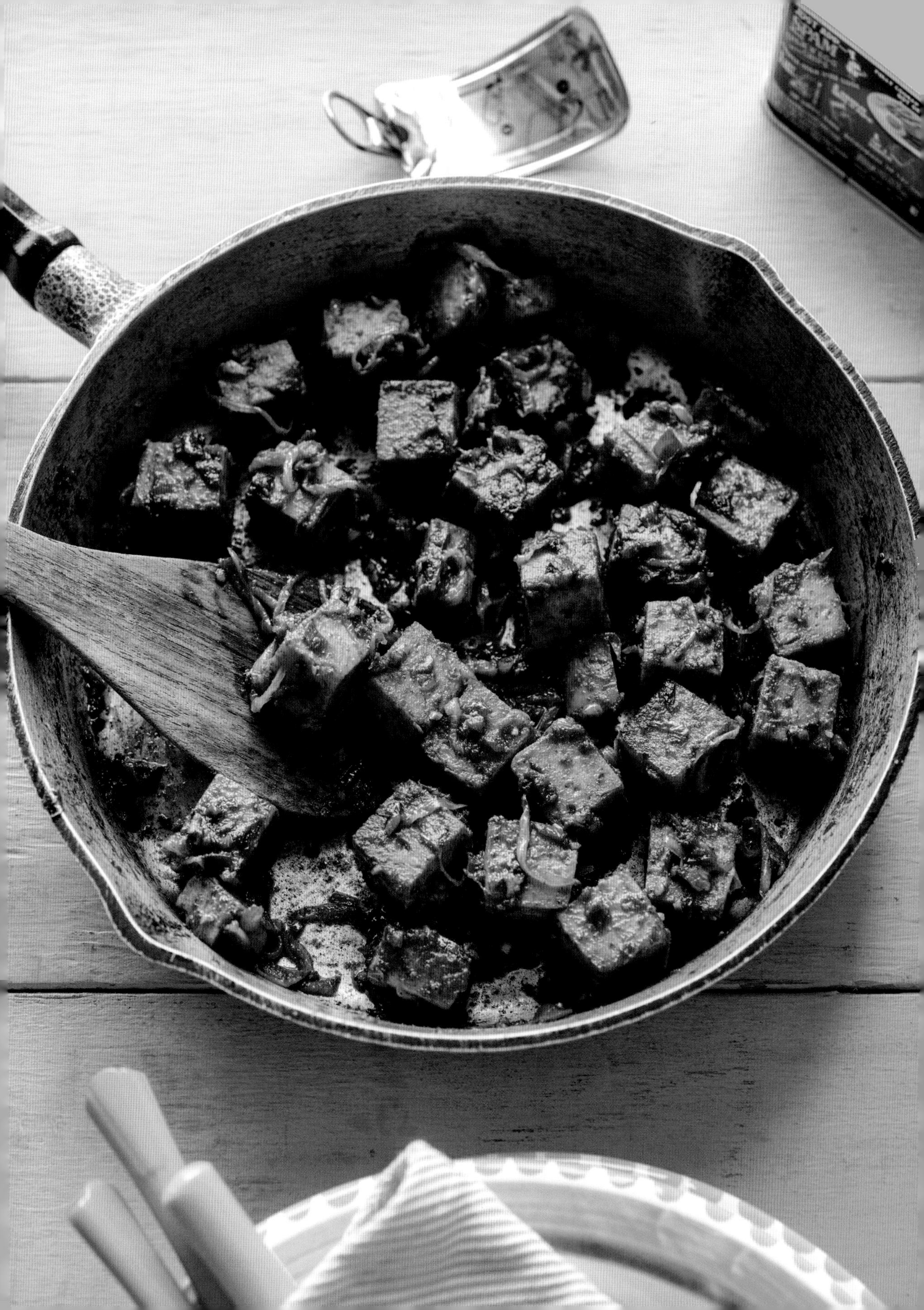

SERVES: 4
PREP: 1 HR 10 MINS
COOK: 40 MINS
CALORIES: 247

HAWAI-IAN CHICKEN

This recipe comes from my good friend and personal trainer Ian, who promises it'll delight and astound you. But then he also promises he hasn't had Botox, yet mysteriously can't blink in unison. You've met Ian if you own our previous *Sunday Times* instant bestseller (sorry, it's muscle memory at this point), *Dinner Time*. I wanged on about his drag performances, but it's as my personal trainer that he really deserves recognition. See, without wanting to be hyperbolic (usually happens when I do squats on a hot day), Ian is a literal walking miracle. A couple of years ago he fell down a flight of stairs, snapped his neck, and was told he would never walk again. Anyway, just as nobody puts Baby in the corner, nobody tells Ian what to do, including his own body. After a year or so of looking at the ceiling and getting RSI from sending his standard 3,000-word WhatsApp messages, he started getting some feeling back in his legs. That progressed to walking with crutches, then to one crutch, then to getting back into the gym and building his strength again. That's when he became my personal trainer and we haven't looked back since, unless there's an especially fit bloke to gawp at. That's enough blowing of his trumpet though, he'll only get a big head. Try his chicken!

- 900g (2lb) chicken drumsticks
- 5 tablespoons cider vinegar
- 3 tablespoons soy sauce
- ¼ teaspoon black pepper
- 1 teaspoon honey
- 4 cloves of garlic, crushed
- 2.5cm (1 inch) piece of ginger, grated
- 1 × 400g (14oz) tin of pineapple chunks, drained

In a bowl, toss together the chicken, cider vinegar, soy sauce, black pepper, honey, garlic and ginger, then leave to marinate in the fridge (covered) for an hour.

Once marinated, carefully pour the liquid into a jug and keep aside, and shake off any excess marinade from the chicken.

Spray a large frying pan with a little oil and place over a medium-high heat. Add the chicken (in batches if needed) and cook until golden (8–10 minutes, then flip and cook for another 8–10 minutes), then remove to a plate and keep warm.

Reduce the heat to medium, then put all the chicken back into the pan. Add the reserved marinade along with 60ml (2fl oz) of water, and stir gently.

Cover with a lid and simmer for 15 minutes.

Stir in the pineapple and cook for 2–3 minutes more, then serve.

Note: We've used chicken drumsticks for this one, but any chicken will do – just make sure it's cooked through properly!

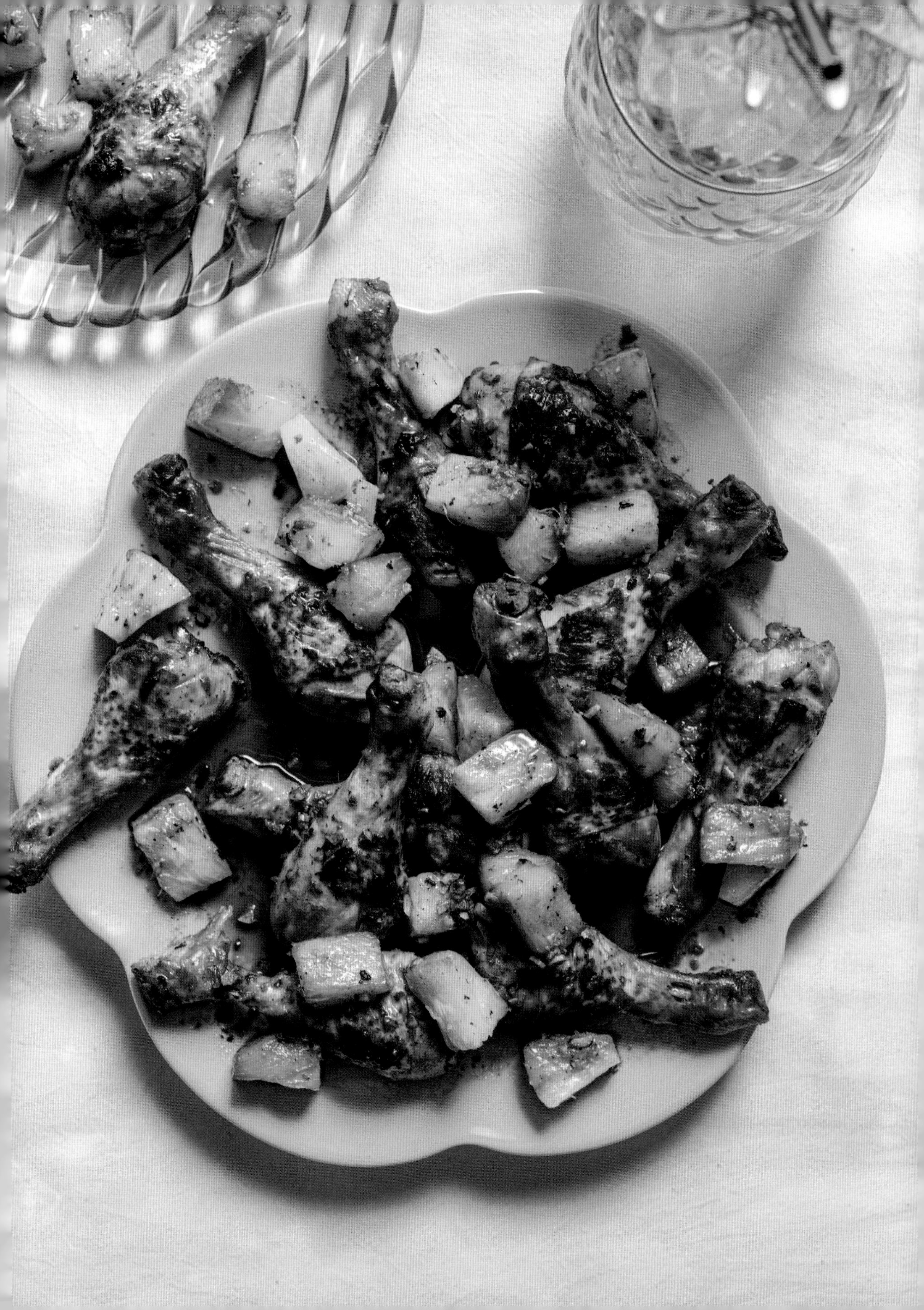

SERVES: 4
PREP: 10 MINS
COOK: 90 MINS
CALORIES: 347

30 mins · freezable · family · GF · DF

SUPER SIMPLE LAMB CURRY

Clearly this curry is wonderful: we wouldn't put it in the book if it wasn't, so instead of extolling its virtues, I'm going to use this space to publicly call out my husband for stealing my tattoo idea. See, for years we've both wanted tattoos, and **my idea** was to have something pertaining to significant places we've visited: Eiffel Tower for Paris, Mickey ears for Disney, a sleeve of doxycycline tablets for each visit to Germany . . . We dithered for ages, then on Instagram I spotted @its_stabbyjoe, who had the exact style we were after. Plus, he's bearded and fit, which may have sweetened the deal. I had Homer from *The Simpsons* tattooed on my arm and it didn't hurt *and* looked great, so Paul booked himself in. He came home with SEVENTEEN tattoos up his arm and you know what? I couldn't even stay mad because they look incredible. Our tattooist really does have a massive talent. I've since had two large leg tattoos done and I absolutely love them. If you're wanting a tattoo but you're put off by the thought of pain, don't give it a second thought. Obviously I'm as hard as nails because the pain barely registers (it helps that I have such leathery skin), but even Paul didn't complain, and he's soft as clarts. Finally, like we said, do give @its_stabbyjoe a follow and a look. He really is gifted. Oh aye, the lamb curry recipe, I do apologise!

- 1 teaspoon cumin seeds
- 2 brown onions, chopped
- 4 cloves of garlic, crushed
- 5cm (2 inch) piece of ginger, grated
- 2 tomatoes, chopped
- 500g (1lb 2oz) diced lamb
- 1 teaspoon ground coriander
- 1 teaspoon ground turmeric
- 1 teaspoon garam masala
- 1 teaspoon hot chilli powder
- a handful of fresh coriander leaves, roughly chopped

Spray a large pan with a little oil and place over a medium-high heat. Add the cumin seeds and let them sizzle for a few seconds, then add the onions and cook until golden.

Add the garlic and ginger and cook for another minute, then add the tomatoes and cook until softened.

Add the lamb and cook until browned all over, stirring frequently.

Add the coriander, turmeric, garam masala and hot chilli powder and mix well. Pour in 125ml (4fl oz) of water and bring the boil, scraping any burnt bits off the bottom of the pan, then reduce the heat to low, cover with a lid and simmer for 45–60 minutes.

Serve with the fresh coriander sprinkled over the top.

Notes: You can substitute curry powder for the cumin, coriander, turmeric and garam masala, if you prefer!

We use frozen diced lamb for this, defrosted in the fridge overnight, as it's much cheaper.

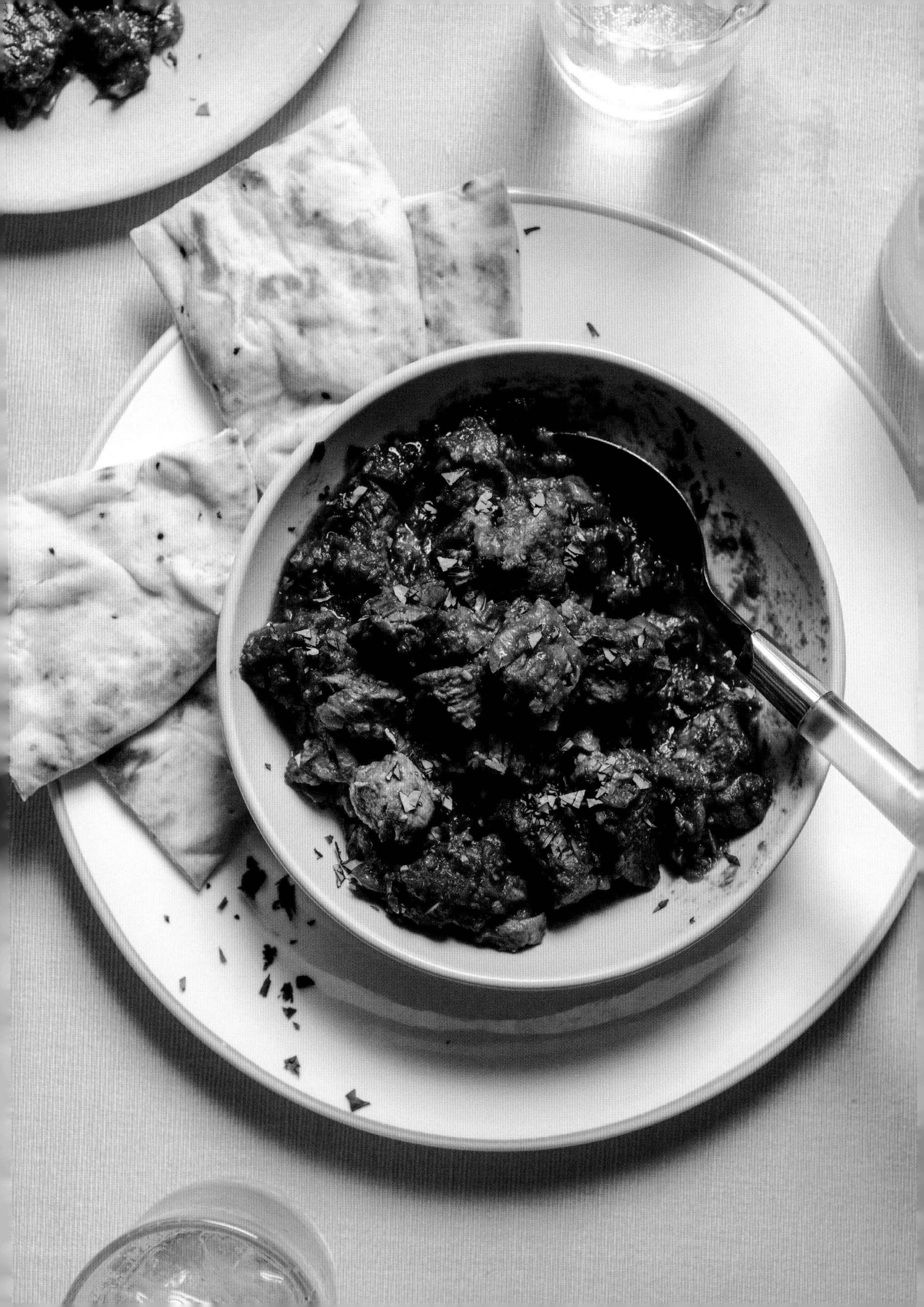

SERVES: 4
PREP: 15 MINS
COOK: 40 MINS
CALORIES: 379

- 60g (2¼oz) fat-free natural yoghurt
- 2 cloves of garlic, crushed
- 1 teaspoon mint sauce
- 200g (7oz) lamb mince
- 1 onion, roughly chopped
- 1 teaspoon ground coriander
- 1 teaspoon garam masala
- 1 teaspoon salt
- ½ teaspoon black pepper
- 8 slices of bread
- 80g (3oz) reduced-fat Cheddar cheese, grated
- ¼ red cabbage, sliced

DONER KEBAB TOASTIE

The second of our toastie recipes, and you may be forgiven for thinking we've got a bloody nerve, sticking toastie recipes in a cookery book. We at twochubbycubs admire your candour but in our defence, this recipe is more about the creation of the doner meat – the cheese toastie we built around it is just the vessel that carries it forth. A friend of mine cooks his puck of lamb mince in a slow cooker on a bed of onions for a good 8 hours. I can testify, as someone who has tried his meat on more than one occasion, that this method works perfectly well. You can even drain and mush the onions afterwards and add them to your toastie / pitta.

Preheat the oven to 180°C fan/400°F/gas mark 6.

In a bowl, mix together the yoghurt, garlic and mint sauce and set aside.

In a separate bowl, mix together the lamb mince, onion, coriander, garam masala, salt and pepper until well combined, then roll into a ball and slap into a loaf tin, spreading it out as much as you can.

Cook in the oven for 20–30 minutes, then remove and allow to cool. Once cool, slice thickly.

Spread the yoghurt mix over half the bread slices and sprinkle over the grated cheese.

Add the slices of doner meat and cabbage, and top with the remaining slices of bread.

Preheat the grill to high. Place the sandwiches under the grill and toast for 4–5 minutes each side, or to your liking.

Notes: We use fresh lamb mince for this one, but the frozen stuff, properly defrosted, works just as well. You can even use diced lamb or steaks if you prefer, just make sure to blitz them in a food processor first to give that 'mince'-like texture. Beef mince also works!

Use any toppings you like in this, it's all good.

You can also slap these into a good sandwich toaster instead!

It still gives me a giddy thrill to be called Big Man or Boss by the lovely chaps in our local takeaway. All for it.

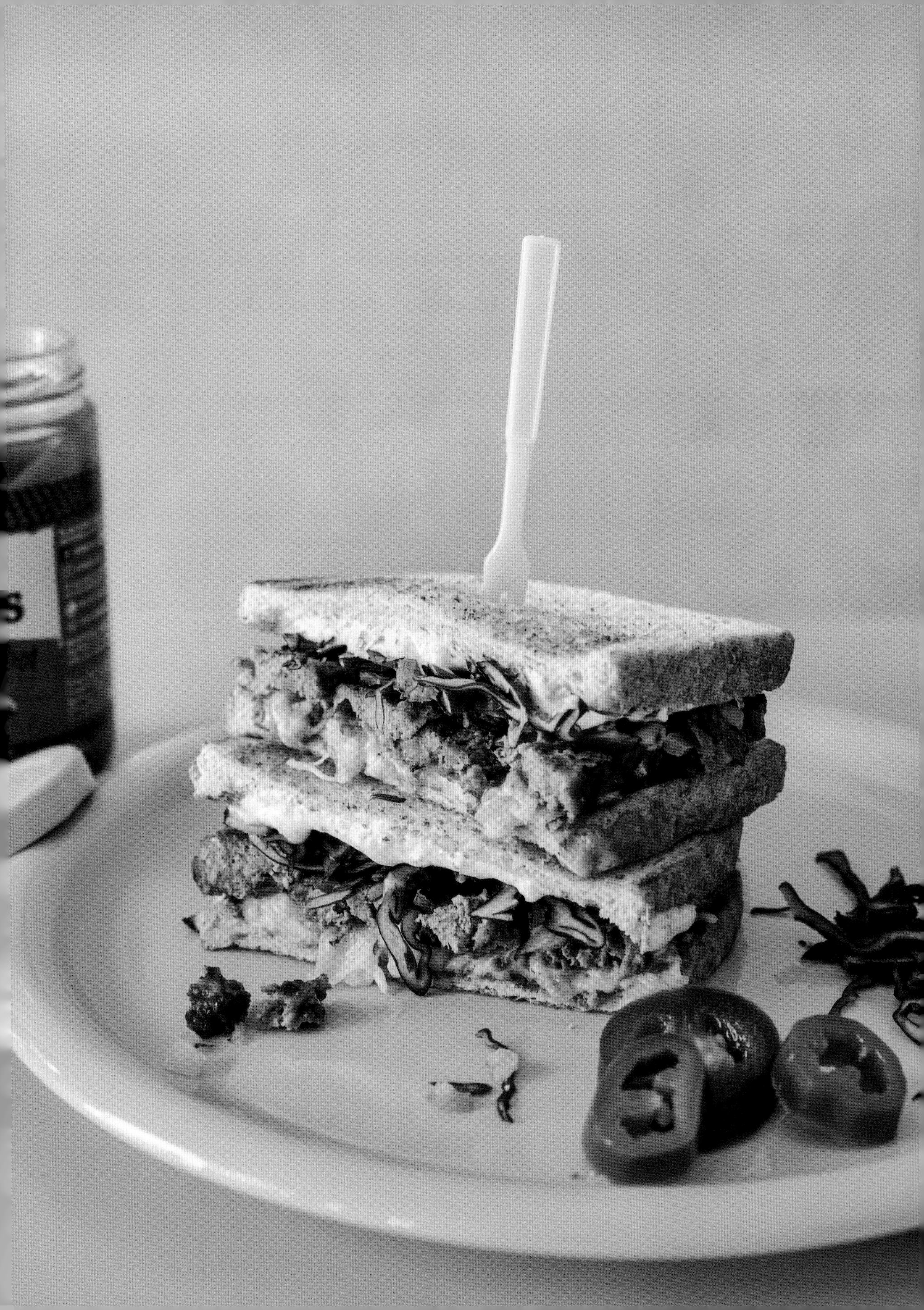

SERVES: 4
PREP: 10 MINS
COOK: 25 MINS
CALORIES: 226

30 mins · DF

ONION BHAJI CURRY

This absolutely works, even if you think it sounds suspicious. For me, it reminds me of the best part of an Indian takeaway: when you're as full as a bull's bum, you've got slicks of sauces on your plate, and you've saved the bhaji and the naan for the mopping up. It does require some deep-frying in oil though, which I know alarms a lot of people, not least me. I have to leave the room when Paul does it, because I grew up on a diet of 999 and *Casualty* and I know we are one drop of water away from a raging inferno. And listen, Paul wears a lot of polyester and Right Guard: he'd go up like a Roman candle. But the risk is worth the reward, because if your bhajis are crunchy, it adds so much to the dish. If we really can't persuade you to fry, that's fine: you can bake the bhajis in the oven until they're crunchy on the outside, though they'll be doughy inside. Still good, but not the best they could be.

- 1 large brown onion, sliced
- 50g (1¾oz) plain flour
- ½ teaspoon ground turmeric
- ½ teaspoon chilli powder
- 1½ teaspoon curry powder
- ½ teaspoon salt
- 2 tablespoons olive oil
- 1 × 400g (14oz) tin of chopped tomatoes
- 1 × 400g (14oz) tin of chickpeas, drained and rinsed
- 250ml (9fl oz) vegetable stock

In a bowl, mix together the onion, flour, turmeric, chilli powder, curry powder, salt and 60ml (2fl oz) of water until they form a thick batter.

Heat the oil in a frying pan over a medium heat. Once hot, drop spoonfuls of the onion batter into the pan and fry until golden brown, turning once, then remove from the pan and set aside.

In a blender or food processor, purée the tomatoes until smooth. Add them to the frying pan with the chickpeas and vegetable stock, and simmer for 10 minutes.

Return the bhajis to the pan and stir to combine.

Serve.

Note: This is perfect with rice or a naan you could dam a lake with.

Freeze the bhajis and the sauce separately.

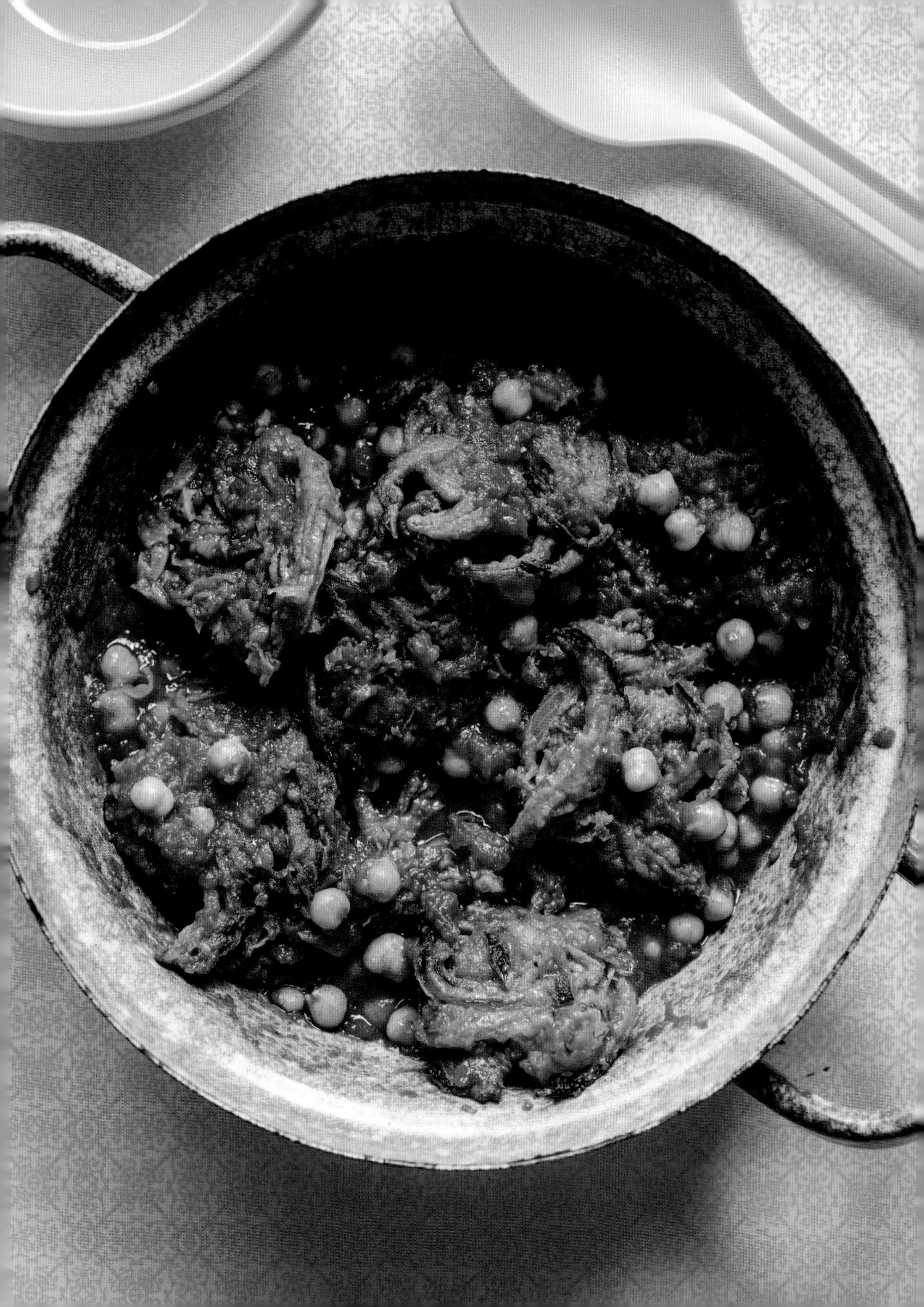

SERVES: 4
PREP: 10 MINS
COOK: 30 MINS
CALORIES: 497

30 mins, freezable, family, DF

- 500g (1lb 2oz) turkey mince
- 5 tablespoons green curry paste
- 4 cloves of garlic, crushed
- 3 spring onions, sliced
- 2 teaspoons ground coriander
- 3 tablespoons soy sauce
- 200g (7oz) long-grain rice
- 1 brown onion, chopped
- 5cm (2 inch) piece of ginger, grated
- 300ml (10fl oz) reduced-fat coconut milk
- 1 lemongrass stalk
- a handful of fresh coriander, chopped (optional)

THAI GREEN CURRY MEATBALLS

In one of our previous books we gave a recipe for making a beautiful green curry paste. If you have the time, dig it out and make it fresh, but know this: there's absolutely no shame in using jarred curry paste. Especially these days, when the quality of the good bought stuff is through the roof. A note on turkey mince: supermarkets sell it, but it can be quite hard to find. It is worth digging out though: this isn't a recipe you could swap out for beef mince, it would be too rich. At a push you could try pork mince, but make an effort here. I gave you an easy time with the jar suggestion, you can't have it all! Oh! One more tip. If you're having trouble cooking the rice, we recommend a rice cooker. We have spent years guiltily tipping burned or undercooked rice into the bin and eating naan instead: don't be like us. Once we caved and bought a little countertop rice cooker we never looked back: they can be picked up for around thirty quid if you're so inclined. Anyway: try our meatballs, they're green!

In a bowl, mix together the turkey mince, 1 tablespoon of green curry paste, 2 cloves of garlic, the spring onions, ground coriander and 2 tablespoons of soy sauce. Roll the mixture into about 28 balls and set them aside on a plate.

Put the rice into a pan with about 1.5 litres (2¾ pints) of cold water and bring to the boil, then cover and simmer for 15–18 minutes. Drain, then return the rice to the pan and keep warm.

Meanwhile, spray a large pan with a little oil and place over a medium-high heat. Add the onion, the remaining garlic and the ginger to the pan and cook for 30 seconds.

Add the meatballs (in batches if necessary) and cook, turning frequently, until browned on all sides.

Add the rest of the curry paste, along with the coconut milk, the rest of the soy sauce and the lemongrass, and simmer gently for 15–20 minutes.

Serve the meatballs with a sprinkle of fresh coriander (if using) and rice.

Notes: Make the meatballs as big or as little as you like, just make sure they're cooked! Paul prefers giant meatballs you could play cricket with, I prefer tiny little meatballs so it feels like you're at an IKEA. Sometimes I start an argument about the kitchen cupboards just to complete the scene.

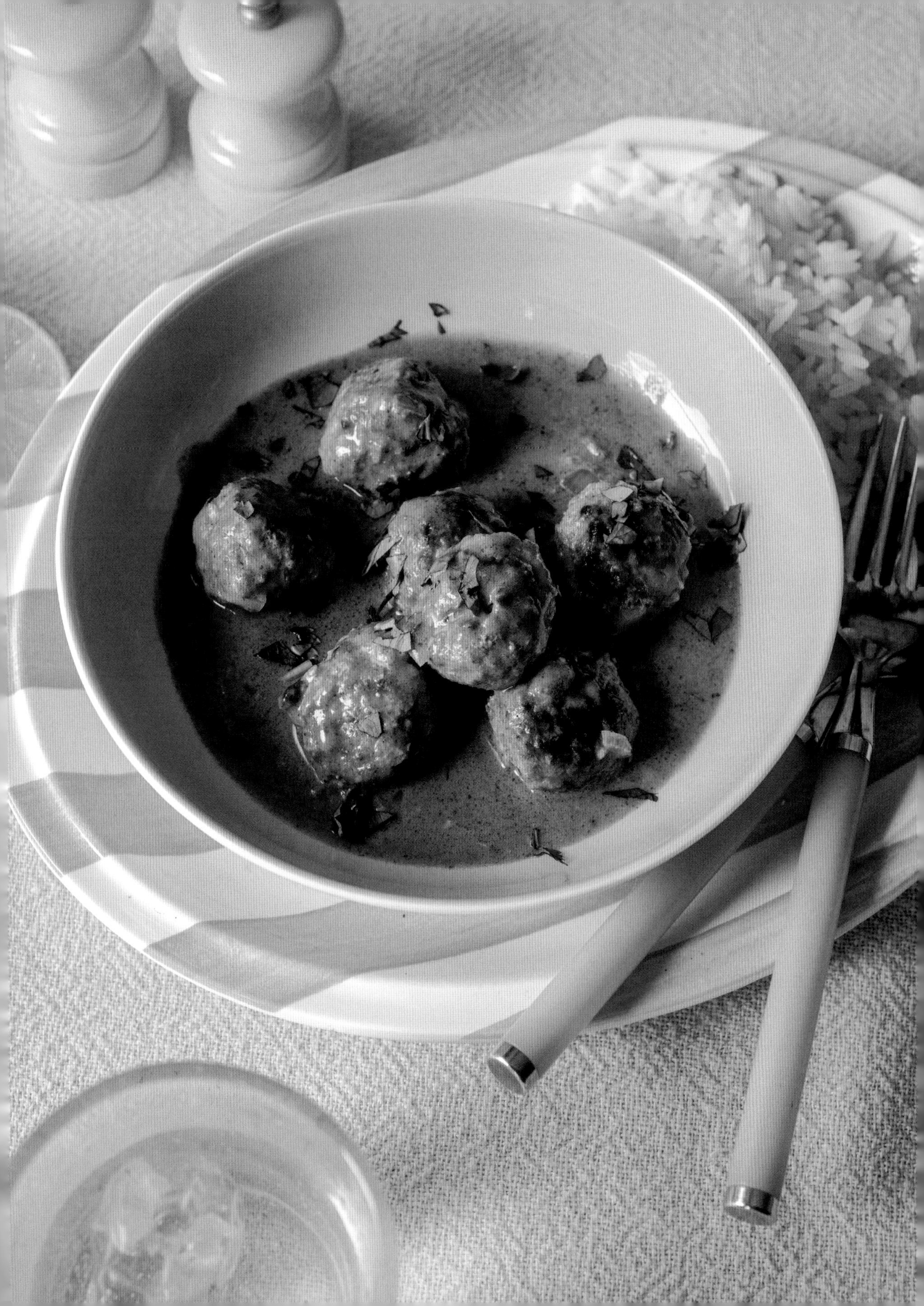

SERVES: 4
PREP: 10 MINS
COOK: 1 HR
CALORIES: 496

30 mins · DF

- 6 boneless chicken thighs
- 1 brown onion, diced
- 2 cloves of garlic, crushed
- 2 tablespoons curry powder
- 1 tablespoon plain flour
- 1 tablespoon honey
- 1 tablespoon soy sauce
- 350g (12oz) frozen vegetable mix (broccoli, cauliflower, carrots)
- 4 potatoes, peeled and cut into chips

CHIPPY TEA CHICKEN CURRY

Paul, perhaps under the impression it'll reduce the calories a little, suggests serving this chicken curry with oven-baked chips. I'm staging an intervention: do them the way we usually do: olive oil, beef stock cube, whack them in the air-fryer with a little garlic salt. Honestly, that boy of mine. This is a very close approximation of the classic chip shop chicken curry, although we've toned down the startling 90s rave yellow hue a little. We have made one key adjustment: we use chicken thighs rather than whatever the chip shop near us is passing off as chicken. This is my go-to order in a chip shop, slopped all over enough chips to keep an army advancing. Mind, that's only if there's not a spam fritter: if they're brave enough to do those, I'll take two, with a pickled egg just to show my stomach I mean business. Paul, forever an adventure in beige, will have fish, chips and scraps.

Preheat the oven to 190°C fan/400°F/gas mark 6.

Spray a large pan with a little oil and place over a medium heat. Open out the chicken thighs, add them to the pan, and cook for 5 minutes on each side. Then remove to a plate and keep warm.

Add the onion and garlic to the pan and cook for about 5 minutes, stirring occasionally.

Add the curry powder and flour and stir for 1 minute, then add the honey, soy sauce and frozen veg, along with 750ml (1¼ pints) of water, and stir to combine.

Put the chicken back into the pan and bring to the boil, then reduce the heat to low and simmer for 45 minutes, stirring occasionally.

Meanwhile, spray the potatoes with a little oil and sprinkle them with salt and pepper. Spread them out on a lined baking sheet and cook in the oven for 35–40 minutes, turning them halfway through.

Gently stir the cooked chips through the curry, and serve.

Notes: We use frozen veg for this but of course fresh is fine – 2 sliced carrots, ¼ cauliflower and ¼ broccoli should do it. Oh, and throw some peas in. If you really want to be Captain Flash, you'd slice the carrots with a crinkle cutter.

In a rush? Well, and keep this strictly between us, that Instant Curry Mix you can buy in your local tat emporium does the job just perfectly. Ssssh.

Only freeze the chicken curry.

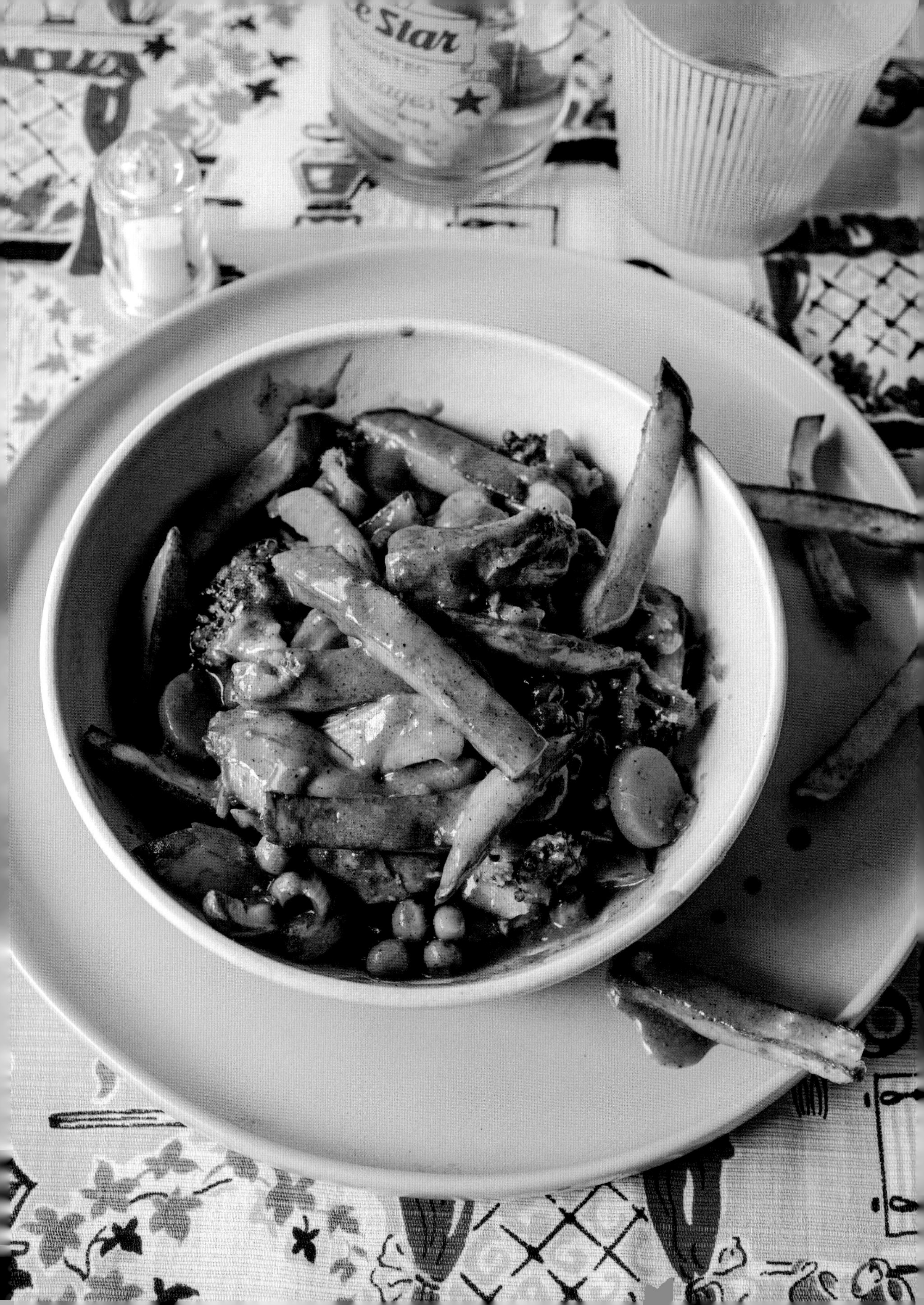

SERVES: 4
PREP: 15 MINS
COOK: 1 HR 25 MINS
CALORIES: 213

- 500g (1lb 2oz) boneless chicken thighs
- 1 large brown onion, finely diced
- 2 cloves of garlic, crushed
- 5cm (2 inch) piece of ginger, grated
- 1 teaspoon ground cumin
- 1 teaspoon ground coriander
- ½ teaspoon ground turmeric
- ½ teaspoon garam masala
- ½ teaspoon chili powder
- 120g (4oz) low-fat natural yoghurt
- 120ml (4fl oz) light coconut milk
- a handful of fresh coriander, chopped

CHICKEN PASANDA

I wish I could regale you with some romantic tale of eating this dish in a beautiful, exotic setting, but alas, no: it's served in our local (whisper it, aghast) chain pub. Now clearly we've upgraded it by adding flavour and not serving it scorching hot on the outside and cold as a well-digger's bum in the middle, but see, we're thoughtful like that. We have two local pubs within stumbling vicinity of Chubby Towers: one is the place we referenced above, which isn't too bad as long as you don't mind *Now That's What I Call a Hen Party 34* (now with extra Anastasia) playing. The other? Well, we're not brave enough to visit. Judging by all the accounts in our local paper, it's very much an 'in through the door and out through the window' sort of place, and, as we very much value having a full set of teeth, we're happy staying away. Pity really, because they probably do an even better pasanda. Sigh.

Cut the chicken into bite-size pieces and set aside.

Put the onion, garlic, ginger, cumin, coriander, turmeric, garam masala, chili powder, yoghurt and coconut milk into a blender or food processor, and blend until smooth.

Spray a large pan with a little oil and place over a medium heat. Add the chicken and cook for about 5 minutes, until browned all over.

Add the blended sauce to the pan and stir, then bring to a simmer and cook for 10 minutes.

Reduce the heat to low, cover and simmer for 1 hour, stirring occasionally.

Remove the lid and simmer for another 10 minutes, to thicken.

Sprinkle over the coriander and serve.

Note: If you have the time to let this simmer for longer over a lower heat, it's absolutely worth it.

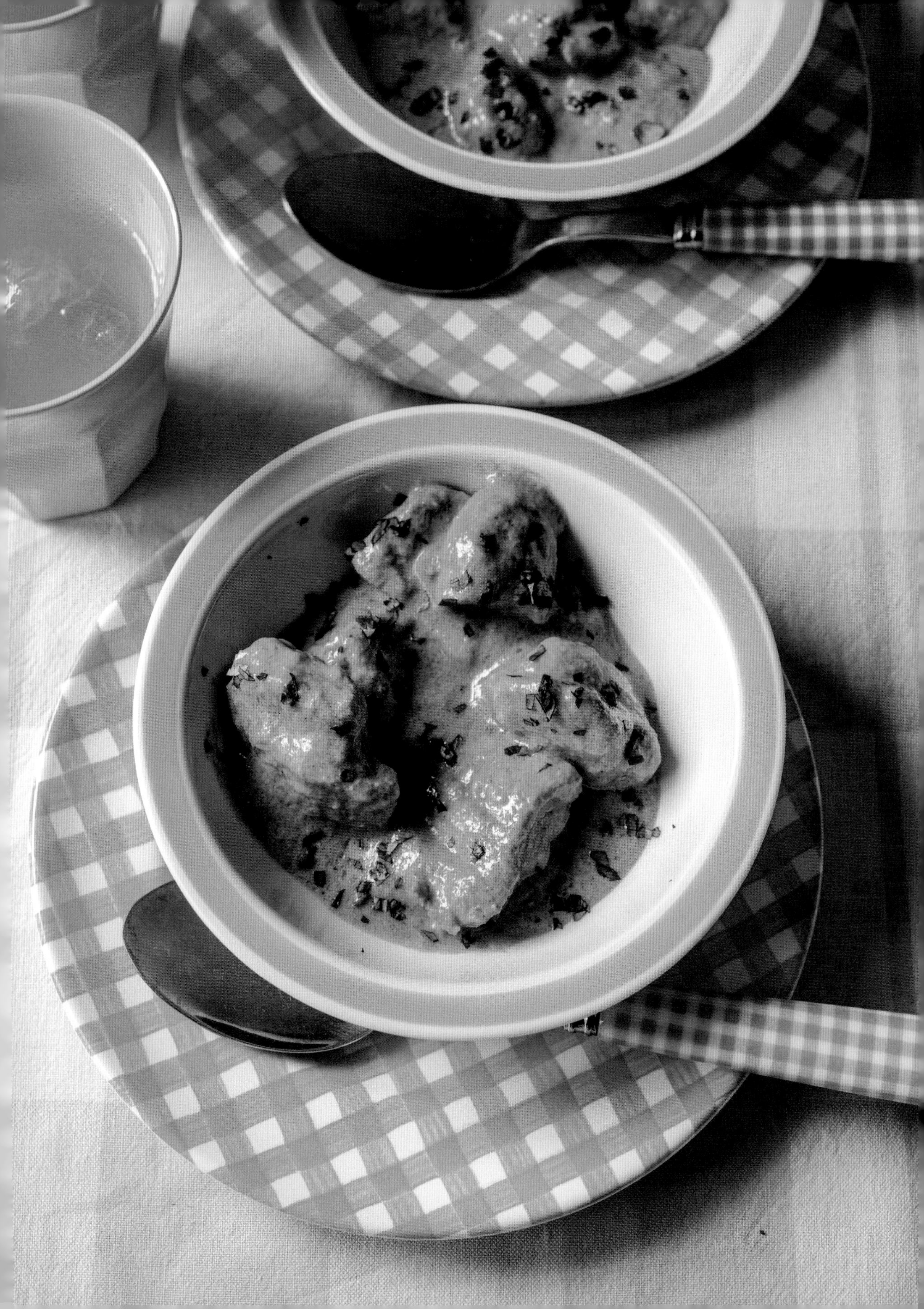

SERVES: 4
PREP: 15 MINS
COOK: 25 MINS
CALORIES: 499

30 mins · DF

POSH AS F*CK POKÉ BOWLS

One thing I do miss terribly from my previous job working in a city centre law firm – aside from flirting outrageously with the IT department and going home with a rucksack full of pilfered Lotus Biscoff biscuits from the meeting rooms – was being able to saunter into town and find somewhere nice for lunch. There's only so much excitement you can muster up for your fifth supermarket meal deal of the week, after all. Happily, Newcastle has always been an amazing place to eat, with a very definite swing towards 'healthy' lunch places. It was on one of my many tramps around the city centre that I discovered poké bowls: super healthy bowls of deliciousness. I'd recommend my favourite place to you, but when I did that in a previous book it shut down two weeks before publication, so I fear I may be cursed. I'll keep schtum. See notes for a quick tip, though. Finally, if you're not a fan of tuna and salmon, it's absolutely fine: some grilled chicken will sit here just tickety-boo.

- 280g (10z) brown rice
- 3 tablespoons rice vinegar
- 1 tablespoon sugar
- ½ teaspoon salt
- 1 avocado
- 1 tablespoon soy sauce
- 1 tablespoon sesame oil
- 1 teaspoon sriracha
- 110g (4oz) salmon fillet, cut into small cubes
- 110g (4oz) tuna steak, cut into small cubes
- ½ cucumber, diced
- 50g (1¾oz) edamame beans
- 1 teaspoon black sesame seeds

Bring a large pan of water to the boil, and while that's boiling, rinse the rice well. Add the rice to the pan and bring back to the boil, then reduce the heat and simmer, covered, for 22–25 minutes.

In a bowl, stir together the rice vinegar, sugar and salt until the sugar has dissolved.

When the rice has cooked, drain well and return to the pan (off the heat), then stir through the vinegar mixture and allow the rice to cool to room temperature.

Halve the avocado and remove the stone, then scoop out the flesh and dice.

In a small bowl, whisk together the soy sauce, sesame oil and sriracha and set aside.

In another bowl, gently toss together the salmon, tuna, avocado, cucumber and edamame beans.

Divide the rice between four bowls. Top with the fish and vegetable mixture, and drizzle the soy sauce mixture over the top.

Sprinkle over the sesame seeds, and serve.

Notes: No edamame beans? Butter beans, chickpeas or peas are fine to use instead.

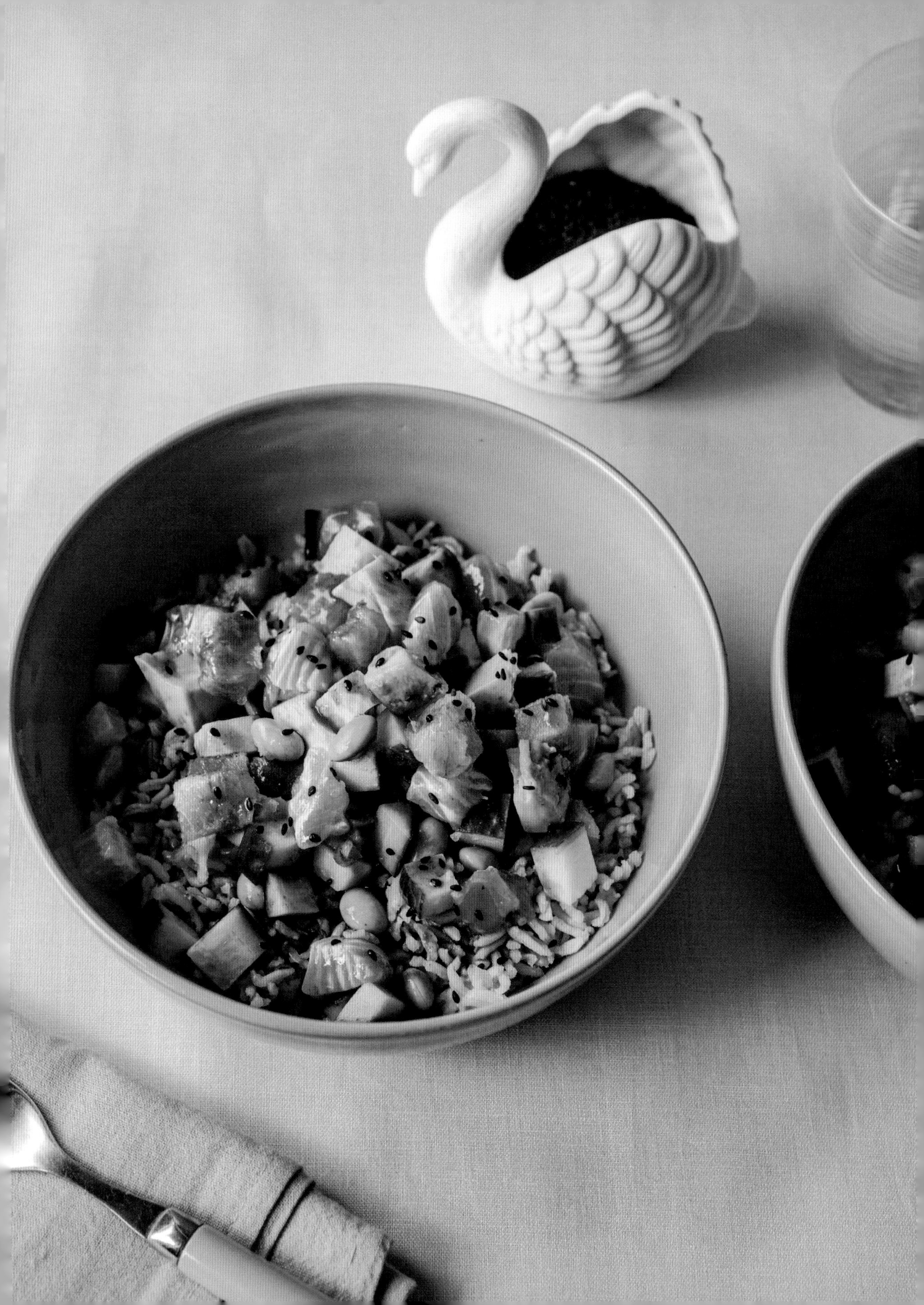

SERVES: 4
PREP: 20 MINS
COOK: 50 MINS
CALORIES: 481

30 mins, family, V, DF

- 450g (1lb) firm tofu
- 8cm (3 inch) piece of ginger, peeled
- 2 teaspoons ground turmeric
- 2 green chillies, sliced
- 1 brown onion, quartered
- 1.2 litres (2 pints) vegetable stock
- ½ teaspoon salt
- 350g (12oz) udon noodles
- 5 spring onions, sliced
- 2 teaspoons sesame seeds
- ¼ teaspoon black pepper

GINGER TOFU NOODLES

We're determined to make you try tofu, aren't we? If the thought leaves you cold, swap it out for cooked chicken. But with that caveat ringing in your lugs, we still encourage you to try this as we intend, because it's utterly scrumptious. If you develop a taste for it, try our chocolate mousse later in the book, although you'll need silken tofu for that. We tend to use ginger paste (and garlic paste, for that matter) in our recipes, but here is a rare exception: when it is one of the core ingredients of the meal, you want it fresh. That said, there's nothing stopping you buying a big knob of it and keeping it in the freezer until it is called into action. And although we suggest peeling it here, the world won't end if you roughly grate it, skin and all.

Wrap the tofu in kitchen paper and place a heavy object on top in order to squeeze out as much liquid as you can. Leave for 15 minutes, then unwrap and cut into 2.5cm (1 inch) cubes.

Meanwhile, spray a large pan with a little oil and place over a medium heat. While the pan is heating up, chop the ginger roughly and smash gently with the bottom of a mug or the side of your knife, then set aside.

Add the ginger, turmeric, chillies and onion to the pan and cook for 1–2 minutes, until darkened.

Add the stock and bring to the boil, then reduce the heat, add the salt, and simmer for 20–30 minutes.

Strain the mixture through a sieve and discard the solids. Return the liquid to the pan and keep warm over a low heat.

Bring a large pan of water to the boil. Add the noodles and cook according to the packet instructions, then drain and divide between four bowls.

Add the spring onions and tofu to the simmering liquid, keeping a few bits of spring onion for garnish, and cook for 5–10 minutes.

Serve the soup over the noodles and sprinkle with the remaining spring onions and the sesame seeds.

Notes: Apologies for the use of scrumptious, but I'm running out of synonyms for 'delicious'!

No apologies for the use of 'big knob', though.

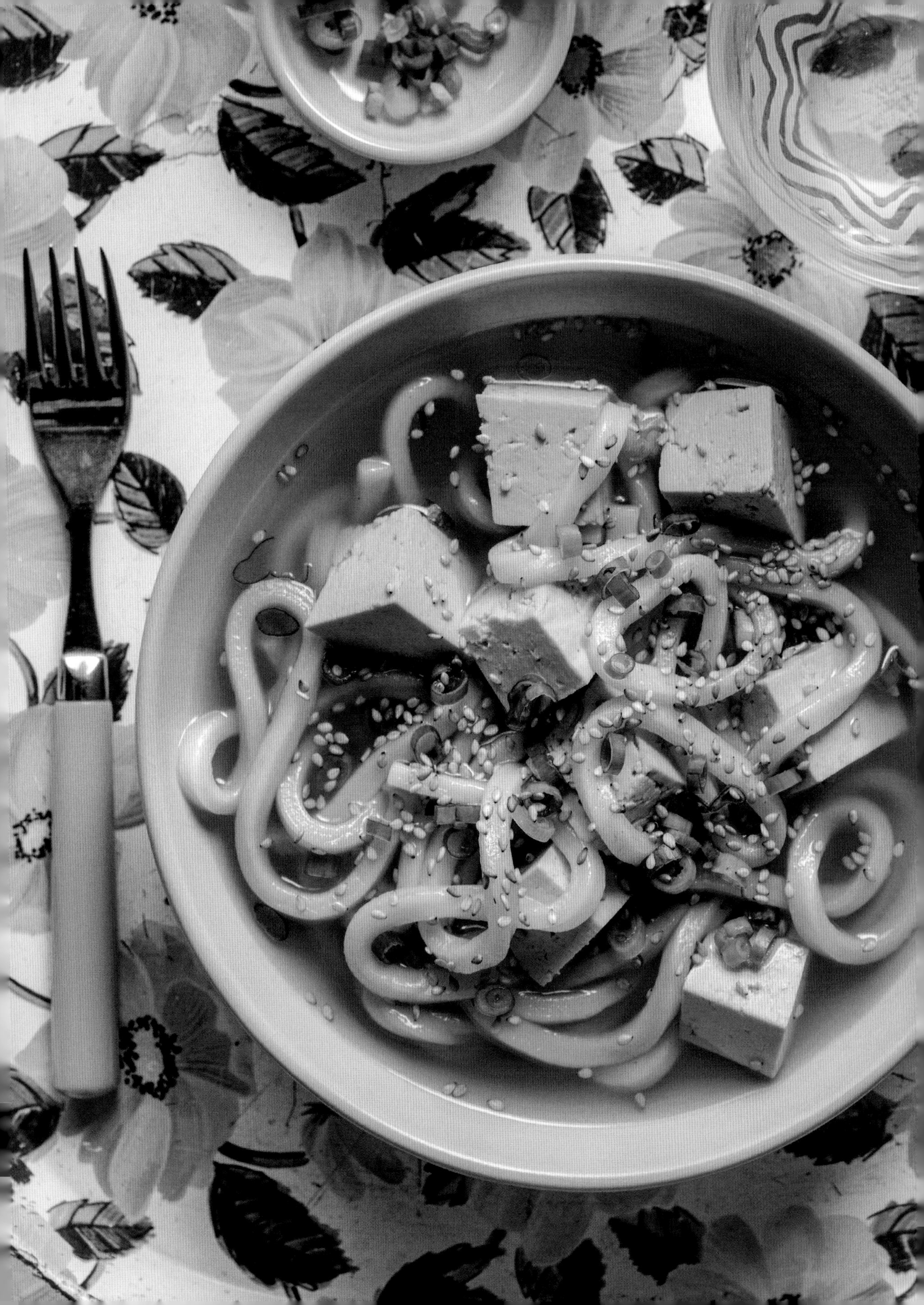

SERVES: 4
PREP: 10 MINS
COOK: 8 HRS
CALORIES: 499

- 110g (4oz) green or brown dried lentils
- 350ml (12fl oz) vegetable stock
- 1 small tin of sweetcorn, drained
- ½ × 400g (14oz) tin of black beans, drained
- 2 green peppers, deseeded and sliced
- 1½ teaspoons ground cumin
- ½ teaspoon dried oregano
- ½ teaspoon paprika
- 2 teaspoons cider vinegar
- ½ teaspoon salt
- 8 mini tortillas
- 4 handfuls of chopped lettuce
- 4 tablespoons tomato salsa
- 4 tablespoons sour cream
- 50g (1¾oz) sliced jalapeños
- 1 small avocado, peeled, stoned and diced
- 50g (1¾oz) reduced-fat Cheddar cheese, grated
- 2 tablespoons sriracha

VEGGIE TACOS

Growing up, tacos always seemed terribly fancy and delicious, despite actually being a very simple dish that is everywhere in America. I blame *The Simpsons* for this: growing up square-eyed in front of the TV left me with a deep yearning for all the cartoon food I saw: the giant sandwich I can't stay mad at, a fancy hat made with nachos, even the birthday cake for sweet little Magaggie. Seeing Comic Boy Guy wobbling out with his wheelbarrow of tacos gave me hope for a tasty future, and as a result, tacos have become a regular visitor to our house. Here's our recipe. And, rather like Springfield Elementary's gym mats, there's very little meat in these tacos. And by little, we mean none – they're entirely vegetarian. Bonus! Enjoy with a cool glass of Malk.

Put the lentils, stock, sweetcorn, beans and green peppers into a slow cooker. Add the spices and salt, and stir well to combine.

Cook on high for 3–4 hours (or low for 7–8 hours).

Divide the mixture between the tortillas and top with the lettuce, salsa, sour cream, jalapeños, avocado, Cheddar and sriracha.

Notes: We use mini tortillas for ease, but the big ones are just fine – 1 or 2 each should do it.

Top these with whatever you like, and feel free to tinker with the amounts of lentils and beans to your preference – you can't really go wrong.

Switch the sour cream and Cheddar to vegan options.

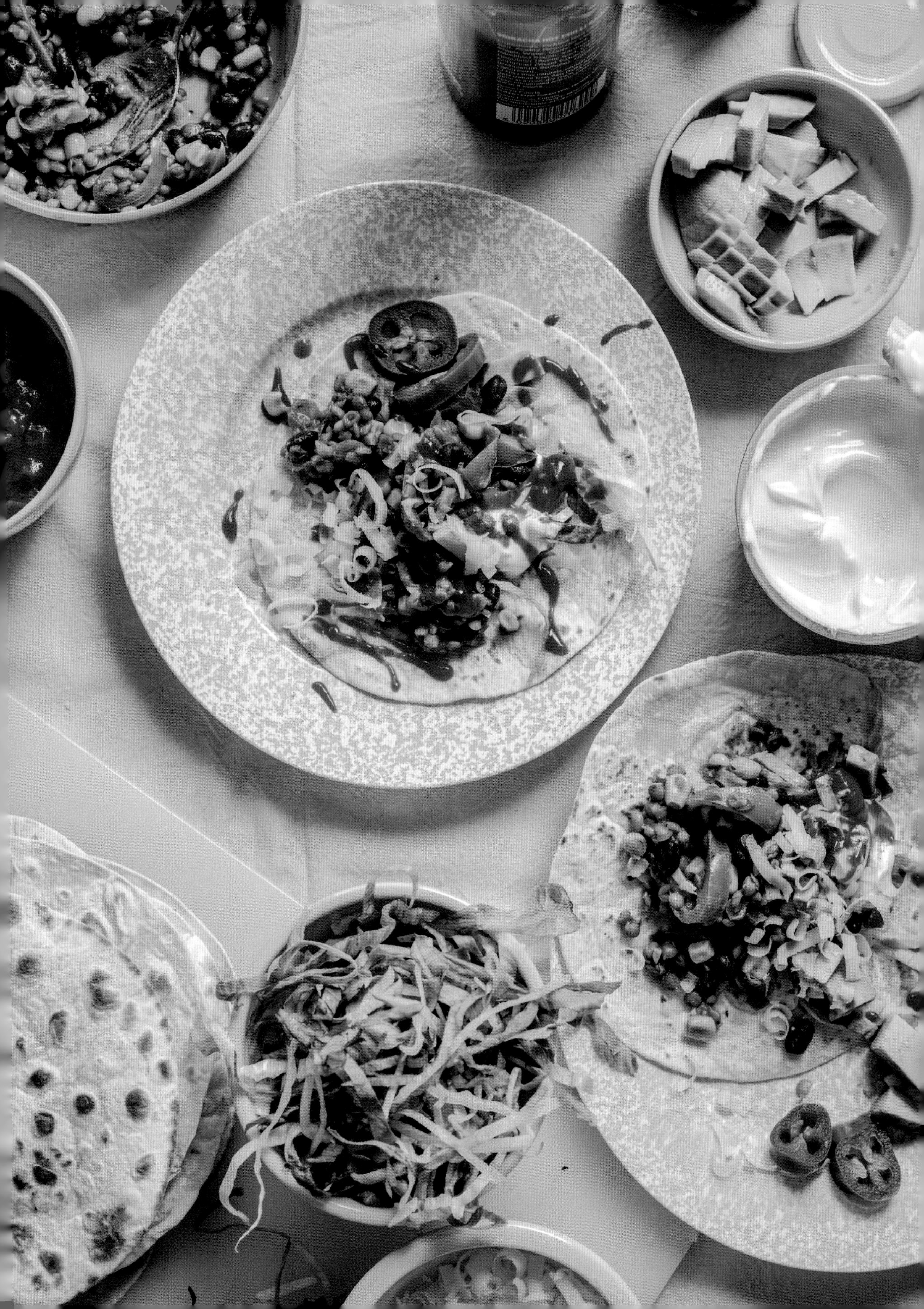

SERVES: 4
PREP: 15 MINS
COOK: 30 MINS
CALORIES: 381

30 mins · GF · DF

SPICY ORANGE CHICKEN

Oh my! There's an ingredients list that will give you pause, we know – but listen here, you'll have most of those ingredients in the cupboard. Hopefully not the chicken thighs though, because they belong in the fridge. This is simple kitchen basics and we shouldn't have to explain these things to you. Now in each of our books we have made the same supplication to you, our fabulous readers: don't be put off by chicken thighs. We know there are those out there who panic at the thought of them, but you must overcome: thighs are gamier, tastier *and* they always make me think of chickens wearing jeans, which in turn makes me laugh. And if you're laughing in the kitchen, that's never a bad thing.

- 2 oranges
- 750g (1lb 10oz) skinless, boneless chicken thighs, diced
- ¾ teaspoon salt
- ¼ teaspoon black pepper
- 4 tablespoons cornflour
- 2 tablespoons cider vinegar
- 2 tablespoons sherry
- 2 tablespoons brown sugar
- 1 tablespoon honey
- 1 tablespoon sesame oil
- 170g (6oz) mushrooms, sliced
- 5cm (2 inch) piece of ginger, grated
- 2 cloves of garlic, grated
- 2 red chillies, finely diced
- 4 spring onions, sliced

Zest and juice the oranges, and set both aside.

Place the chicken in a large bowl. Add the salt and pepper along with 3 tablespoons of cornflour and toss well.

In another bowl, mix together the orange zest and juice, cider vinegar, sherry, brown sugar, honey and sesame oil, and set aside.

Spray a large pan with a little oil and place over a medium-high heat. Add the chicken and cook for 5–6 minutes on each side, until golden brown, then remove to a plate. Make sure the pan isn't too crowded, and cook in batches if you need to.

Spray the pan with a little more oil, then add the mushrooms and cook for 4–5 minutes, until lightly golden all over, stirring frequently. Once cooked, remove from the pan and add to the chicken.

Spray the pan with a little more oil again, then add the ginger, garlic, chillies and half the spring onions and cook for 1 minute.

Pour the sauce into the pan and bring to the boil, then reduce the heat to medium-low and cook for 4–5 minutes, stirring frequently until thickened.

Add the chicken and mushrooms to the pan and toss in the sauce. Serve with the remaining spring onions sprinkled over.

Note: This goes great with rice, of course, but is also very tasty indeed when folded into a pitta bread or a wrap, with as much salad as your heart desires. Which is to say, if you're anything like us, none.

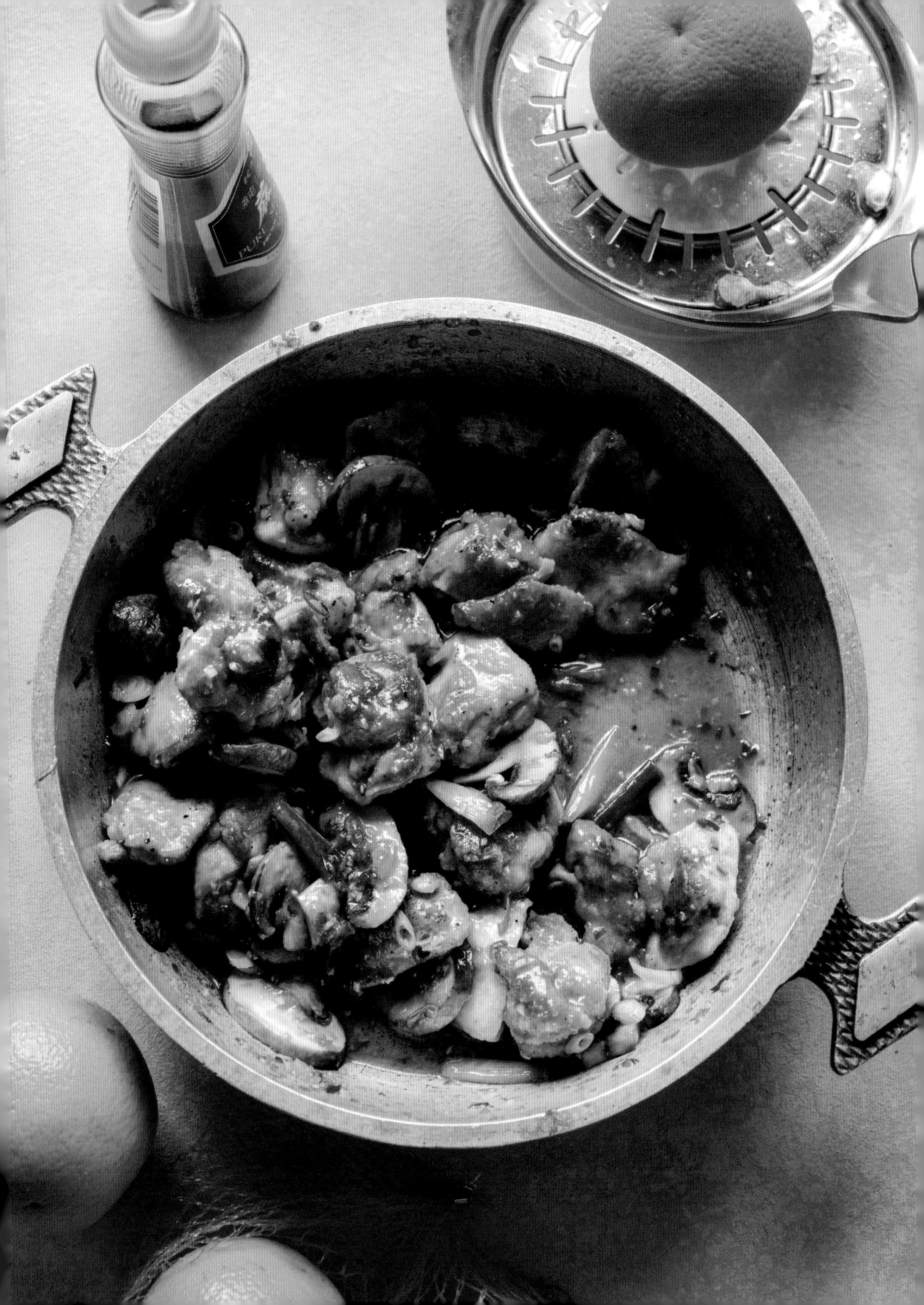

PAST

& G

A, RICE
RAINS

SERVES: 4
PREP: 5 MINS
COOK: 20 MINS
CALORIES: 450

EASY CHICKEN & TOMATO PASTA

We always like to include a good simple pasta recipe or two in our books because, well, who doesn't like pasta? Miscreants, that's who, and we don't listen to them. This is very much one of those recipes to throw together at the end of a busy day with minimal attention needed, so it's a winner for us. Of course, we ask that you keep an eye on the hob, as no one needs a house fire. Trust us, we know. Paul and I have settled into a lovely groove when it comes to cooking: he comes home from a day at work and an hour-long HIIT class, I spend ten minutes telling him how terribly tired my fingers are from typing, and he disappears into the kitchen, makes lots of noise, and emerges thirty minutes later with something delicious. I'll do all the cleaning, so it balances out, I'm sure, and anyway, Paul can't make himself a bowl of cereal without finding a reason to use nine pans, the potato ricer, fourteen spatulas and scatter food on the floor – therefore I can confidently say I do my fair share. Speaking of a fair share, you'll not want to share this chicken and tomato pasta, so feel free to do what I know Paul does and have yourself a little extra portion before serving up. I'll keep it between us.

- 225g (8oz) pasta
- 4 chicken breasts, diced
- ½ teaspoon salt
- ¼ teaspoon black pepper
- 4 cloves of garlic, crushed
- 1 × 400g (14oz) tin of chopped tomatoes
- 2 tablespoons tomato purée
- ¼ teaspoon dried chilli flakes
- 1 teaspoon dried mixed herbs
- ½ bunch of fresh basil, chopped
- 2 tablespoons balsamic vinegar
- ½ teaspoon onion granules
- 2 tablespoons green pesto

Bring a large pan of salted water to the boil and cook the pasta according to the instructions on the packet, then drain and set aside.

Meanwhile, spray a large pan with a little oil and place over a medium-high heat. Add the chicken, sprinkle over the salt and pepper, and cook for 5–7 minutes until cooked through. Remove to a plate and keep warm.

Return the pan to the heat. Add the garlic and cook for 1 minute, then add the chopped tomatoes, tomato purée, chilli flakes, mixed herbs, basil, balsamic vinegar and onion granules and stir well. Simmer for 10 minutes.

Slice the chicken, add it to the sauce, and stir well to mix.

Serve the pasta on plates, top with the chicken mixture, and drizzle over some pesto. Top with any remaining basil leaves.

Notes: This works great with sausages instead of chicken if you prefer, or with no meat at all!

As ever with us, use whatever pasta you fancy. It makes little difference.

Only freeze the sauce.

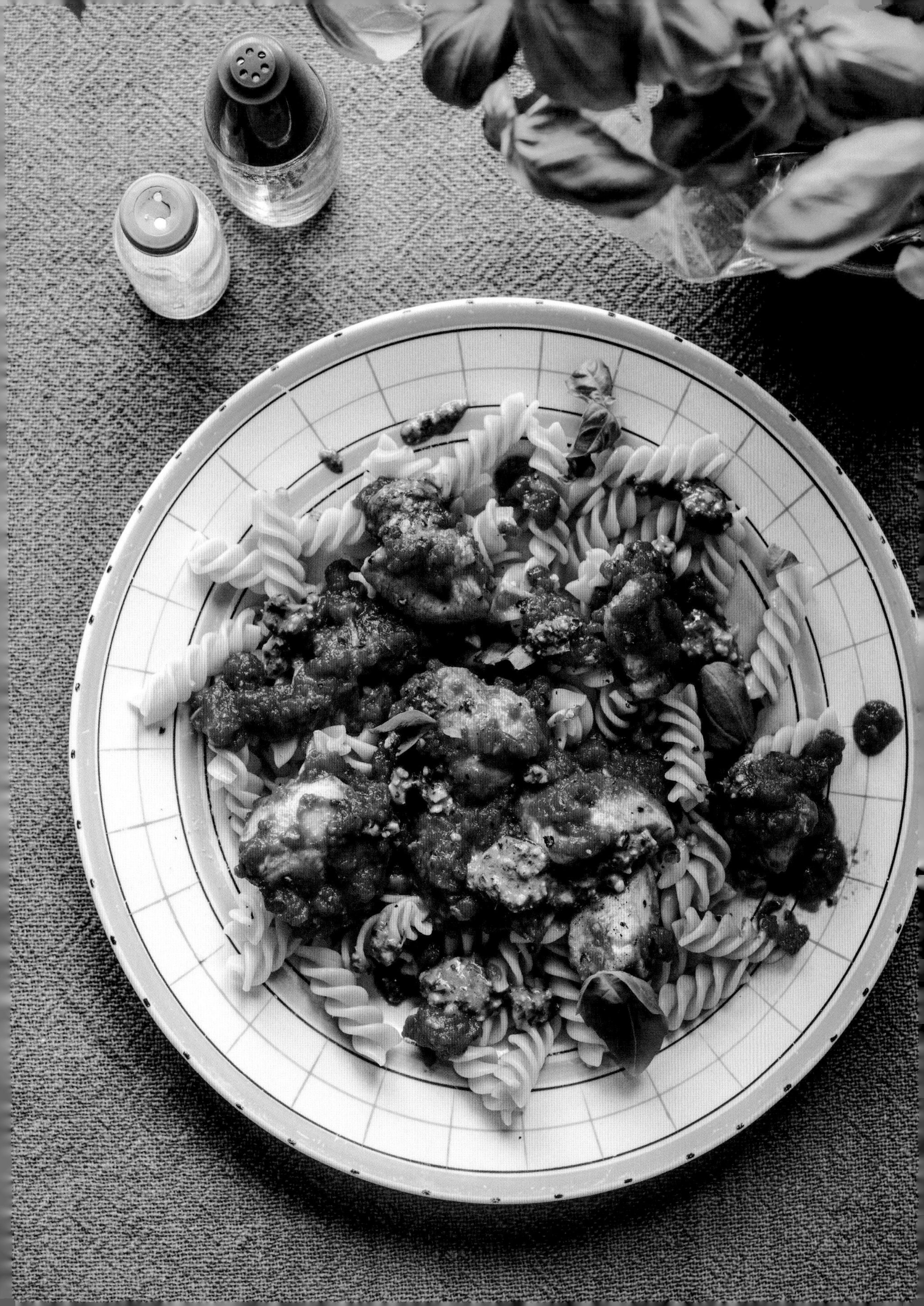

SERVES: 4
PREP: 5 MINS
COOK: 5 MINS
CALORIES: 329

GNOCCHI POUTINE

We need to apologise on two fronts here. First, our sincerest apologies go to Canada for this absolute affront to your poutine ways. We know that this is far from poutine, which is usually made with chips and cheese curds. We ask that you don't write to us, although if you're a beautifully handsome mountain man who wants us to visit and apologise in person, you're exempt from that request. Second, to Down The Hatch in Edinburgh. This isn't anything like any of your delicious poutine recipes, but it was in your wonderful restaurant that Paul had the idea for this 'quick' take, if only to use up the packaged gnocchi we invariably have sitting around in the fridge. We don't apologise for that, though, but rather the tinnitus your serving staff may have suffered as a direct result of us visiting with six of our friends, all terribly hungover and shrieking accordingly. Paul and I were visiting for an event called BearScots, where folks who (usually):

- play for our team;
- have a beard and a shaved head; and
- have a credit account with Jacamo

all descend on Edinburgh for a weekend of polite mingling. Now you might be thinking it's some raunchy event (because, I mean, it's us), but actually no, it's just the most brilliant time and raises lots of money for local LGBT+ charities. We love it. Anyhoo – should you find yourself equally fuzzy-headed after a night on the liquor, and you sensibly don't want to risk putting the chip pan on, try this.

500g (1lb 2oz) gnocchi
1 × 125g (4½oz) ball of reduced-fat mozzarella
120ml (4fl oz) chicken gravy
2 spring onions, sliced (optional)

Bring a large pan of salted water to the boil and add the gnocchi. Cook for about 2–3 minutes, or until they float to the surface, then drain and divide between four plates or bowls.

Drain the mozzarella and roughly chop, then sprinkle it over the gnocchi.

Pour over the gravy and top with the spring onions (if using).

Notes: Of course, you can swap the gnocchi for chips. You could also fry some bacon and crisp the gnocchi up in the bacon fat. Heck, you could even order a pizza. You're a sassy, independent person, after all.

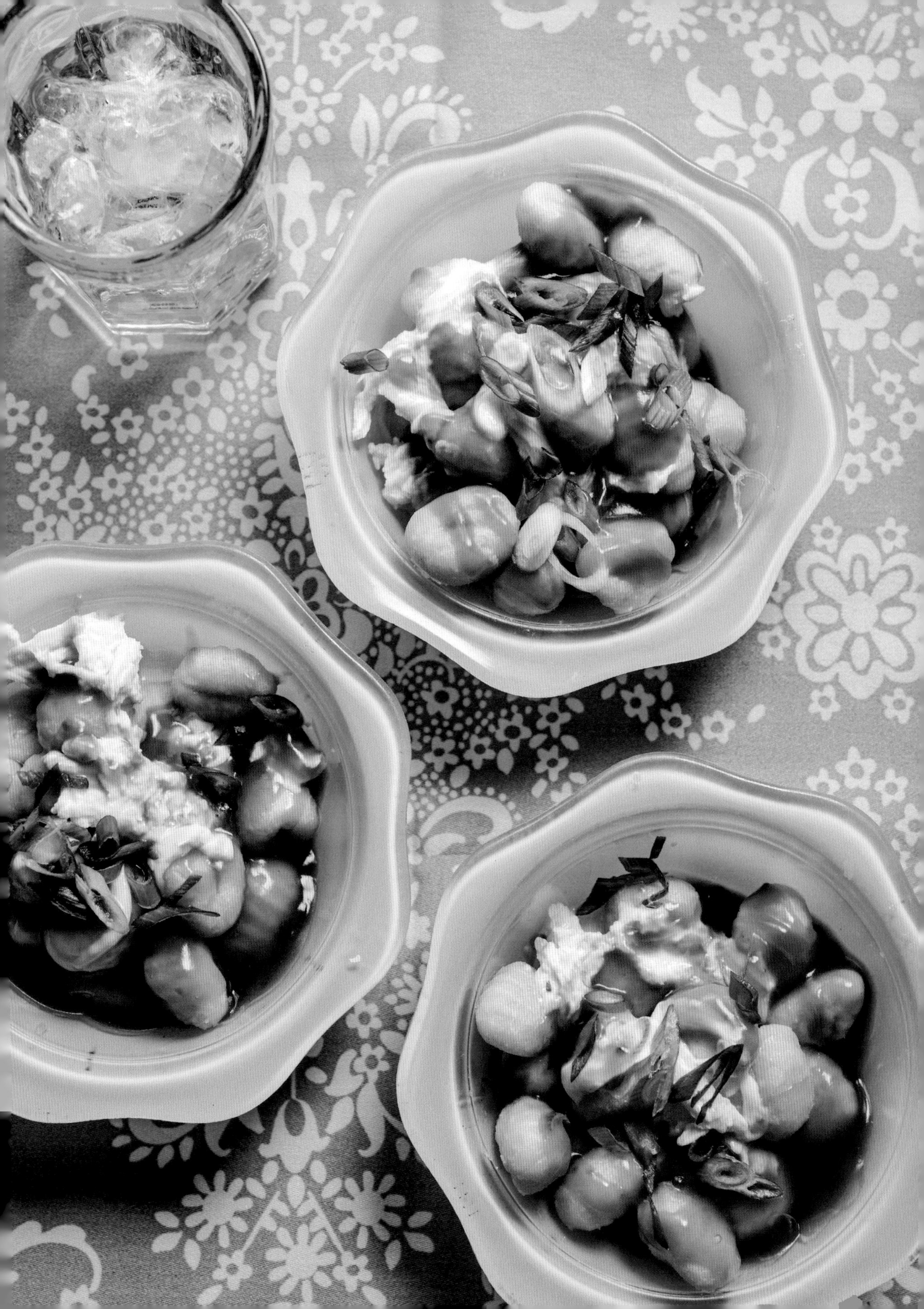

SERVES: 4
PREP: 10 MINS
COOK: 15 MINS
CALORIES: 454

PASTA OF THE SEA

Pasta of the sea is a somewhat grandiose name for a simple pasta supper with some anchovies mixed in, but if we called it anchovy and broccoli pasta we would run the risk of everyone zipping past, because anchovies have no place in a civilised society. Listen, I'm with you, they're salty and smell awful. Paul loves them, but he's also started wearing flip-flops to do the food shop, so we can't look to him as an astute arbiter of taste. However, as you will see in the notes below, you can swap anchovies for tuna and we won't tell a soul. We only ask for one thing in exchange for our service as your confidante: please buy pole-and-line-caught tuna where you can. It is a little more expensive, yes, but you look Flipper in the eye and tell him you don't care. Of course, this expostulation only works if you love dolphins – I'm less enthused: I've always found them a little clicky.

- 400g (14oz) pasta
- 400g (14oz) broccoli, cut into florets
- 2 cloves of garlic, crushed
- ½ tin of anchovies, drained and chopped
- 1 tablespoon capers
- 12 green olives, pitted and chopped
- ¼ teaspoon dried chilli flakes
- 2 tablespoons Parmesan cheese, grated

Fill a large saucepan with water and bring to the boil. Add the pasta and the broccoli and cook for about 10 minutes, then drain.

Meanwhile, spray a pan with a little oil and place over a medium heat. Add the garlic, anchovies, capers, olives and chilli flakes and cook for 3–4 minutes, stirring frequently.

Remove from the heat and stir through the cooked pasta.

Serve, sprinkled with the Parmesan.

Notes: As ever with us, any pasta will do here, though we rather like rigatoni, as the capers and olives can hide inside and play peek-a-boo.

Not a fan of anchovies? Tuna also works well!

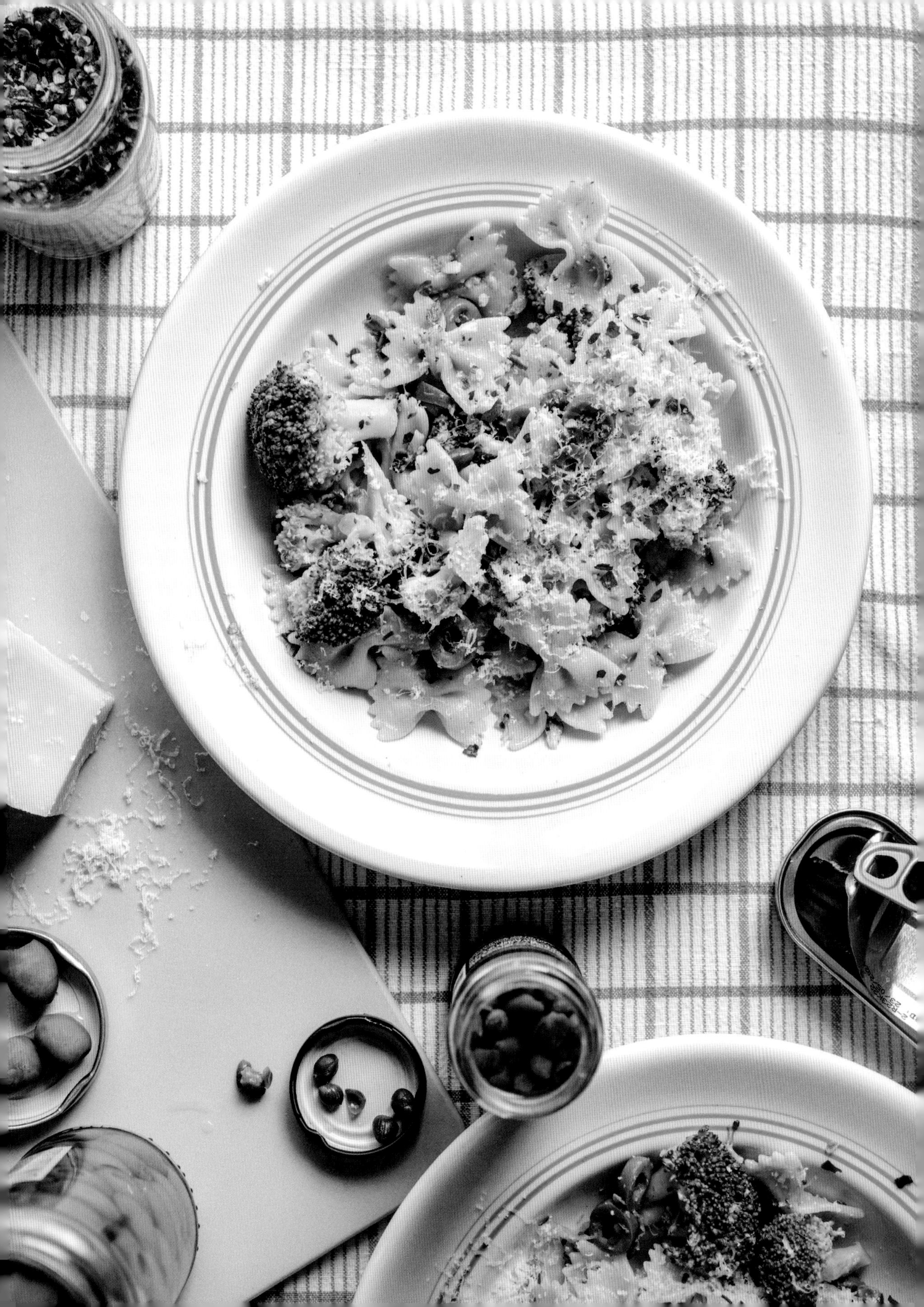

SERVES: 4
PREP: 5 MINS
COOK: 45 MINS
CALORIES: 498

30 mins · GF

- 1 large bulb of garlic
- olive oil
- 4 boneless chicken thighs
- 2 tablespoons butter
- 240g (8½oz) risotto rice
- 1 litre (1¾ pints) chicken stock

CHICKEN KYIV RISNOTTO

Now this recipe absolutely hinges on whether you like garlic: we won't try and hide the fact that if you're not a fan of having breath that could bring back the dead (and then, as per vampiric law, kill them off again), you'll be better turning the page. However, if you're garlic mad, keep reading. It's a very simple recipe – essentially all the bits of a chicken Kyiv, made into a bowl of starchy sticky wonder. Although we have used a bulb of garlic, wild garlic, if you can find it, makes this dish absolutely pop. Wild garlic grows plentifully in the spring in damp soil, so you'll usually find massive patches of it along woodside walks. Pick the long green leaves and chop them into the risotto as you go.

Preheat the oven to 190°C fan/400°F/gas mark 6.

Slice through the garlic bulb horizontally, exposing the cloves, and place on a roasting tray cut side up. Brush with oil (or butter if you're feeling decadent), then roast in the oven until the garlic is softened and sticky.

Spray a large ovenproof dish with a little oil and add the chicken thighs. Cook for 5 minutes on each side, then remove from the pan and set aside.

Add the rice to the pan and cook for a further minute, stirring constantly until all the grains are coated. Add the stock and stir until well combined.

Squeeze in the roasted garlic cloves and stir. Bring to the boil, then reduce the heat to low, cover with a lid and place in the oven. Cook for 30 minutes, then stir in the remaining butter.

Five minutes before the end, pop the chicken into the oven on a tray to heat it through.

Serve the risnotto and top with the chicken.

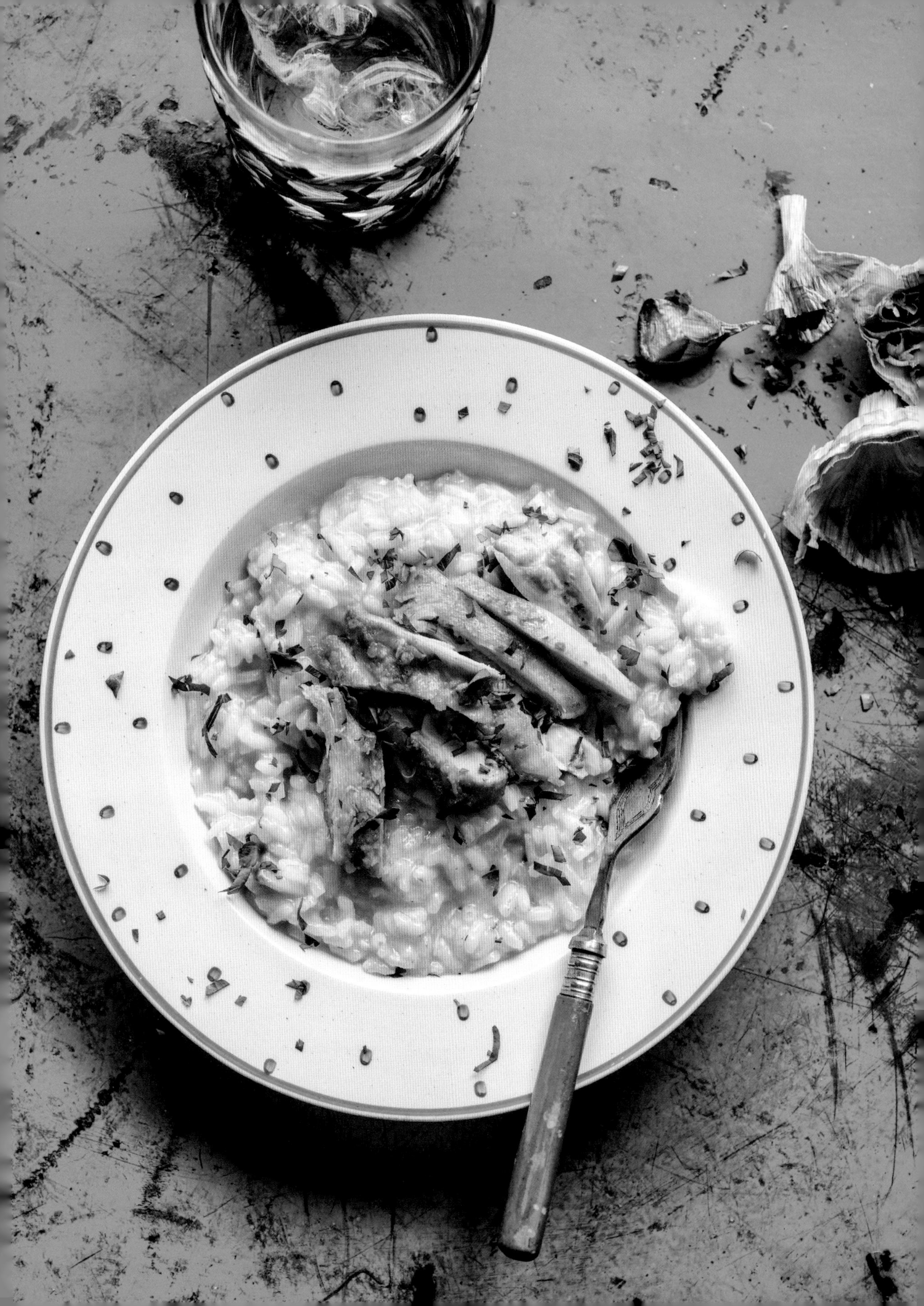

SERVES: 4
PREP: 5 MINS
COOK: 55 MINS
CALORIES: 269

BAKED ORZO

Every now and then I'll get a fit of the vapours and decide that Paul and I need to produce more video recipes and bits for the internet. It seems like a good idea until you remember that we're both hurtling towards forty and, perhaps more importantly, both have the on-screen presence of a potato. Stick a camera in front of Paul and it's like asking a baby to explain nuclear fusion. Of course, humour is subjective, but no one needs subjecting to our humour. Unless you paid for this book, in which case, we thank you. I only mention it because we did a full video tutorial of this for YouTube and it worked very well, but we only received about ten views. I can't help but think it was my stubborn refusal to pose with a shocked face and a crying emoji as the thumbnail, or perhaps it was not calling it 'BAKED ORZO SHOCK: can I EVER get a THICK SAUCE'. I don't know: as I say, we're old. Either way, we can't let such a good recipe go to waste, so please enjoy it with our regards.

- 120g (4oz) orzo
- 60g (2oz) frozen peas
- 60g (2oz) ham, chopped
- 100g (1¾oz) reduced-fat green pesto
- 50g (1¾oz) natural yoghurt
- 50ml (2fl oz) semi-skimmed milk
- 60g (2oz) low-fat soft cheese
- 40g (1½oz) Parmesan cheese

Preheat the oven to 190°C fan/400°F/gas mark 6.

Bring a large pan of water to the boil. Add the orzo and cook for 10–12 minutes, adding the frozen peas for the last 4 minutes, then drain.

Mix together the drained orzo and peas, ham, pesto, yoghurt, milk, soft cheese and half the Parmesan and tip into a small ovenproof dish.

Sprinkle over the rest of the Parmesan, cover with foil and bake in the oven for 30 minutes, then remove the foil and bake for another 10 minutes.

Serve.

Notes: This is perfect for using up leftover boiled ham – we will often pressure-cook a yellow-stickered ham joint, shred it, then use it in dishes like this. You can always freeze what you don't need. Thrifty!

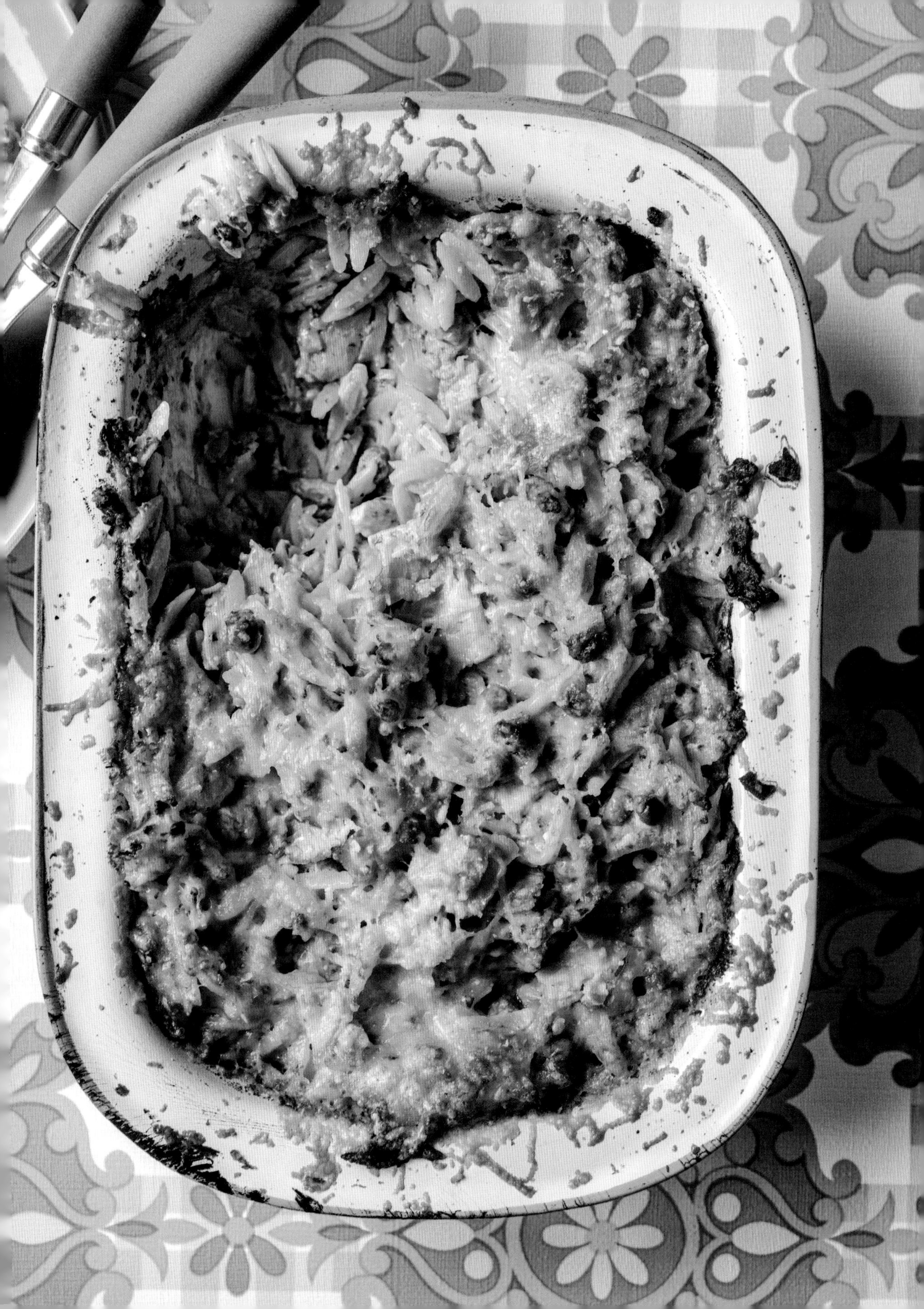

EASY COUSCOUS 'N' COD

SERVES: 4
PREP: 10 MINS
COOK: 30 MINS
CALORIES: 295

DF

There's a biennial event at Chubby Towers guaranteed to lead to the creation of some weird and wonderful recipes: the clearing of the freezers. One freezer is for leftovers, the other is for ingredients. As you can perhaps imagine, the leftovers freezer never really fills up. No such joy with the ingredients freezer, though. I can't resist a yellow sticker, I just can't. Knock 29p off a pack of out-of-date sausages and they'll be in my trolley before you can say acute gastroenteritis. Each trip to the supermarket yields mysterious treasure which I secrete in the freezer. So Paul will go to put away our actual shopping only to find a frozen wall of chicken fillets or gammon joints or party packs that still make reference to the Queen's Jubilee. He'll huff and fuss and I'll rashly promise to use up every ingredient before buying more, and I'll take over cooking for a couple of weeks. As a result, simple little recipes like this are born. In my defence, this is bloody tasty.

- 1 onion, finely diced
- 3 cloves of garlic, crushed
- 160g (5¾oz) couscous
- 4 sun-dried tomatoes, chopped
- 60g (2¼oz) pitted green olives, halved
- 400g (14oz) cod fillets (see notes)
- a handful of fresh parsley, chopped
- ½ lemon

Spray a large pan with a little oil and place over a medium-high heat. Add the onion and cook for 5 minutes, stirring occasionally, then add the garlic and cook for another minute.

Add the couscous, sun-dried tomatoes and olives and stir. Pour in 350ml (12fl oz) of boiling water and bring the lot to a simmer.

Carefully place the fish fillets on top of the couscous and sprinkle over half the parsley.

Reduce the heat to low, cover with a lid, and simmer for 12–15 minutes.

Remove the lid, squeeze over the lemon juice, and serve.

Notes: Any white fish will do here, haddock, cod, pollock – all are fine to use.

We tend to use frozen fish fillets for this as it's much cheaper – just be sure to defrost them in the fridge overnight before cooking.

Not a fan of Satan-Grapes / olives? Leave them out, and up the amount of tomatoes instead.

Little does he know I'm using the leftovers freezer to keep boxes of raspberry sorbet lollies in.

Please don't think of us as awful braggarts with our dual freezers: one came with the house, the other is part of the fridge.

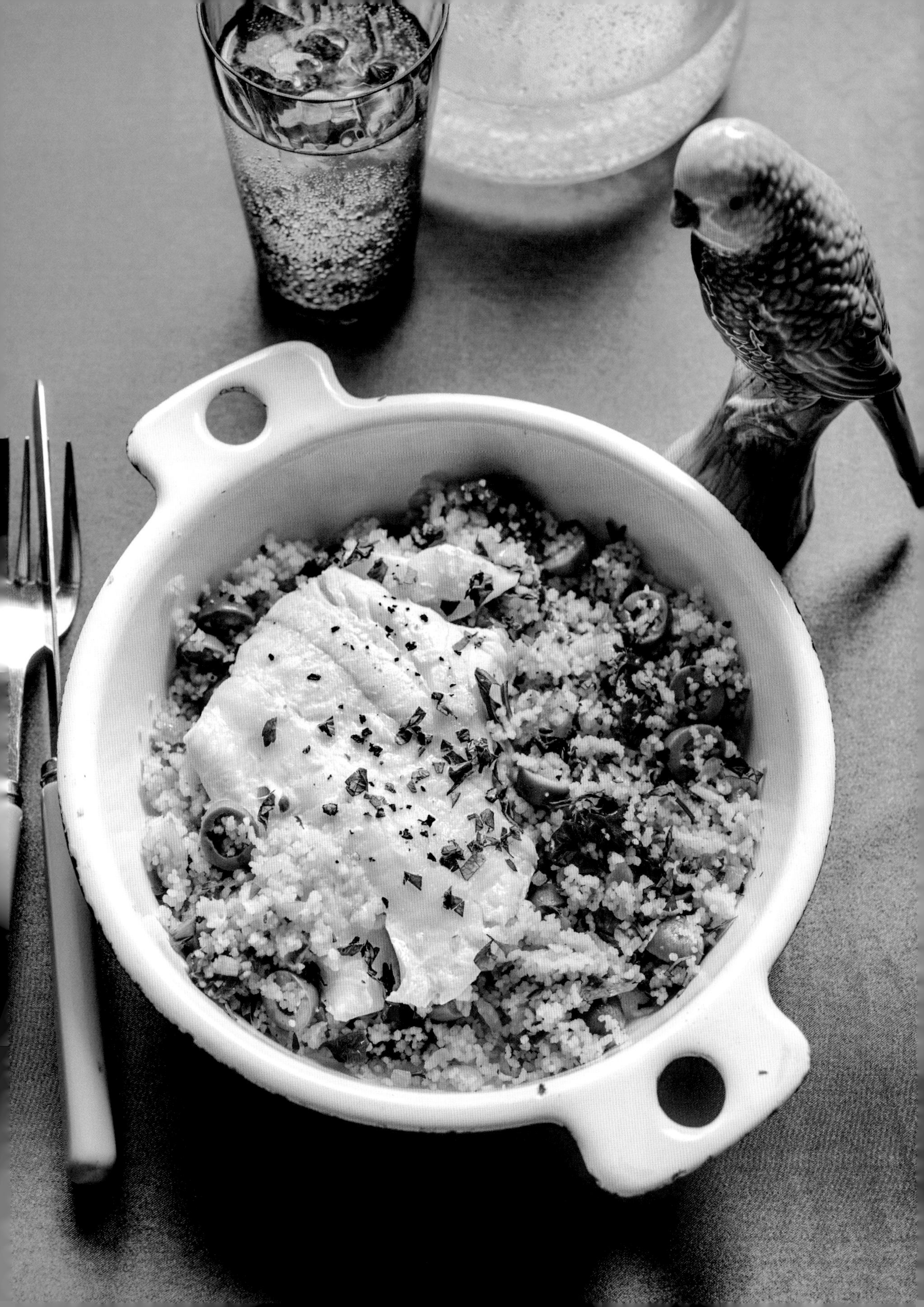

SERVES: 4
PREP: 50 MINS
COOK: 50 MINS
CALORIES: 214

- 1 vegetable stock cube
- 200g (7oz) instant polenta
- a small handful of fresh flat-leaf parsley, roughly chopped
- a handful of fresh chives, chopped
- 1 clove of garlic, crushed
- 2 courgettes, halved lengthways and sliced
- 25g (1oz) Parmesan cheese (or vegetarian alternative), finely grated
- 200g (7oz) cherry tomatoes, quartered
- ½ red onion, finely chopped
- 4 sun-dried tomatoes, finely chopped
- 1 tablespoon capers, drained
- a handful of black olives, chopped
- 1 tablespoon balsamic vinegar
- a handful of rocket
- 1 × 150g (5½oz) ball of low-fat mozzarella, drained and thinly sliced

LOADED POLENTA WITH TOMATO SALSA

I remember the very first recipe we ever did with polenta, back in the olden days when we went to a church hall for an hour a week to listen to how Sandra was getting on with her bowel movements. That, and to learn about slimming and nutrition. Cough. We had followed a healthy recipe and made polenta cakes, only for the whole hall to look smug as we were told we had used twice as many 'points' as we were allowed that day. There was an awful amount of judgement coming from someone who measured her milk allowance out in a washing powder cup, I can tell you. Since then, despite having moved towards being sensible with calories and realising that nothing is off limits, we've still had a curious relationship with it. Well, no more! This loaded polenta is stodgy but tasty, filling but fabulous: everything you want in a gorgeous vegetarian recipe. Note the calories: perfectly healthy. Take that, Sandra! Hope you've at least managed a small one this week.

Line a 20 × 20cm (8 × 8 inch) brownie tin with clingfilm and spray with a little oil. Dissolve the stock cube in 800ml (1½ pints) of boiling water, pour into a pan, bring back to the boil, then slowly add the polenta, stirring continuously for 5 minutes until it is smooth and thick.

Beat in the parsley, chives and garlic. Tip into the brownie tin and spread out into an even layer. Leave to cool and firm up in the fridge for about 30 minutes.

Preheat the oven to 200°C fan/425°F/gas mark 7.

Spray a baking tray with some oil, then add the courgettes in a single layer. Cook in the oven for 20 minutes or until golden and soft, turning them halfway through.

Meanwhile, remove the polenta from the tin. Cut it into quarters, then cut each quarter into 6 fingers. Transfer the fingers to a lined baking sheet and sprinkle over the Parmesan. Cook in the oven for 25 minutes, until really crisp and starting to take on some colour.

Mix the cherry tomatoes, red onion, sun-dried tomatoes, capers, olives and balsamic vinegar together in a bowl, toss in the rocket, season and set aside.

Divide the polenta between plates, pile on the courgettes, followed by the tomato and rocket salad, then tear over the mozzarella and serve.

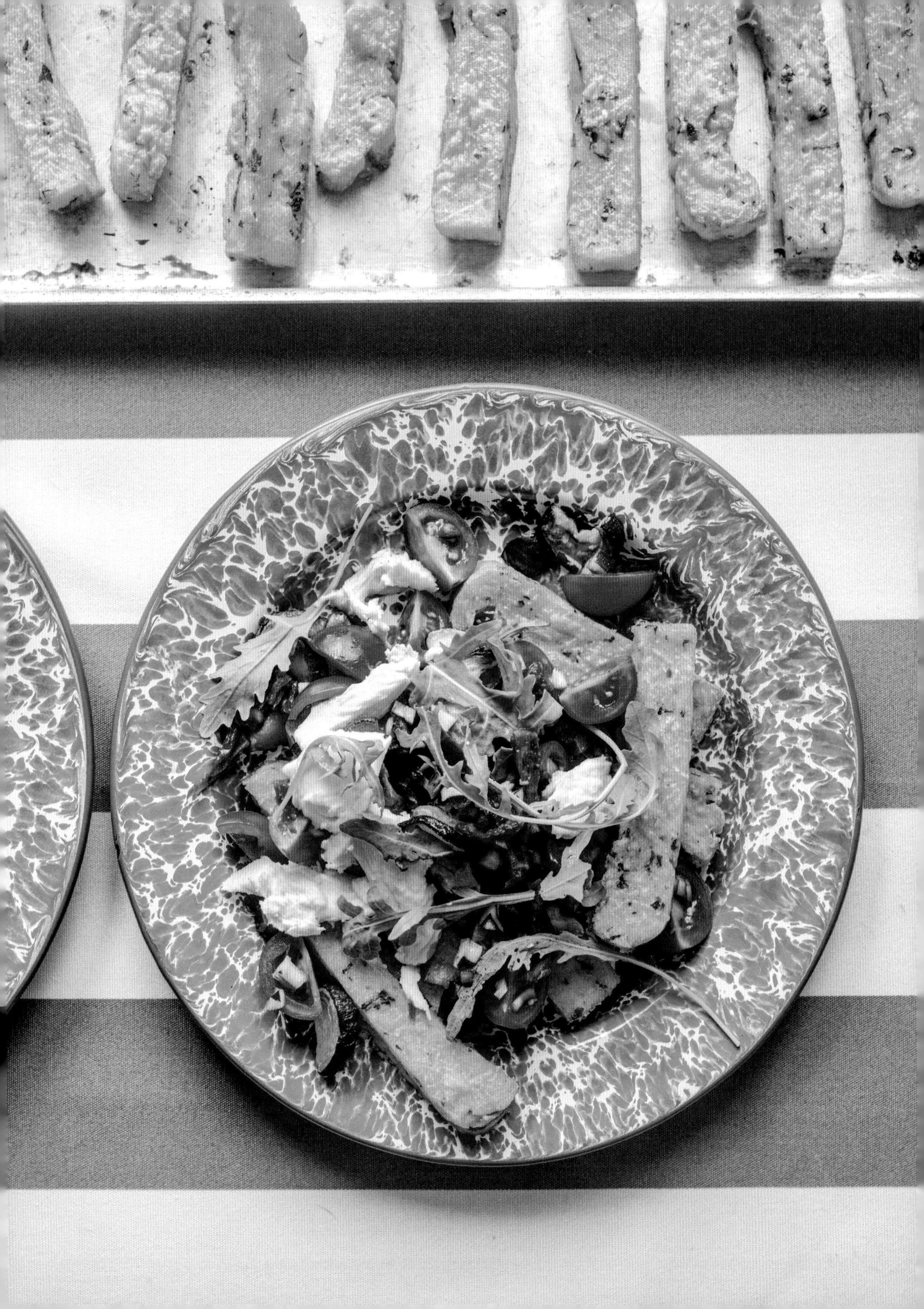

SURF & MIRTH CARBONARA

SERVES: 4
PREP: 10 MINS
COOK: 35 MINS
CALORIES: 496

Again, not entirely sure what Paul is doing with the title, but he does like a laugh, so maybe that's it. The surf bit makes sense, certainly, on account of the prawns, but the mirth? If you have prawns leftover from our Prawn Cocktail recipe on page 180, chuck them in here. Previous experience of us posting a carbonara recipe has told us it will elicit all manner of angry responses for not being a purist take on the dish. That's fair, but at least we didn't stir through a load of Quark. Pop the pitchforks down: this is delicious, filling and a wonder to make. What more can you ask?

- 1 brown onion, diced
- ½ red pepper, deseeded and diced
- 12 cooked jumbo prawns, peeled and deveined
- 1 clove of garlic, crushed
- 6 bacon medallions, diced
- 1 chicken breast, diced
- 1 large egg, beaten
- 30g (1oz) plain flour
- 20g (¾oz) panko breadcrumbs
- 200g (7oz) tagliatelle
- 3 egg yolks
- 70g (2½oz) Parmesan cheese
- a handful of fresh parsley, chopped

Preheat the oven to 190°C fan/400°F/gas mark 6.

Spray a large pan with a little oil and place it over a medium-high heat. Add the onions and red pepper and cook for 5–6 minutes, until starting to soften, then remove from the heat and set aside.

Add the prawns to the pan along with the garlic and a pinch of salt and pepper. Cook for about 3 minutes, until they're pink all over, then remove to a plate and keep warm.

Put the pan back on the heat and add the diced bacon. Cook until crispy, then remove to a plate and keep warm.

Dip the diced chicken first into the beaten egg, then into the flour, then roll it in the panko. Spread the chicken out on a lined baking sheet and bake in the oven for 15–20 minutes.

Meanwhile, cook the pasta according to the instructions on the packet. Drain, keeping aside half a mug of the cooking water for later.

Whisk the egg yolks in a bowl with the Parmesan and set aside.

When the pasta is cooked and drained, transfer it to the frying pan and stir it through the egg mixture until well coated. Loosen with a splash of the pasta water if needed.

Stir through the onions and peppers and serve in bowls, topped with the chicken, prawns and bacon. Finish with the chopped parsley.

Notes: This has quite a few steps, so be sure to read the recipe through and have everything ready and to hand.

We use tagliatelle here, but really, any pasta will do.

In retrospect, we ought to have called this recipe 'Surf and Oeuf', given the chicken and egg, but what can you do?

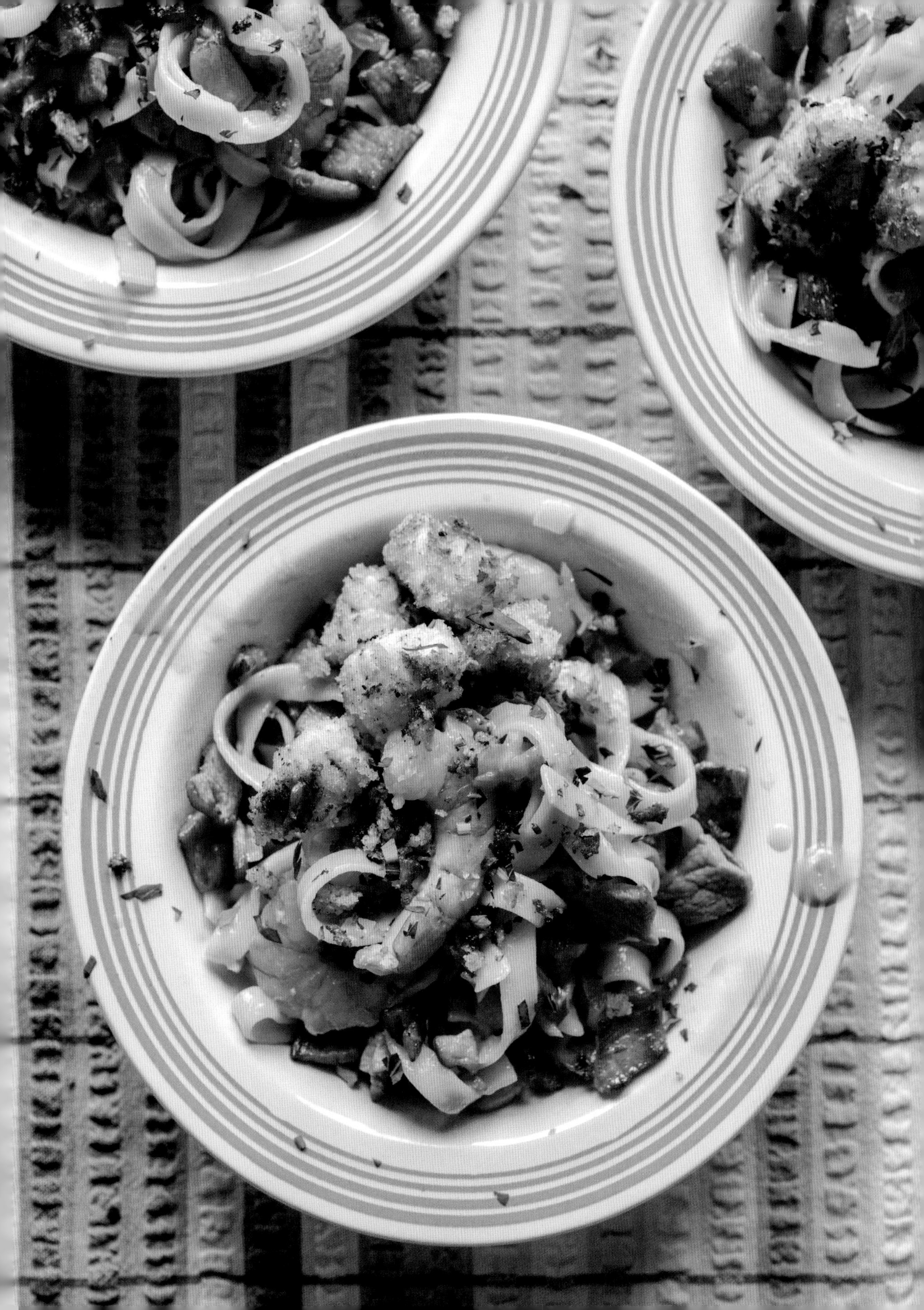

SERVES: 4
PREP: 10 MINS
COOK: 35 MINS
CALORIES: 378

30 mins · serves · 10 · GF

SMOKED SALMON RISOTTO

Our continued drive to bring you risotto dishes that [checks the young person dictionary] 'slap' continues at a pace with this salmon risotto. As mentioned elsewhere in this book, Paul prepares a lunchbox for his work each day, and part of that is nearly always a salmon and cream cheese sandwich. At the end of the week we're always left with leftover salmon trimmings (I know, it's a surprise we sleep at night), and this dish was created to use them up. We genuinely do try to be 'zero waste' at Chubby Towers – it's very important to us – although the five separate jars of pickled onions containing one solitary onion in our fridge right now might suggest otherwise. Speaking of leftovers, check the notes. We're conscious that we have two risotto recipes in this book, so in the notes we've included a bonus recipe to use up leftover risotto, although it is a trifle high in calories. But you know what: you've earned this!

- 1 small brown onion, finely diced
- 2 cloves of garlic, crushed
- 200g (7oz) arborio rice
- 125ml (4fl oz) white wine
- 1 litre (1¾ pints) vegetable stock
- 120g (4oz) smoked salmon trimmings
- 30g (1oz) Parmesan cheese, grated
- 2 tablespoons butter
- fresh dill fronds

Spray a large pan with a little oil and place over a medium heat. Add the onion and garlic and fry for about 4–5 minutes.

Add the rice and stir for 2–3 minutes, then add the wine and continue to stir until it's absorbed by the rice.

Add the stock, a ladleful at a time, stirring the rice continuously until absorbed, and keep repeating until the rice is cooked but still slightly firm, which will take about 20–25 minutes.

Remove the pan from the heat, stir through the salmon, Parmesan and butter, and serve sprinkled with dill fronds.

Notes: If you're like me, dill is one of those tastes that leave you cold. If so, swap it out for chopped chives.

Leftover risotto can be turned into arancini very easily: whisk a couple of eggs in a bowl. Pop some fine breadcrumbs into another bowl, and fill a third bowl with plain flour mixed with ground pepper. Shape your risotto into balls, dredge with the flour, follow it up with the egg, then roll in the breadcrumbs. Fry in oil until golden. Beautiful!

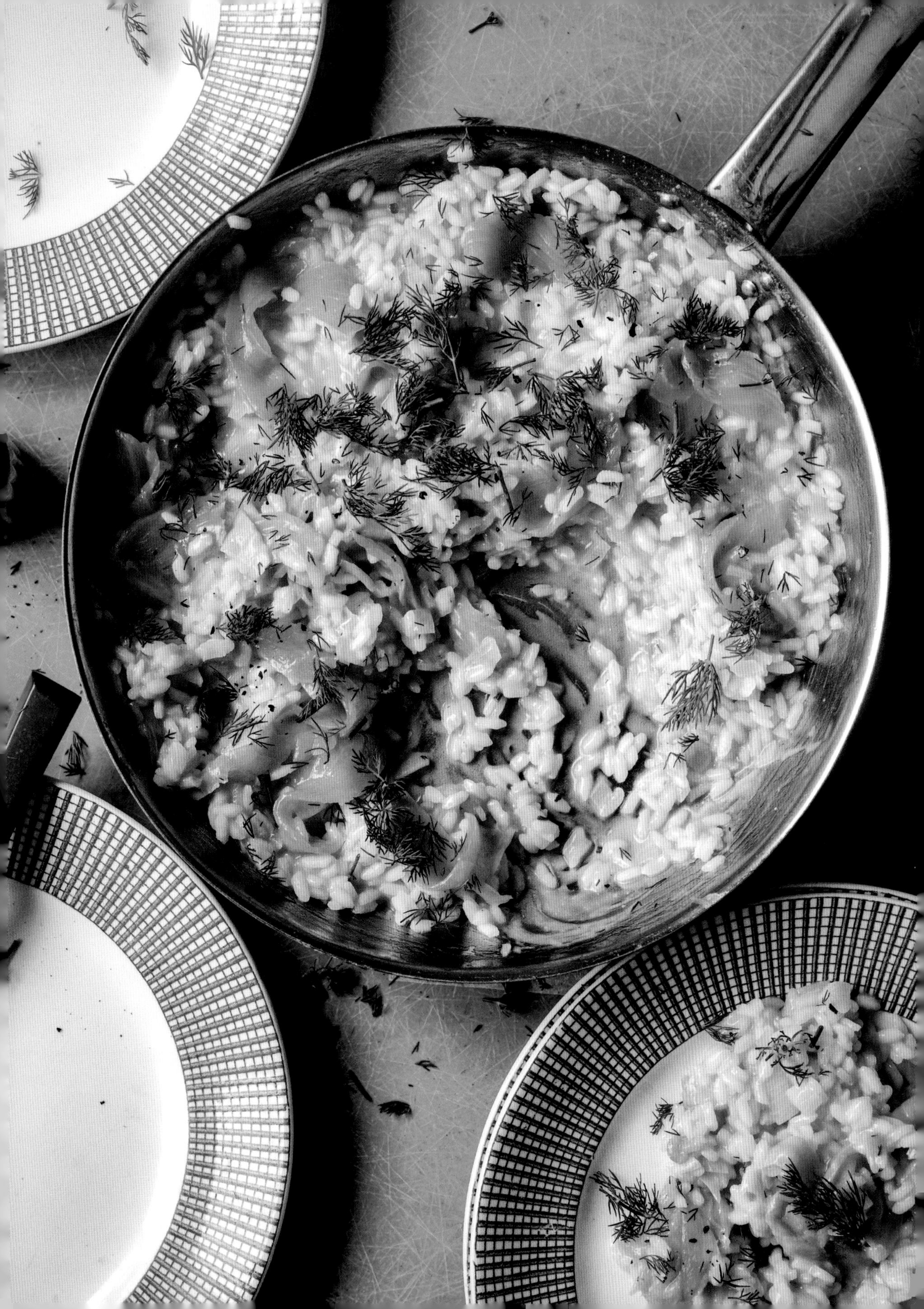

SERVES: 4
PREP: 10 MINS
COOK: 45 MINS
CALORIES: 380

300g (10½oz) long-grain rice
1 brown onion, finely diced
4 cloves of garlic, crushed
450g (1lb) baby spinach, washed and chopped
20g (¾oz) fresh dill, chopped
20g (¾oz) fresh parsley, chopped
125ml (4fl oz) passata
juice of ½ lemon
80g (3oz) feta cheese, crumbled
a handful of fresh mint leaves, torn

SPANAKORIZO

Readers of the previous books will remember our 'lighter spanakopita', a lovely and healthier take on one of our favourite Greek dishes. I described spanakopita as one of the most wonderful words to say with a Geordie accent, and now I must amend that – spanakorizo sounds even better! And quite right too: this is an utterly fantastic dish: entirely vegetarian, totally tasty. A note on the rice washing – we have always been one for washing rice before cooking it, as apparently it removes the excess starch and makes for a less 'clumpy' end result. We're not entirely sure of the science – our expert knowledge extends to watching a few episodes of *How 2* – but it seems to work for this dish.

Rinse the rice in a sieve until the water is almost clear, then set aside.

Spray a large pan with a little oil and place over a medium heat. Add the onion and garlic and cook until soft, about 5 minutes or so.

Add the spinach, dill, parsley and passata and stir to combine.

Add the rice, along with 1 litre (1¾ pints) of water, season with salt and pepper to taste, and bring to the boil. Reduce the heat to low, cover with a lid and cook for 20–25 minutes, until the rice is tender.

Remove the lid from the pan and leave to rest for 5–10 minutes.

Add the lemon juice, crumble over the feta, sprinkle over the mint leaves, and serve.

Note: Although this is terrific when served hot, it's another one of those dishes that will only get better if you leave it for lunch the next day.

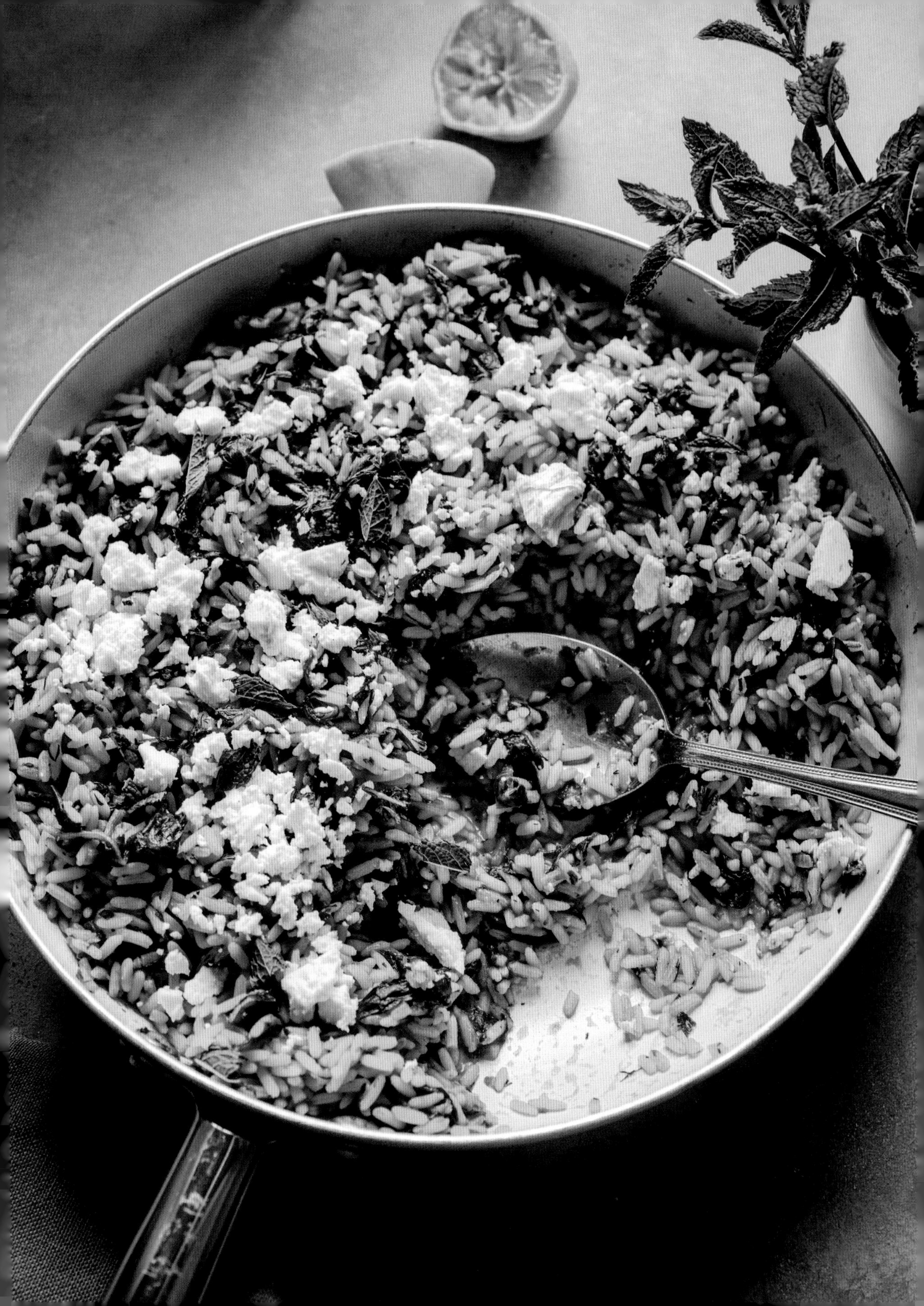

SERVES: 4
PREP: 5 MINS
COOK: 50 MINS
CALORIES: 423

FRENCH ONION GNOCCHI

Long time readers will have spotted that, over the years, we have worshipped at the altar of a French onion base many times. We make no apology for it: onions are so cheap and terrific that it just makes perfect sense to plan a new recipe around them. The thinner the slices of onion, the better this recipe will be, and so that leads us to our usual recommendation and warning around the use of a mandoline slicer. This natty little gadget will make thin slices of anything an absolute breeze, but what applies to thinly sliced apple and onion also encompasses your fingertips. The blade on a mandoline could slice through diamond without a blink, and your fingers are no match. Most models come with a little guard to prevent you from cutting yourself: don't do what I did and consider yourself too sensible to use it – my middle finger still looks like it hasn't fully rendered. Rather takes the impact out of sticking my finger up at errant drivers, I can tell you. Anyhoo, let's get to this terrific little bake – a low-prep, high-taste wonder!

- 500g (1lb 2oz) gnocchi
- 2 tablespoons butter
- ½ teaspoon salt
- ¼ teaspoon black pepper
- 2 teaspoons sugar
- 2 large brown onions, thinly sliced
- ½ teaspoon dried thyme
- 125ml (4fl oz) beef stock
- 25g (1oz) panko breadcrumbs
- 25g (1oz) Parmesan cheese, grated
- a handful of fresh parsley, finely chopped

Preheat the oven to 200°C fan/425°F/gas mark 7.

Place the gnocchi in an oven dish and spray with a little oil, toss, then cook for 25 minutes to crisp up.

Meanwhile, place a large pan over a medium heat. Add the butter, salt, pepper and sugar, and stir until melted. Add the onions and thyme and cook for about 30 minutes, stirring occasionally.

Once the onions are nicely caramelised, add the beef stock and simmer for 5 minutes.

Stir the onions through the gnocchi and top with the panko and Parmesan, then bake in the oven for 5 minutes.

Serve.

Note: If you're ordering a mandoline, make sure you spell it correctly. The last thing anyone needs as you cook is someone prancing around the kitchen twanging away and singing.

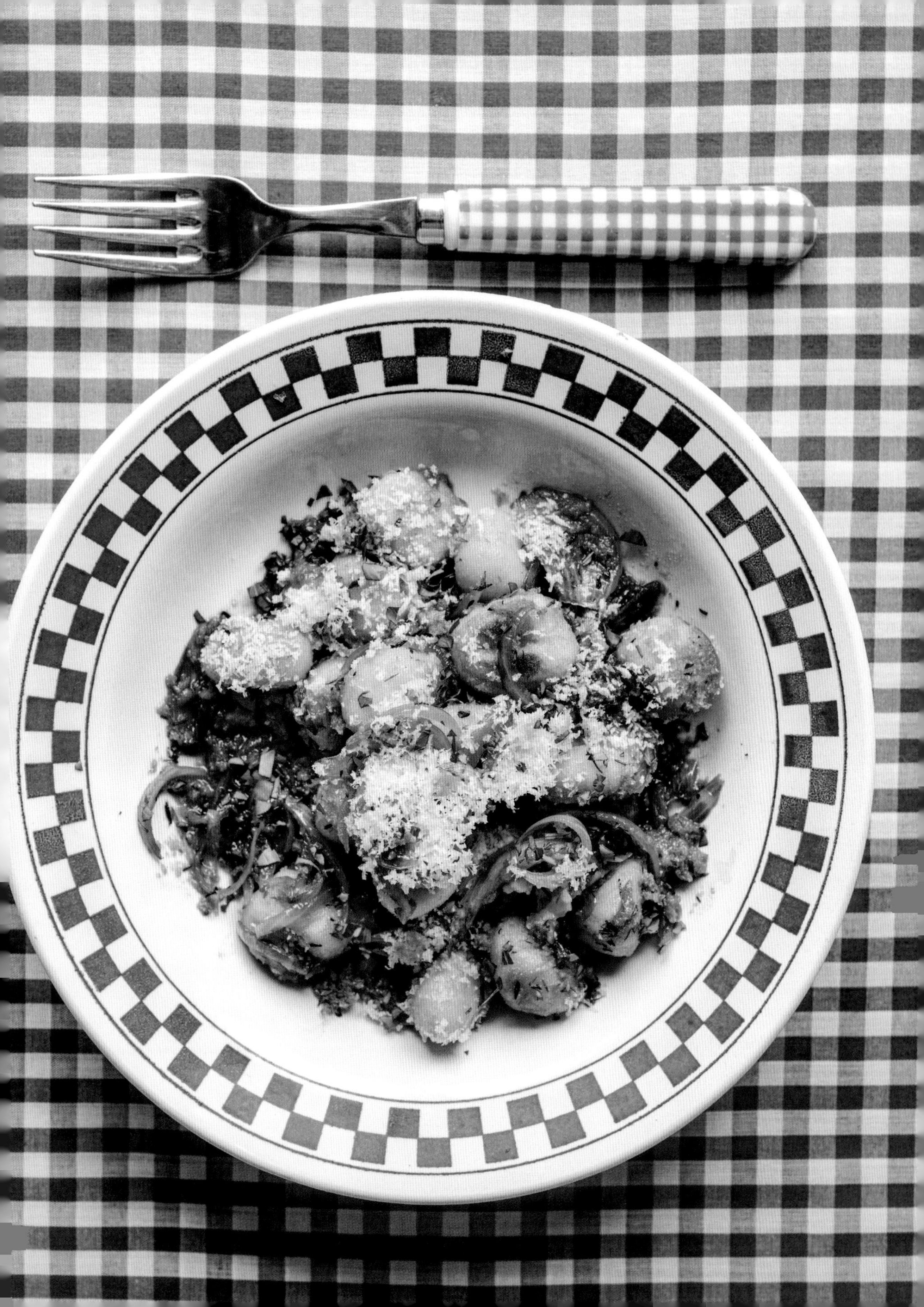

SERVES: 4
PREP: 10 MINS
COOK: 1 HR 10 MINS
CALORIES: 499

30 mins · ❄ · GF

BANGIN' CHICKEN & RICE

Protein-packed and ever-so-filling, bangin' chicken and rice will keep you right when days are dark. Plus, if you're making it, the chicken part can be baked in big hearty batches, cubed and then frozen for when you need it. Top tip: great scattered into a wrap. We say batch cooking as though we do it all the time: honestly, we wish we did. We have nothing but admiration and praise for those who can studiously prepare their lunches for the week ahead on a Sunday, but we're too flighty for such business. I get bored halfway through blinking. If you're far more disciplined than we ever could be, then this is the one for you, and more power to your elbow.

- 4 boneless skinless chicken thighs
- 2 tablespoons melted butter
- 70g (2½oz) light mayonnaise
- 70g (2½oz) low-fat natural yoghurt
- 3 tablespoons sriracha
- 1 teaspoon hot chilli powder
- ½ teaspoon paprika
- ¼ teaspoon garlic granules
- ¼ teaspoon black pepper
- 1 tablespoon cider vinegar
- 180g (6oz) long-grain rice
- 1 celery stalk, finely chopped
- 45g (1½oz) reduced-fat feta cheese, crumbled
- 3 spring onions, sliced

Preheat the oven to 200°C fan/425°F/gas mark 7.

Put the chicken thighs and butter into a dish and toss well until coated. Sprinkle with a little salt and bake for 20 minutes.

Meanwhile, mix together the mayonnaise, yoghurt, sriracha, chilli powder, paprika, garlic granules, black pepper and cider vinegar in a bowl and set aside.

Once the chicken is cooked, remove from the dish to a plate. Pour the cooking juices into a jug and top up with water to make 400ml (14fl oz). Pour into a saucepan and add the rice. Bring to the boil, then reduce to medium-low, cover with a lid and simmer for about 15 minutes. Remove from the heat and leave to stand for another 10 minutes.

Tip the rice into the baking dish and even out, then top with the celery.

Cut the cooked chicken into small cubes and coat with the mayonnaise mixture. Spread the chicken on top of the rice and sprinkle over the feta.

Bake in the oven for 15–20 minutes, and serve sprinkled with the sliced spring onions.

Notes: Don't be tempted to forgo the celery, unless it absolutely brings you out in hives: it's good for what ails you.

Also don't be tempted to use black rice for this: we did that once, and accidentally created one of the least appetising meals we've ever had.

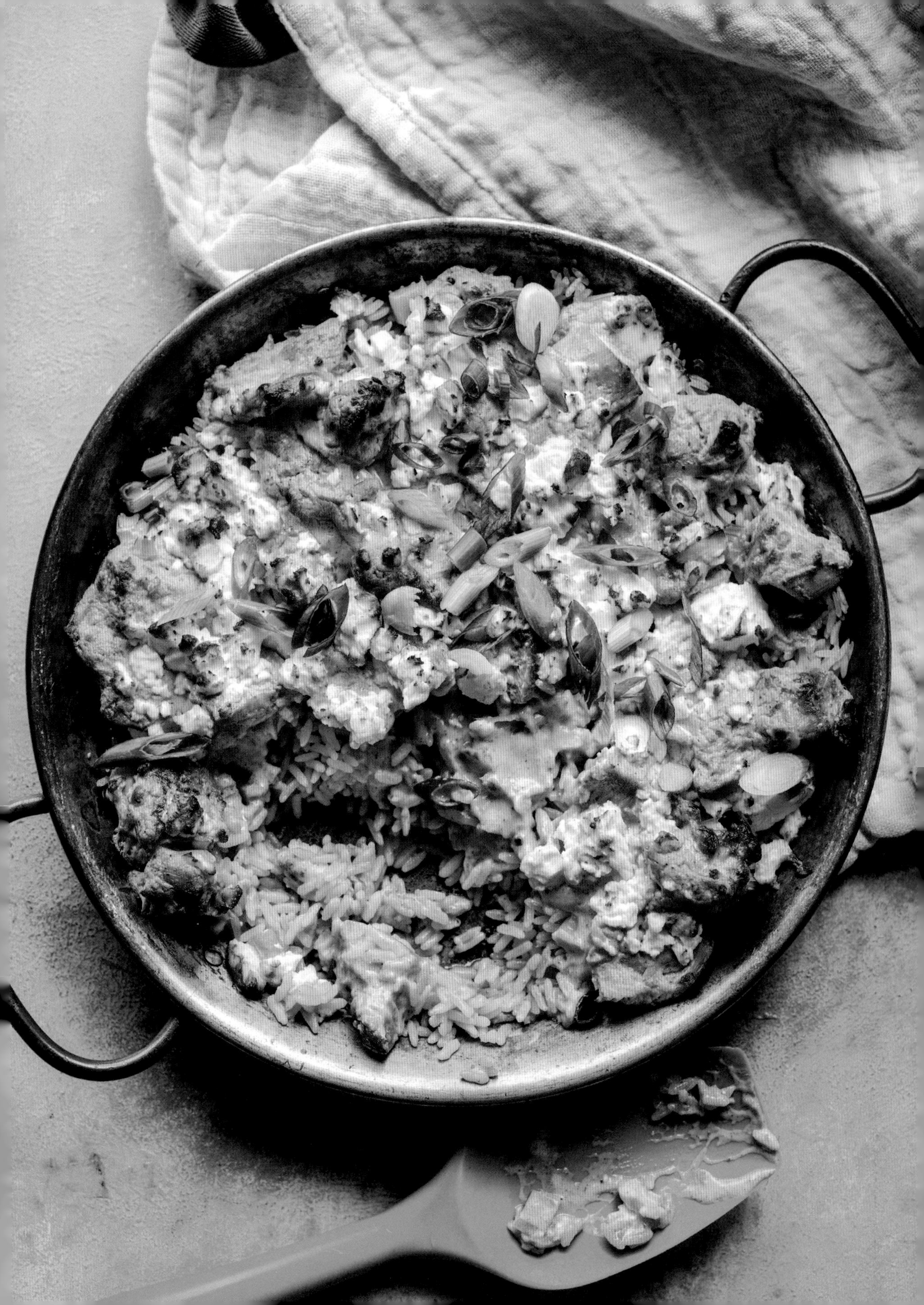

SERVES: 4
PREP: 15 MINS
COOK: 30 MINS
CALORIES: 499

BACON & TOMATO RIGATONI

Paul and I have been making this dish, or variations thereof, ever since we moved in together so many moons ago. Only the aubergine is a recent addition, born from having green-fingered neighbours who send us their surplus. Although Chubby Towers is very much our home (until we bugger off to Canada), our first home holds many precious memories, one of which unexpectedly bubbled up to the surface just the other day when I hired a carpet cleaner. Way back when, a work colleague set up her own business cleaning carpets. As Paul and I were sloppy little souls living in a rented flat, we hired her to give the carpets a deep clean. Well, she certainly made them wet. It was as if she had used a pressure washer to rinse everything down. Being British, trying to be good friends, and more than a bit scared of her, we agreed that she had done the most terrific job, sent her on her way, then spent the next two weeks trying to dry those sodden carpets out. She gave up that business a few weeks later (presumably liquidated, ayoo!).

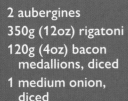

- 2 aubergines
- 350g (12oz) rigatoni
- 120g (4oz) bacon medallions, diced
- 1 medium onion, diced
- 2 cloves of garlic, sliced
- ½ teaspoon dried chilli flakes
- 1 × 400g (14oz) tin of chopped tomatoes
- 300g (10½oz) plum tomatoes, halved
- 80g (3oz) reduced-fat feta cheese, crumbled

First, preheat your grill to high and bring a large pan of salted water to the boil.

While those are heating up, halve your aubergines lengthways, then slice each half into 1cm (½ inch) wide strips, then slice the other way for cute little 1cm (½ inch) cubes.

Spread the aubergine cubes on a baking sheet in a single layer. Spray with a little oil, and sprinkle with a little salt. Place under the grill and cook for about 10 minutes, then turn and cook for another 10 minutes.

While that's going on, cook the pasta according to the instructions on the packet.

Meanwhile, spray a large frying pan with a bit of oil and place over a high heat. Add the bacon and cook for 5–6 minutes, until crispy. Reduce the heat to medium-high. Add the onion and cook until soft (about 4 minutes, stirring frequently). Add the garlic and the chilli flakes, stir, and cook for another minute. Add the tinned tomatoes and stir, then reduce the heat to medium and simmer for about 8 minutes, stirring occasionally.

Once the aubergine is cooked, stir it into the sauce.

Meanwhile, place the plum tomatoes on the same tray you used for the aubergine, spray with a bit of oil, and crumble over the feta. Pop under the grill for 4–5 minutes.

When the pasta is cooked, drain it and stir it into the tomato sauce along with the grilled plum tomatoes and feta.

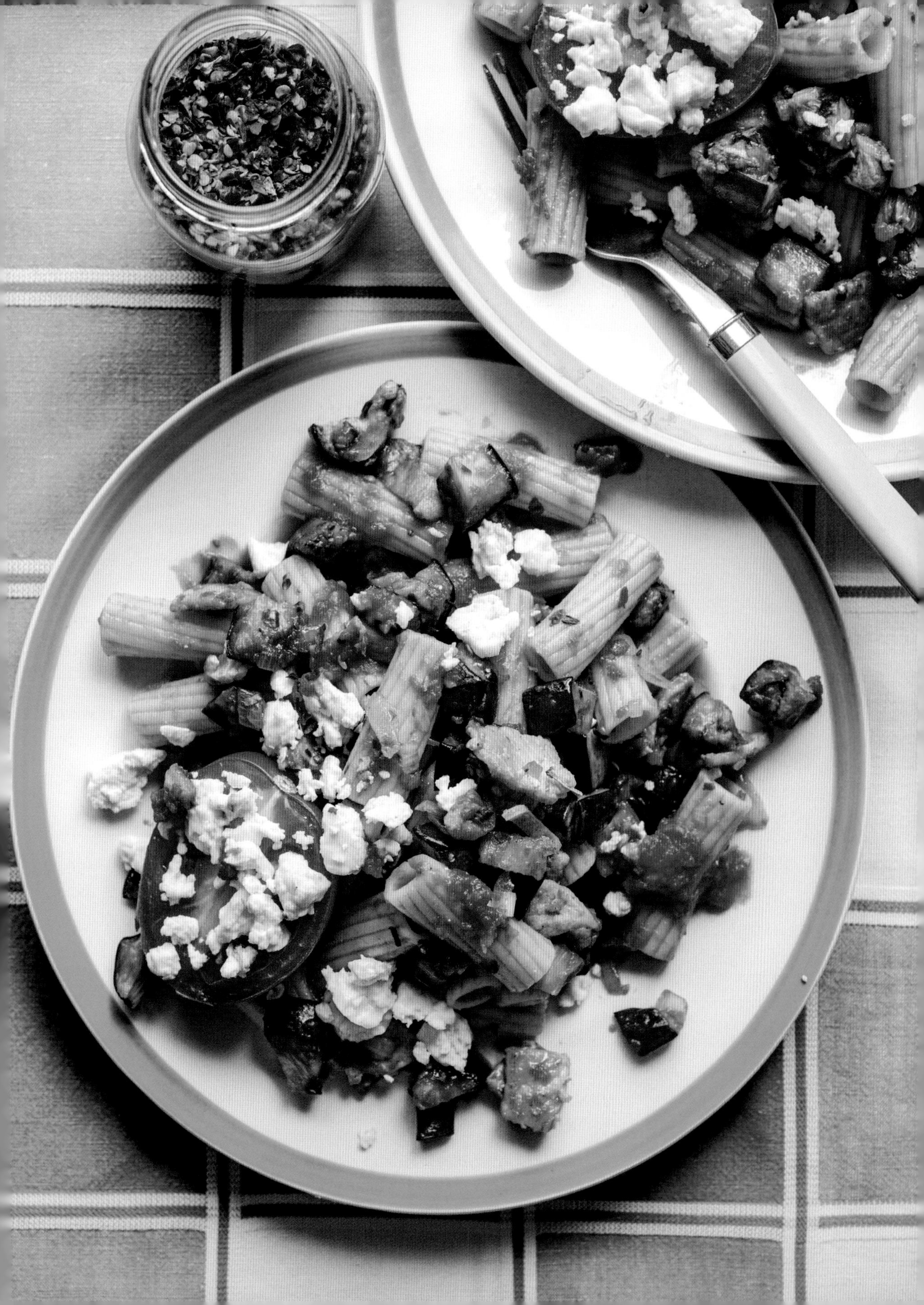

SERVES: 4
PREP: 5 MINS
COOK: 15 MINS
CALORIES: 304

QUICK CREAMY MUSHROOM MACARONI

The key to this recipe is making those mushrooms as small as possible so they tire of sitting in your lunch and decide to head inside the macaroni to get some sleep. That's just science, folks, and you can't argue with it. This is a late addition to the book: we often used to make a version of it in the slimming club days, but as you can imagine, it was Quark that was used, with a matchbox-size block of cheese grated on top. We've learned so much since then, and this vastly improved yet wonderfully simple recipe is the result of that. The old take only came to light when it resurfaced on my Facebook Memories page, which I maintain is one of the most awful features to exist on social media. There's nothing quite like looking at your face over the years and tracking the ravages of time to really make you feel creaky. I tend to look the same: pulling a face like I'm solving a tricky crossword, though the beard length and eye-wrinkles change. I'm always especially aghast when the goatee years roll around: I look like David Brent fell on a tyre-inflator. Not a strong look. Seeing Paul in older photos is even more odd, because he genuinely doesn't look like how I see him now – losing ten stone will do that. Now I think he's beautiful no matter his shape, but seeing him always at the edge of photos or hiding, or that pained look he does when he's uncomfortable, makes me so sad. The best thing about him finally getting his weight under control is seeing his genuinely gorgeous smile in photos again. Aw. That was quite sweet, wasn't it? I promise to do better.

- 220g (8oz) macaroni (see notes)
- 1 brown onion, finely diced
- 3 cloves of garlic, crushed
- 240g (8½oz) mushrooms, diced
- 125g (4oz) reduced-fat soft cheese
- 125ml (4fl oz) semi-skimmed milk
- 30g (1oz) Parmesan cheese (or vegetarian alternative), grated

Cook the pasta according to the instructions on the packet, then drain and set aside.

Spray a large pan with a little oil and place over a medium heat. Add the onion and garlic and cook for about 5 minutes, until softened.

Add the mushrooms and cook until tender and browned, about 10 minutes.

Reduce the heat to low, add the soft cheese, milk and Parmesan, and stir until well mixed.

Add the pasta to the sauce, stir until it's well coated, and serve.

Notes: We tend to use macaroni for this, but any pasta will do!

Mind, the goatee era wasn't the worst: we've also had 90s blonde-tipped me, Abba haircut me, Emo McGee me, red-haired me . . . at least Paul is consistent!

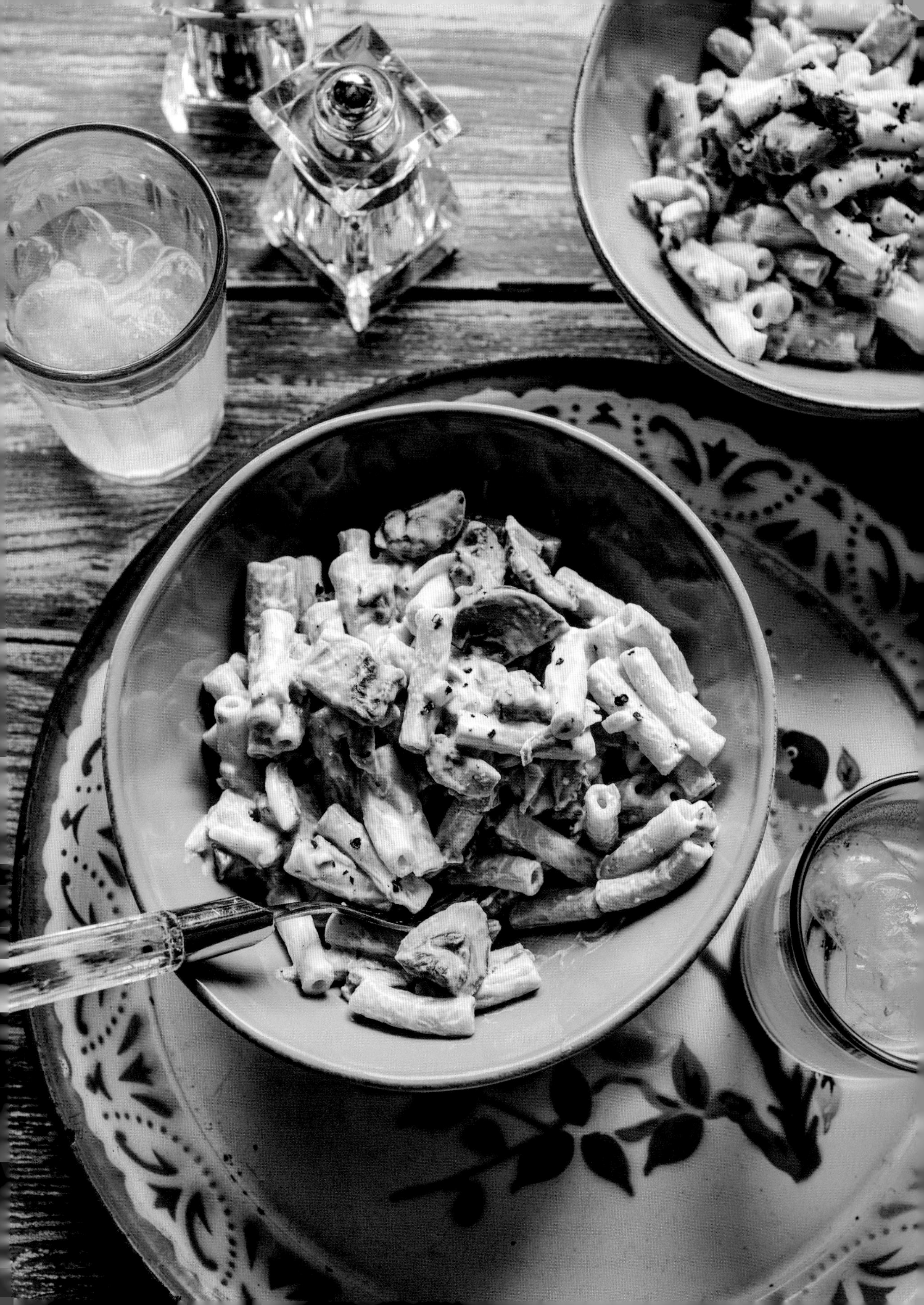

SERVES: 4
PREP: 10 MINS
COOK: 25 MINS
CALORIES: 499

- 1 onion, chopped
- 2 cloves of garlic, crushed
- 1 teaspoon dried oregano
- 150g (5½oz) mushrooms, sliced
- 2 × 400g (14oz) tins of chopped tomatoes
- 1 vegetable stock cube
- 1 teaspoon Worcestershire sauce (or vegetarian alternative)
- 14 dried lasagne sheets, broken into shards
- 500g (1lb 2oz) bag of frozen chargrilled vegetables, defrosted
- 2 tablespoons vegetarian green pesto
- 125g (4½oz) ricotta
- 15g (½oz) Parmesan cheese (or vegetarian alternative), grated

VEGGIE CHEAT'S LASAGNE WITH CREAMY RICOTTA TOPPING

This veggie lasagne is so good, you won't miss meat. Well, no, if you're like me and pull out a packet of bacon to blow your nose on and keep a cooked sausage behind your ear to suck on in times of concentration, it won't be quite as revelatory: but it's bloody good. It's certainly a lot tastier than the lasagne Paul and I had during our Murder Mystery dinner earlier in the year. In a fit of whimsy we had booked a dinner show: you watch Act 1 of the corniest production you'll ever see (so hammy I'm worried our publishers might rescind the veggie symbol on this recipe just for mentioning it), stop for dinner and discussion, then spend Act 2 gasping and oohing as the murderer is revealed. Imagine your school production doing an episode of *Vera* and you're mostly there. I do the whole thing a massive disservice here by being sarcastic – it was actually great fun, not least because the drama was ramped up considerably by being sat at a table with a very 'traditional' couple, the husband of which looked as though he'd part my hair with a shotgun as soon as look at me. That certainly focuses the mind, I can assure you. You, however, should focus exclusively on making this delicious lasagne, and we shall say no more.

Heat a large, shallow, ovenproof casserole dish and spray with a little oil. Add the onion and fry for 3 minutes, until starting to soften, then add the garlic, oregano and mushrooms and stir-fry for 5 minutes, until the mushrooms are cooked.

Tip in the tomatoes, crumble in the stock cube and add the Worcestershire sauce, then fill both tomato tins with hot water and carefully pour into the pan. Bring to a simmer, then drop the lasagne sheets into the pan and cook for 15 minutes, stirring every 5 minutes so the pasta doesn't stick together.

Preheat the grill to high.

Once the pasta is al dente, gently fold through the chargrilled vegetables and the pesto, cook for a few minutes to heat through, and season with plenty of salt and pepper.

Dollop over the ricotta and sprinkle over the Parmesan. Flash under the hot grill for 2–3 minutes, or until golden in places and piping hot.

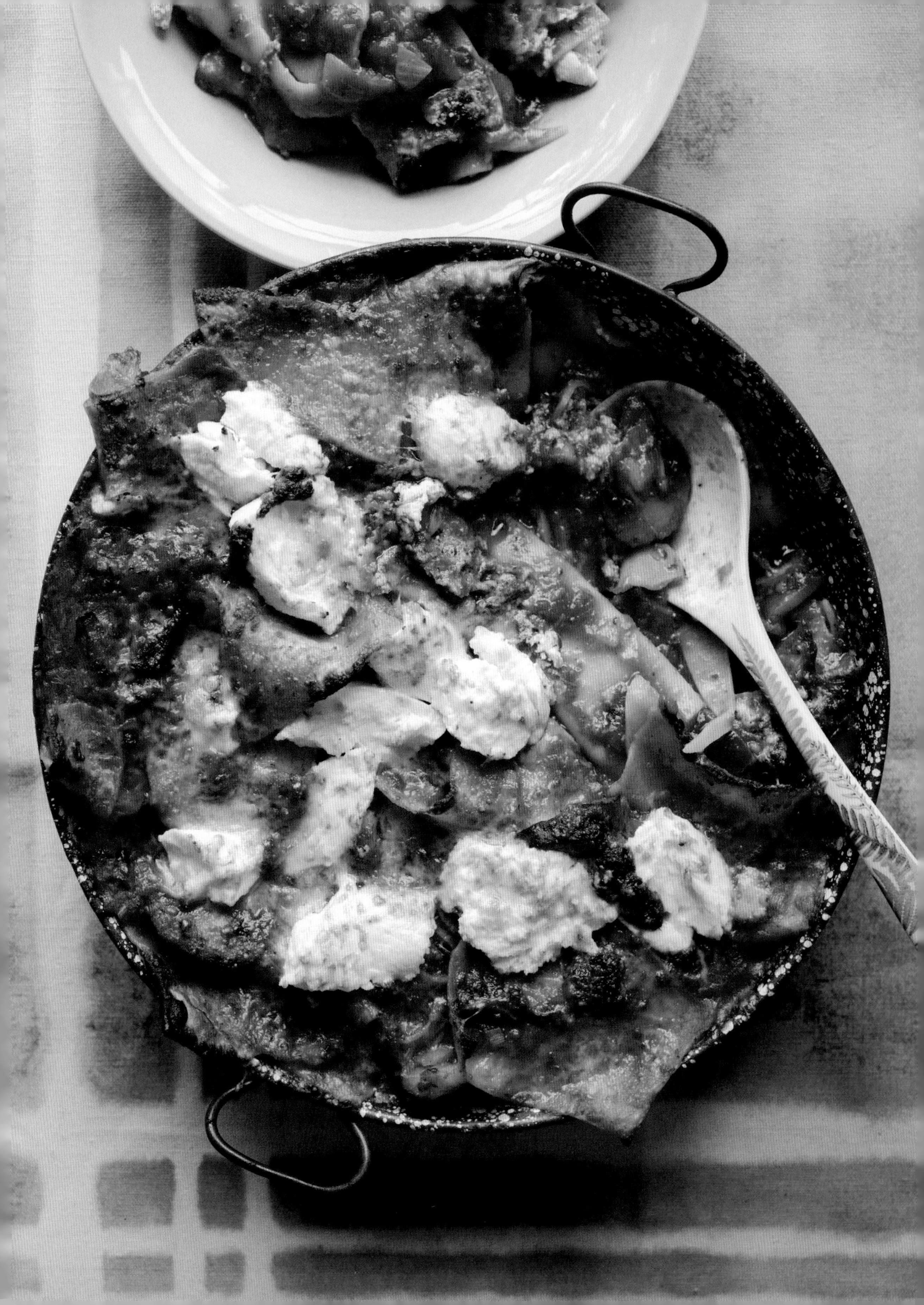

SERVES: 4
PREP: 10 MINS
COOK: 45 MINS
CALORIES: 458

30 mins · DF

180g (6oz) long-grain rice
500g (1lb 2oz) beef frying steaks
1 tablespoon cornflour
2 teaspoons rice wine vinegar
2 tablespoons soy sauce
1 tablespoon sesame oil
5cm (2 inch) piece of ginger, grated
4 cloves of garlic, crushed
1 brown onion, finely diced
1 carrot, peeled and very finely diced
2 eggs
2 spring onions, sliced
a handful of fresh coriander, finely chopped

BEEF CONGEE

Officially one of the meals that I (James) cook when I decide Paul needs a night off from toiling away in a hot kitchen (well, got to give him a chance to clean the bathroom), this tasty beef dish is one for the ages. For all that I endlessly tease him in these books, he truly does work ever so hard. I have the easy life: I sit at home and forget to type up recipes, whereas he goes out and actually grafts. On top of this, since losing his weight, he's taken up all manner of exciting exercises: running, HIIT classes and my personal favourite – becoming a member of the Newcastle Ravens, our regional gay rugby group. Although it does baffle me to think what attracted him to spending so much time around burly blokes in rugby kit, he absolutely adores it – and turns out he's bloody good at it, even if he does (by his own admission) run like an old man hastening to a toilet before he has an accident. It's been great to see, it really has: his confidence is so much higher now. You know, he's earned every gum-shielded mouthful of this congee.

Rinse the rice in cold water until it's almost clear, then drain and set aside.

Dice the beef into small cubes and toss with the cornflour. Add the rice wine vinegar, soy sauce, sesame oil, ginger, garlic and a pinch of salt and pepper and mix well, then leave to marinate for 15–20 minutes.

Bring a large pan of water to the boil and add the rice, onion and carrot, then reduce the heat to low, cover with a lid and simmer for 30 minutes, stirring occasionally.

Once the rice is looking a bit porridge-y, add the beef and cook for about 5 minutes, stirring now and again.

Meanwhile, bring another pan of water to the boil. Add the eggs and cook for 6 minutes, then remove from the pan, cool under running water, and peel.

Serve the congee in bowls, with half a boiled egg per person, and top with the spring onions and coriander.

Note: As you're a decent sort, you will of course be forgoing the coriander. Because nobody needs that soapy adornment in their life.

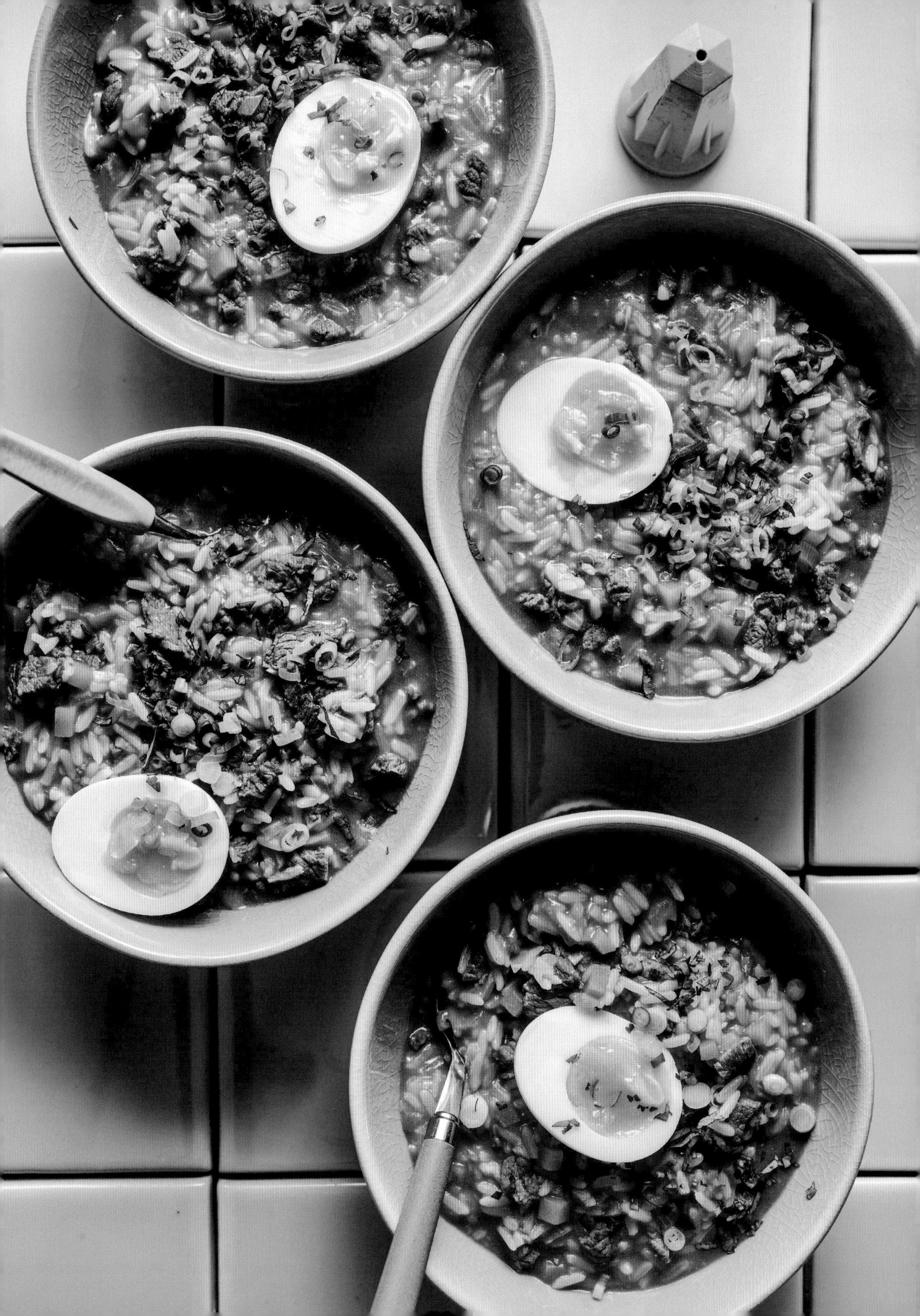

SERVES: 4
PREP: 10 MINS
COOK: 15 MINS
CALORIES: 487

BROCCOLI & BLUE CHEESE SPAGHETTI

Since we finally realised that you can't outrun a poor diet and did the sensible thing of combining exercise with healthy eating, we haven't been quite so susceptible to falling for crazy health kicks. Atkins was fun for a couple of weeks, until people stopped talking to us because our breath smelled like a corpse washed up from the sea. Intermittent fasting is all well and good until you realise you've got an afternoon ahead with a paucity of anything sustaining and all you can think about is a Kinder Bueno. No, calorie counting will do, thank you. That said, we're not averse to being sucked into other nonsense fads if we see a particularly clickbaity article online. My personal favourite from the last year has been Paul's adventure into 'contrast showers', namely a shower where you alternate between hot water and freezing water. Good for all sorts of things apparently, but I only learned of his endeavour on the morning he started his health-kick: there was so much alternate screaming and moaning coming from the shower that I could have reasonably assumed he had a gentleman in there with him. Alas no, unless you count Mr Matey, and we don't because he's a creep who looks at you weeing. This particular health burst lasted exactly one morning, and Paul has since gone back to showering like a normal person. I mention all the above simply to preface this recipe, which came from a period where we were experimenting with organic vegetable deliveries because 'health', and we had a surfeit of broccoli. Luckily, unlike Paul's Adventure through Temperature, it works.

- 300g (10½oz) spaghetti
- 1 head of broccoli, stem chopped, florets broken into bite-size pieces
- 2 cloves of garlic, unpeeled
- 1 tablespoon finely grated Parmesan cheese (or vegetarian alternative)
- 1 egg
- 120g (4oz) semi-soft blue cheese (we love Saint Agur)
- 25g (1oz) hazelnuts, toasted and crushed

Bring a large pan of salted water to the boil, then add the spaghetti, broccoli stalks and garlic cloves and cook for 5 minutes. Add the florets and continue cooking for 5 minutes more. Drain, reserving a ladle of the pasta cooking water, remove the garlic, then tip the pasta and broccoli back into the pan.

Working quickly, push the garlic out of its papery skins into a bowl, add the Parmesan, egg and two-thirds of the blue cheese, season with salt and pepper, then mash everything together until well combined. Add 100ml (3½fl oz) of the reserved hot pasta cooking water. Pour this mixture over the spaghetti and stir until the sauce is clinging to the hot pasta. Add a splash more of the pasta water if it looks too thick.

Divide the spaghetti between bowls, sprinkle over the rest of the blue cheese and the crushed toasted hazelnuts, and serve immediately.

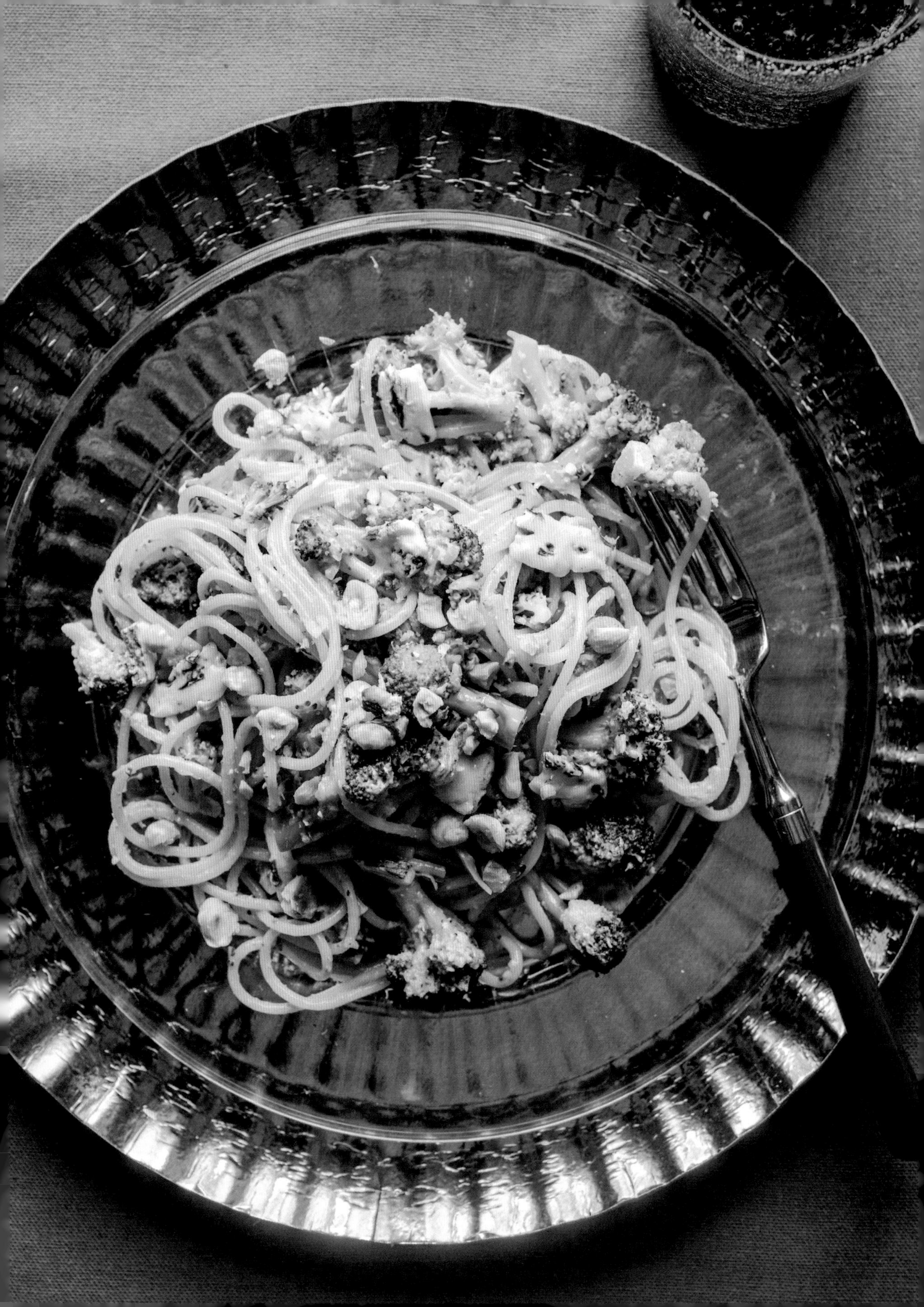

CHICKPEACCATA

SERVES: 4
PREP: 5 MINS
COOK: 40 MINS
CALORIES: 496

Now, as the title of this recipe sounds a shade like 'Chiquitita', I'm naturally going to take the next paragraph to entirely ignore the recipe and implore you to go along and see *ABBA Voyage*. Paul and I were lucky enough – after a year of procrastinating and rearranging – to finally get to see it earlier in the year. It was incredible: it takes a minute or two for your brain to forget they're not actually there in front of you, then it is a solid ninety minutes of pure ABBA goodness. Plus I'm not going to lie, having a 100ft avatar of 70s-era Benny Andersson to look at was a *delight*. Forgive my mushiness for a moment: you know what made it such a great evening? In all our sixteen years together, I don't think Paul and I have ever danced together. Both very self-conscious with good reason – we both have the co-ordinated movement of a large coach careering off an icy mountain road – but all that buggered off for the evening and we were dancing and singing with the rest of the crowd. It was glorious. There's a lot to be said for that – unexpected little moments of delight together. Speaking of surprising moments, do try this recipe. It suffers not a jot for being so stridently vegetarian.

- 2 × 400g (14oz) tins of chickpeas, drained
- 300g (10½oz) pasta
- 1 brown onion, finely diced
- 2 tablespoons capers
- 25g (1oz) butter
- 180ml (6fl oz) vegetable stock
- juice of 1 lemon
- a handful of fresh parsley, finely chopped
- ¼ teaspoon dried chilli flakes

Preheat the oven to 220°C fan/475°F/gas mark 9.

Spread the chickpeas on a lined baking tray and spray with a little oil. Sprinkle over some salt and pepper, toss, and cook in the oven for 25–30 minutes, turning once.

Meanwhile, bring a large pan of salted water to the boil. Add the pasta and cook according to the instructions on the packet, then drain and set aside.

Spray a large pan with a little oil and place over a medium heat. Add the onion and cook for 5–6 minutes, then add the capers and cook for a further minute.

Add the butter and allow to melt, then add the vegetable stock and bring to the boil. Reduce the heat and simmer for 10 minutes, until reduced by about half.

Stir in the lemon juice and add the chickpeas, then toss and cook for a further 3–4 minutes.

Add the parsley to the pan, stir in the pasta, sprinkle over the chilli flakes, and serve.

Notes: No notes for the recipe folks, it's a simple one, so it's left to me to tell you our favourite ABBA songs so you can message Paul and tell him how wrong he is. Mine is 'Lay All Your Love on Me', his is 'Summer Night City'. Pfft, hipster.

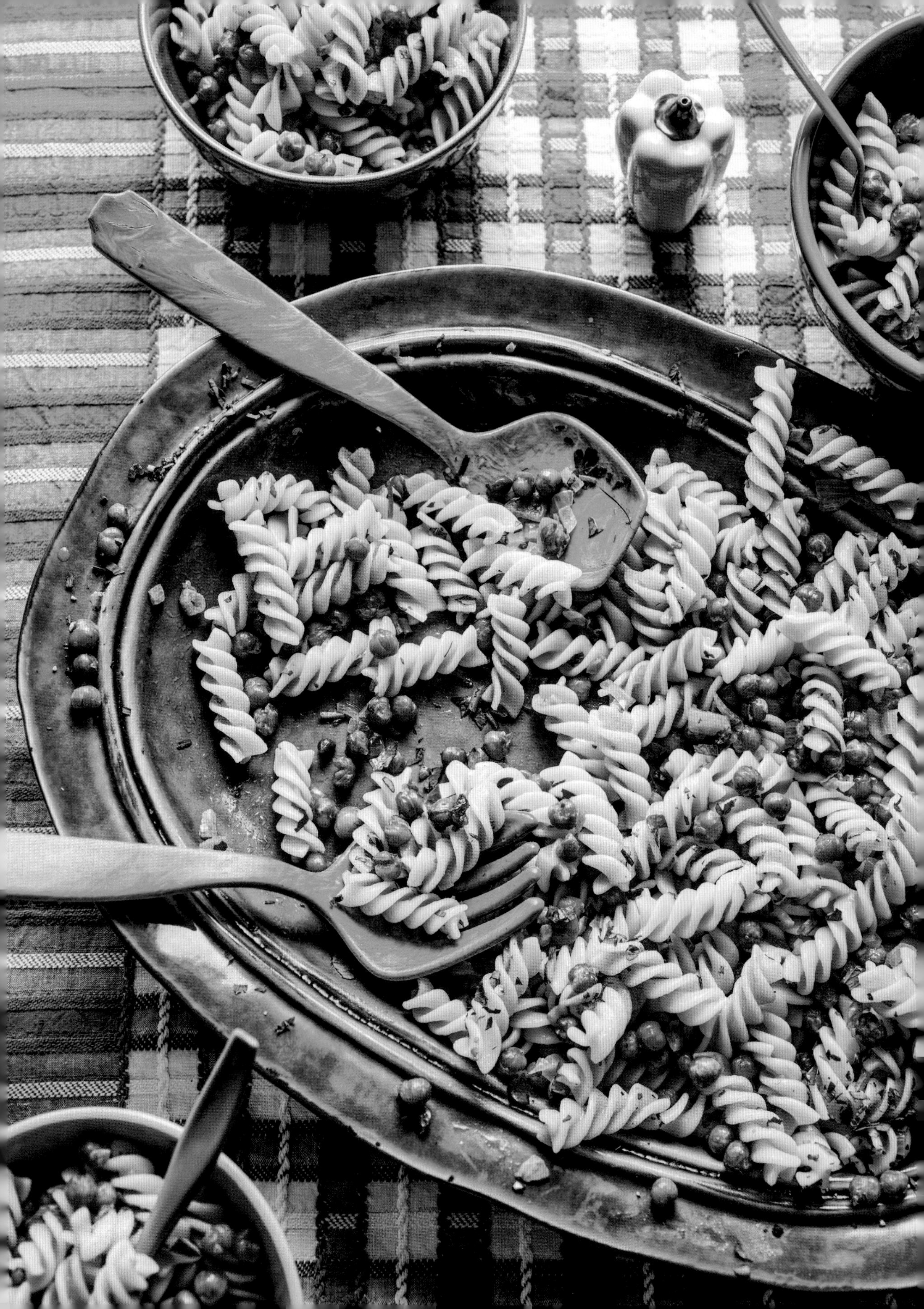

SERVES: 4
PREP: 15 MINS
COOK: 20 MINS
CALORIES: 342

30 mins, V, GF, DF

- 1 bunch of spring onions, green and white parts separated and chopped
- 2 peppers (red and yellow), chopped
- 4 cloves of garlic, chopped
- 1 teaspoon dried thyme
- 2 teaspoons smoked paprika
- 1 vegetable stock cube
- 2 tablespoons tomato purée
- a big pinch of saffron
- 200g (7oz) long-grain rice
- 100g (3½oz) cherry tomatoes, halved
- 100g (3½oz) frozen peas, defrosted
- ½ × 400g (14oz) tin of cannellini beans, drained
- a handful of fresh parsley, roughly chopped
- ½ lemon, cut into wedges

For the smoky aïoli

- 4 tablespoons extra low-fat mayonnaise
- 1 clove of garlic, crushed
- 1 teaspoon smoked paprika
- juice of ½ lemon

SPANISH-STYLE RICE WITH SMOKY AÏOLI

Now as this recipe does pivot a little into the 'list as long as my arm' territory, we'll keep the intro as short and sweet as a little onion. That didn't quite work, but I'm exhausted from making sure I get the spelling of aïoli correct. Just the quickest of tips: one that's a constant throughout our books. Spring onions, as long as you keep about an inch of root, can be grown again by simply putting the root into water. Give it a week or so in sunlight and new greenery will form. The other tip? Don't fret if you aren't King Croesus and don't have access to saffron. It is an expensive addition and although it does add to the dish, please don't buy it especially. A pinch of turmeric will do the job just as well.

First, make the smoky aïoli. Mix together the mayonnaise, crushed garlic, smoked paprika and the lemon juice, season, cover and chill until ready to use.

Spray a large frying pan with a little oil, set over a medium heat and fry the spring onions, reserving a bit of the green part for later. Fry for 5 minutes, or until starting to soften. Tip in the peppers, garlic, thyme and smoked paprika and continue to fry for 5 minutes, stirring often.

Crumble the stock cube into a jug, add the tomato purée, then crush the saffron with your fingers and drop it into the jug. Pour in 700ml (1¼ pints) of boiling water and stir to combine.

Add the rice to the frying pan and stir to coat in the spices, then add the hot stock mixture. Drop the tomatoes on top, cover, and cook for 10 minutes, or until the rice is tender. Remove the lid, and fold in the peas, cannellini beans and parsley. Leave to stand for 5 minutes.

Sprinkle the spring onion greens over the top and serve the rice with a dollop of smoky aïoli.

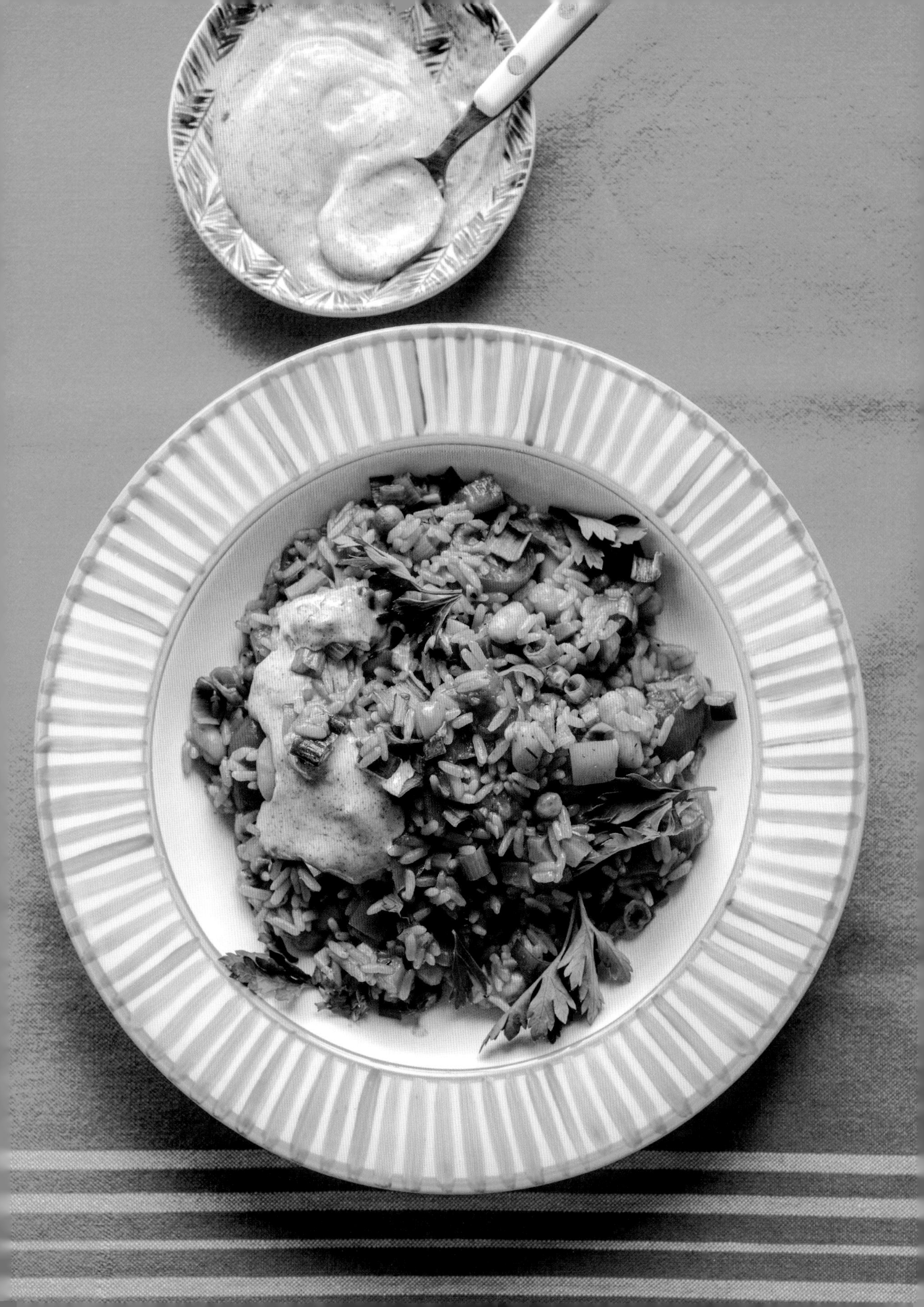

SERVES: 4
PREP: 10 MINS
COOK: 20 MINS
CALORIES: 486

PIZZA PASTA ALL-IN-ONE

Pizza pasta seems like such an obvious combination to us that it's surprising we have never thought to throw them together. Still, there was a wise Doctor Who said, '*Whole worlds pivot on acts of imagination,*' and she was never wrong, so here we find ourselves. Now please, before we get any angry correspondence, you are free to put whatever you like into this recipe: we've included the ingredients below because we know it is a combination we both enjoy. If you want to put pineapple in there, leave out the mushrooms, change up the cheese . . . go for it. The best recipes are those you make your own, and if this isn't the best template to base that on, then whatever is? For the record, the weirdest ingredient we've tried on a pizza was kimchi – and it really, REALLY worked. Perhaps not here though.

- 3 cloves of garlic, crushed
- ½ teaspoon dried chilli flakes
- 3 tablespoons tomato purée
- 300g (10½oz) penne or short pasta of your choice
- 700ml (1¼ pints) passata with herbs
- 150g (5½oz) mushrooms, sliced
- 1 × 150g (5½oz) ball of low-fat mozzarella, drained, patted dry and torn
- 50g (1¾oz) spicy chorizo slices
- 2 roasted peppers from a jar, drained and sliced
- a handful of black olives
- fresh basil leaves

Heat a large, shallow frying pan over a medium heat. Spray with a little oil, then add the garlic and cook for 1 minute. Add the chilli flakes, tomato purée and pasta.

Stir in the passata, then swill out the empty bottle with 300ml (10fl oz) of hot water from the tap, and add to the pan. Bring to the boil and cook, stirring frequently, for 15 minutes.

Meanwhile, spray another frying pan with oil and fry the mushrooms until cooked and golden. Remove from the heat and set aside.

Preheat the grill to high.

Level out the top of the pasta. Scatter over the mushrooms, mozzarella, chorizo slices, roasted peppers and olives, then flash under the hot grill for 1–2 minutes, or until the cheese has melted. Serve cut into wedges and garnished with basil leaves.

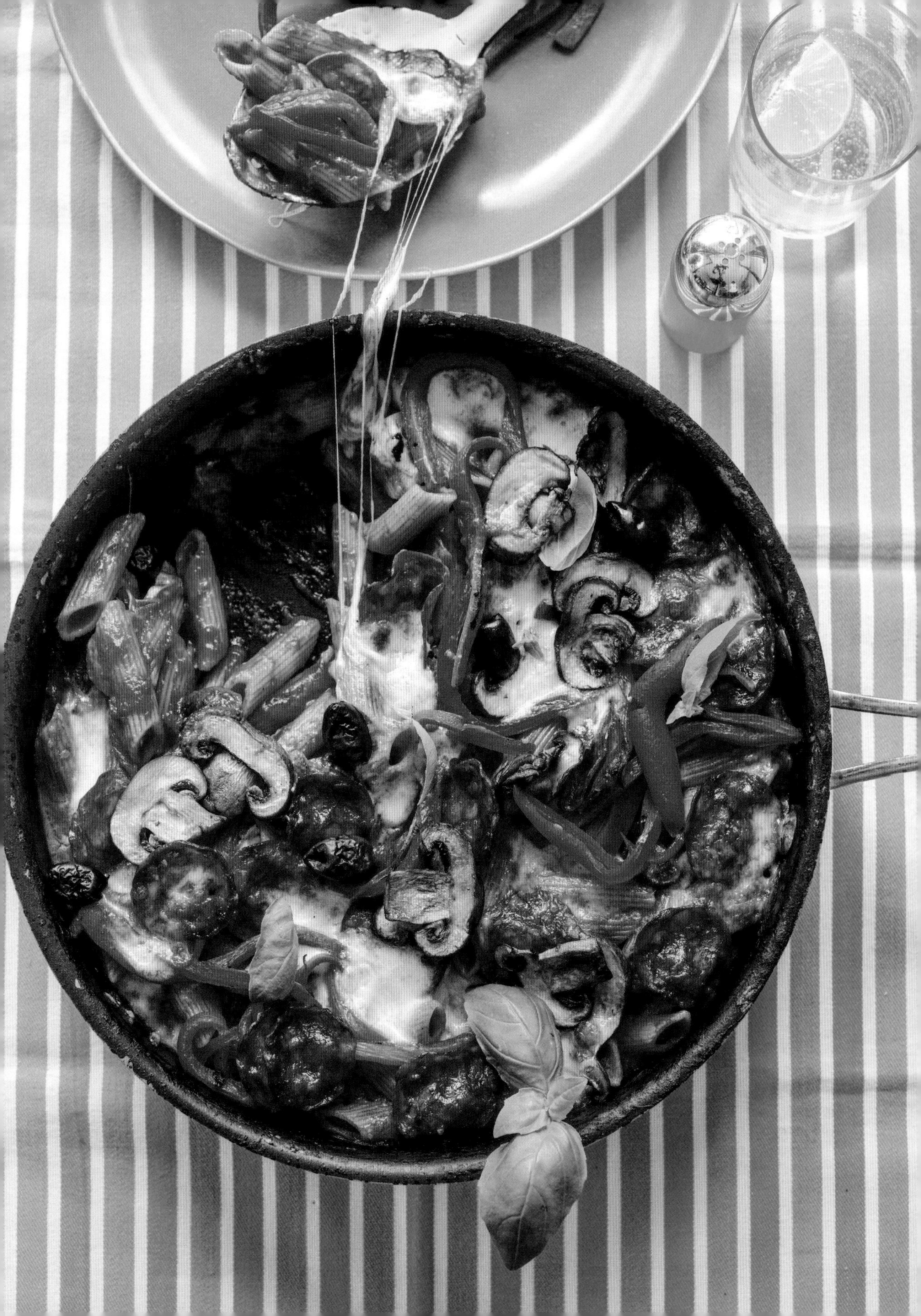

SP
SPL

EDY &

ENDID

SERVES: 4
PREP: 10 MINS
COOK: 5 MINS
CALORIES: 478

30 mins · 10 · GF

- 150g (5½oz) tortilla chips
- 80g (2¾oz) reduced-fat Cheddar cheese, grated
- 500g (1lb 2oz) tuna steaks
- 1 lime
- 15g (½oz) fresh coriander, chopped
- ½ red onion, chopped
- 1 tomato, chopped
- 1 green chilli, sliced
- 1 avocado
- 50g (1¾oz) fat-free Greek yoghurt

TUNA NACHOS

To tell you I love this recipe is to sell the dish massively short: of all the amazing dishes in the book, this is easily my favourite. And mind, it's a fish recipe – and raw fish at that! Wonders will never cease. We actually ordered this accidentally at a restaurant in Universal Studios – we were taking a break to let our ankles steam and had barely a moment to check the menu before a walking smile came over and demanded, in that wonderful well-howdy-do style of waiting staff in the US, that we picked a dish. I panicked and ordered the first thing I saw, which turned out to be this but with a far fancier name, and when it was plonked on the table we both did the British thing of grimacing inside but saying how delightful it looked. Turned out to be one of the best things we put in our mouths that holiday, and that's high praise indeed when you consider we had a gelato station in our hotel that was open 24 hours a day. Honestly, if you're hesitant, trust us – oh, and check the notes.

Preheat the oven to 170°C fan/375°F/gas mark 5.

Spread the tortilla chips on a baking sheet and sprinkle over the grated cheese. Bake in the oven for 5–6 minutes, until the cheese has melted.

Dice the tuna into small cubes and tip into a bowl. Add the juice of the lime, the coriander, red onion, tomato and green chilli and gently combine.

Remove the tortilla chips from the oven and put them on a serving plate. Top with the tuna mixture.

Slice the avocado and remove the stone, then gently spoon out the flesh, dice and sprinkle over the nachos. Drizzle over the yoghurt and serve.

Notes: You don't need to bake the tortilla chips in the oven with the cheese, but we like the ooey-gooeyness of it all. You could just as well scatter the cheese on and stay entirely away from the oven if you so desire.

Add some wasabi mixed with mayonnaise (you can buy the pre-mixed stuff now) for a bit more spice.

Tuna steaks from the supermarket are generally safe to eat raw, but always check the label. Good dark flesh and as fresh as you possibly can. Even better would be those from a decent fishmonger, if you're lucky enough to have one nearby.

If you're really unsure and don't want to spend the money on tuna steaks, try it with good-quality tinned tuna, drained and flaked.

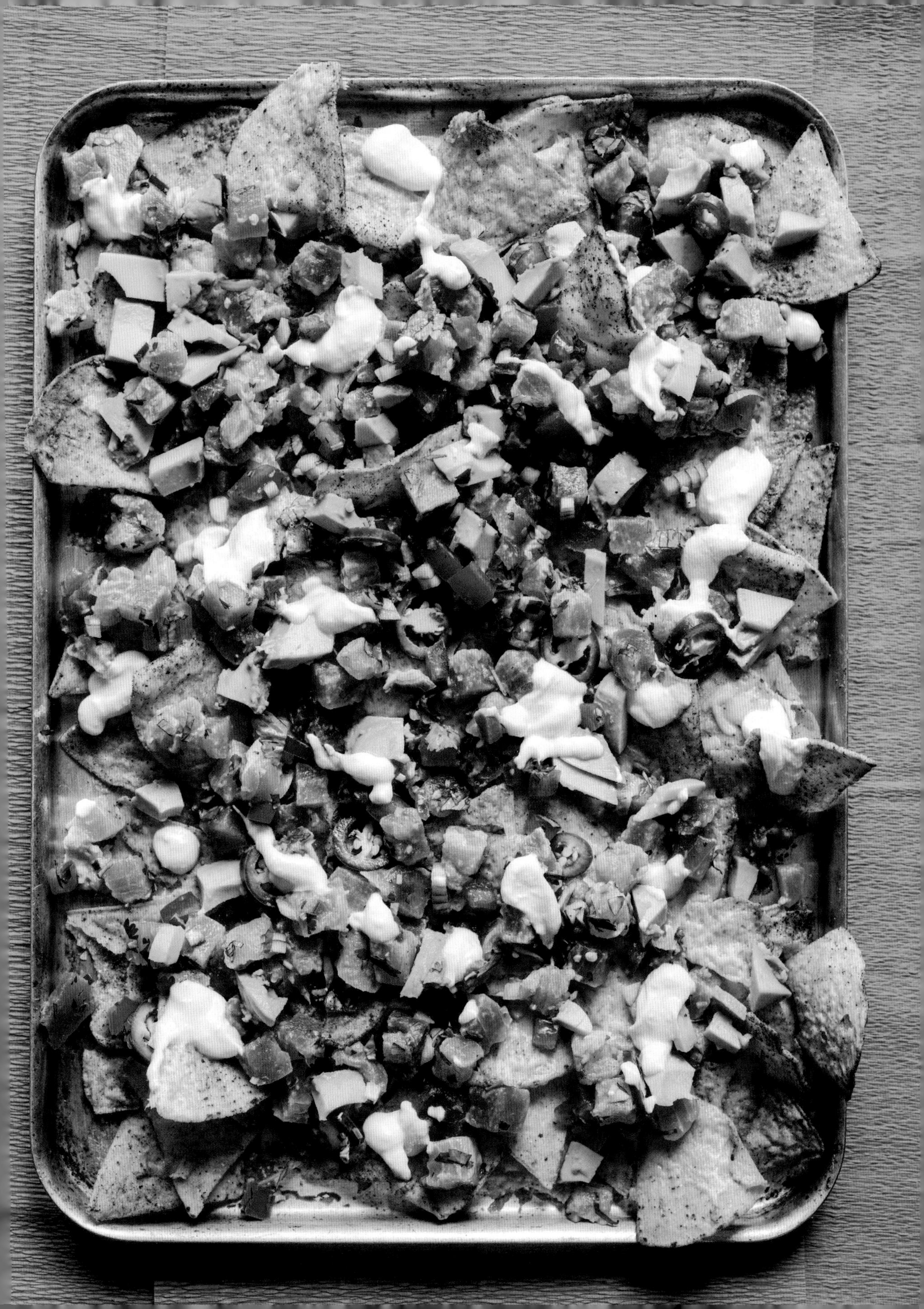

SERVES: 4
PREP: 10 MINS
COOK: 20 MINS
CALORIES: 452

30 mins · DF

- 350g (12oz) diced beef
- 2 cloves of garlic, crushed
- 1 brown onion, chopped
- 1 tablespoon dark soy sauce
- 3 tablespoons hoisin sauce
- 3 tablespoons fish sauce
- 1 tablespoon sriracha
- 1 tablespoon honey
- ½ teaspoon dried chilli flakes
- 300ml (10fl oz) beef stock
- 250g (9oz) dried flat rice noodles
- 200g (7oz) beansprouts
- 3 spring onions, sliced

SPICY BEEF PAD THAI

This is what we call at Chubby Towers an 'emergency' meal. That emergency is usually me driving home after the gym and deciding on a whim that I can't possibly have chips and must have meat, otherwise all the hard work I do gawping at folks and disinterestedly lifting weights will be undone. Luckily, we always have diced beef in the freezer, noodles in the cupboard and a song in Paul's heart, so this is a dish that can be thrown together before I get home. If I'm not calling Paul to politely request Pad Thai, it'll be for two other reasons: to gravely inform him that I'm dying (this happens at least three times a month) or to ask the name of a song he always plays, and which I promptly forget until it starts to rain. 'Rhythm of the Rain' by The Cascades, since you're wondering, but if you forget don't worry: I'll call Paul. We're calling it spicy, but it won't trouble your tum at this level, though you can absolutely leave the chillies out if you like.

Boil half a kettle of water.

Spray a large pan or wok with a little oil and place over a medium-high heat. Add the beef and cook until browned all over, about 5–7 minutes, stirring frequently, then remove from the pan to a plate and keep warm.

Add the garlic and onion to the pan and cook for 30 seconds, stirring continuously. Add the soy sauce, hoisin sauce, fish sauce, sriracha, honey and chilli flakes and stir well.

Add the stock and bring to a simmer, then add the noodles, stirring gently to help them separate out a bit, topping up with more water as needed.

Put the beef back into the pan, along with the beansprouts, and mix well.

Serve on plates and top with the sliced spring onions.

Notes: We like to use beef, but really any meat will do! The fancier among you might even like to combine meats, but let's not get ahead of ourselves.

No honey? Sugar is fine!

Add as much or as little stock to this as you like, it's just as nice 'saucy' as it is 'soupy'.

At this point in the story, do we really need to reassure you about fish sauce? Well, just in case: when you open it, it will smell like something in the room died. And not recently. But cook with it and the stink will burn off, leaving behind a lovely flavour. Peg your nose if you have to.

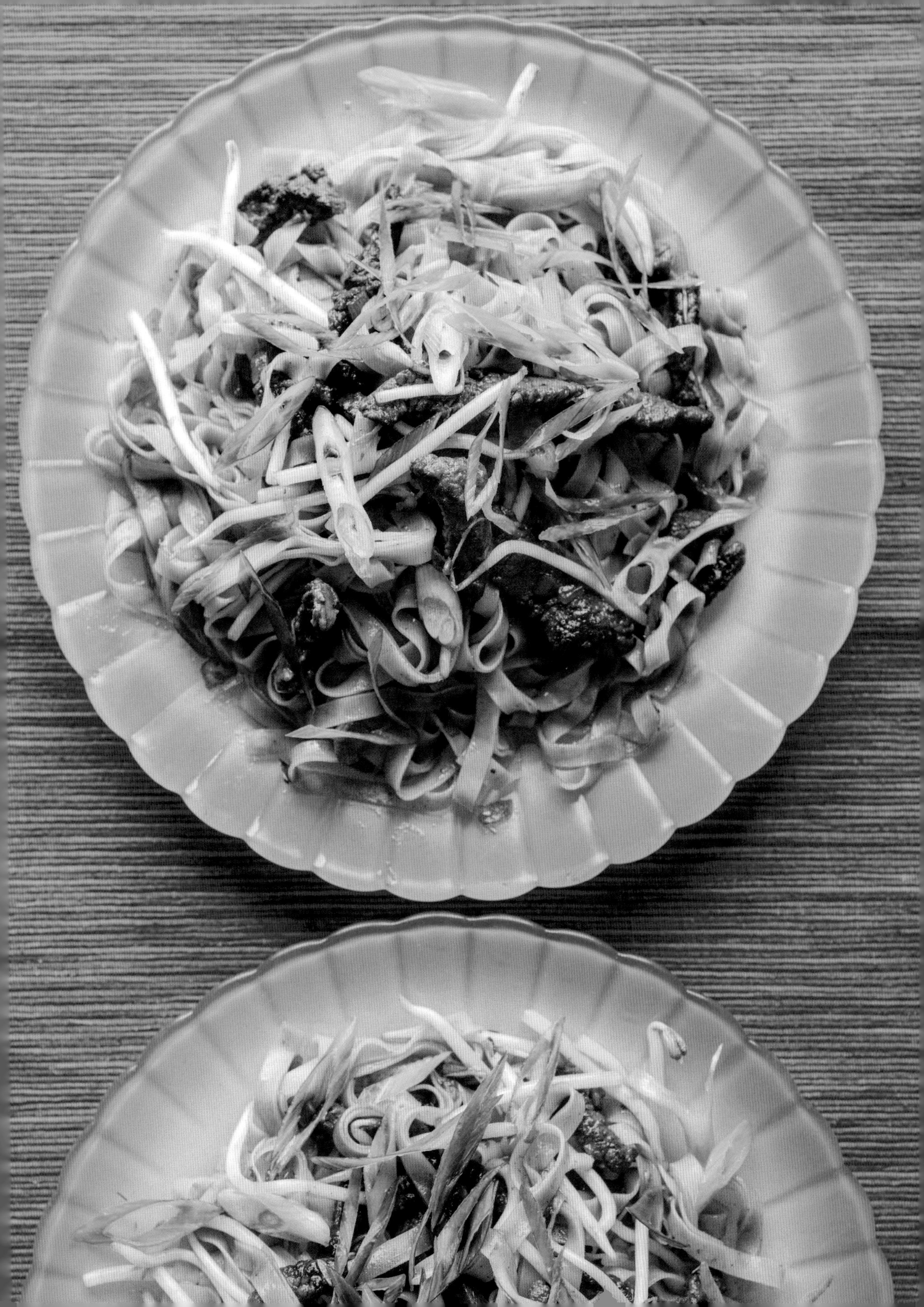

SERVES: 4
PREP: 10 MINS
COOK: 20 MINS
CALORIES: 296

30 mins · Freezer · Family · GF · DF

- 500g (1lb 2oz) pork mince
- 1 brown onion, chopped
- 1 celery stalk, chopped
- ½ green pepper, chopped
- 3 cloves of garlic, crushed
- 1 litre (1¾ pints) beef stock
- 2 tablespoons tomato purée
- 1 teaspoon dried rosemary
- 350g (12oz) frozen cauliflower
- 1 teaspoon salt
- ½ teaspoon black pepper

FREEZER-FIND STEW

Growing up, my dad wasn't much of a cook – he was brilliant in all other ways, don't get me wrong. He certainly doesn't get enough credit for dealing with all my teenage weltschmerz: I was very much your atypical angsty emo for a good couple of years – all long black hair and Sartre novels in lieu of a personality and getting my end away. I cringe when I look back, not least for the sheer amount of cosmic blue hair-dye I ruined my mother's towels with. With the above in mind, he might not seem like a good well to visit for recipe inspiration, but rather like my mother's hotdog recipe in the last book, there was the occasional banger to be brought out when mum was 'resting her head'. This stew, with the less traditional addition of pork mince, is one of those such beauties – but don't be beholden to the pork mince if you would prefer beef. Frozen cauliflower isn't necessary either – feel free to swap it out for fresh – but this is very much a meal of freezer bits. Heck, we would normally use frozen chopped onion for completeness, but times are tight, so here we are.

Spray a large pan with a little oil and place over a medium-high heat. Add the pork mince and cook for 5–6 minutes, until browned, then set aside.

Add the onion, celery, green pepper and garlic and cook for 3–4 minutes, until softened, then add the stock, tomato purée and rosemary and bring to a simmer.

Put the pork mince back into the pan, add the cauliflower, salt and pepper, and simmer for 10 minutes.

Notes: A tin of those little new potatoes in water will add more bulk to this meal, though make sure you rinse all the 'tin' water off. It smells so unpleasant.

If you want to really replicate my teenage years, you'll eat this in your bedroom listening to Placebo and InMe and switching your MSN Explorer status between Appear Offline and Online.

'Crushed Like Fruit' by InMe is still, of course, a certified banger.

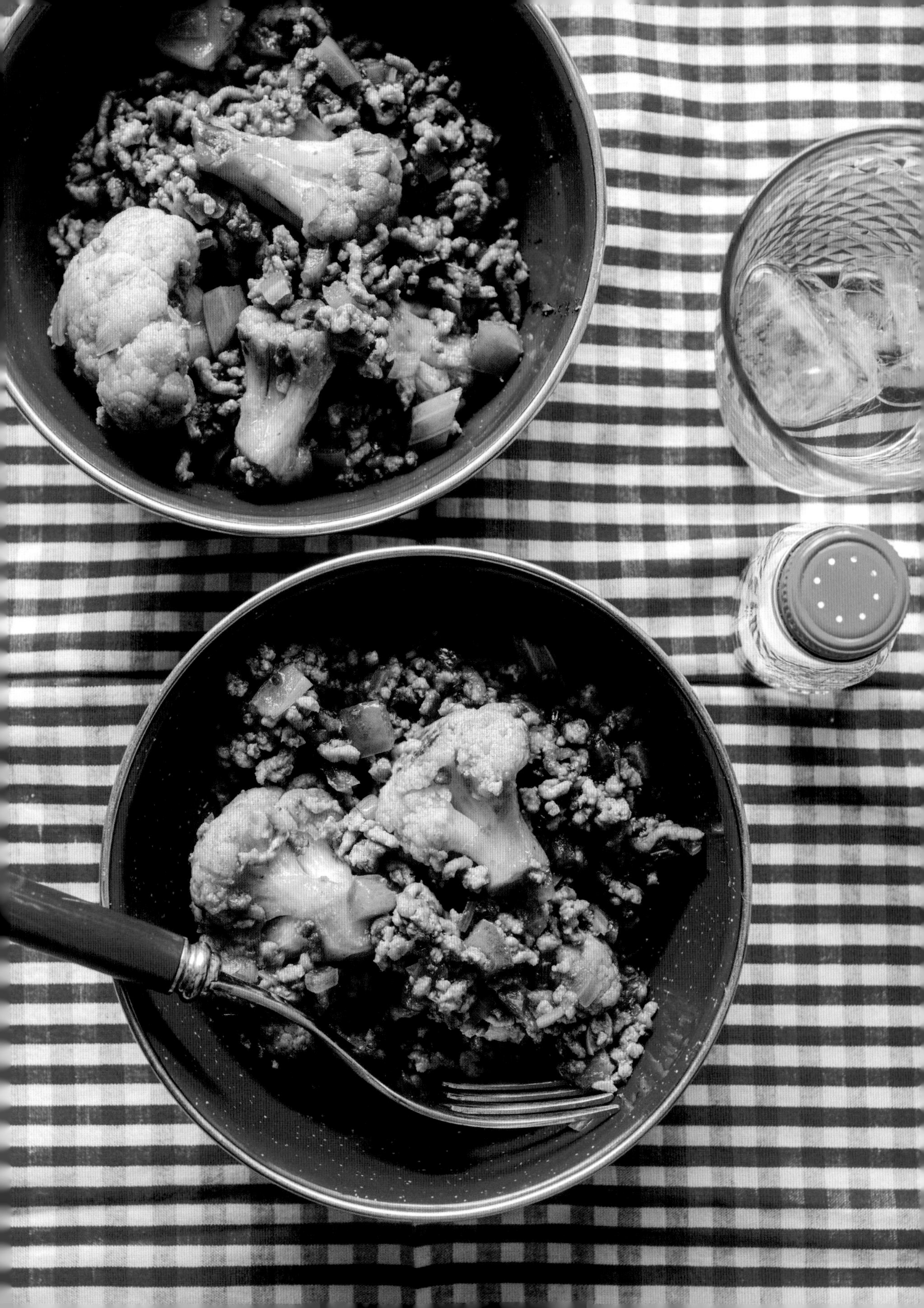

SERVES: 4
PREP: 10 MINS
COOK: 30 MINS
CALORIES: 486

CRUNCHY COWBOY CAVIAR BOWLS

There's truly nothing sexier to find in a recipe than the words 'pickling juice', now is there? It sounds a bit like an olde-worlde affliction you'd expect a spinster to catch a case of. Regardless, it simply means the brine from your jar of jalapeños, so please, calm down. We shan't keep you long up here because the recipe below demands your full attention: it's one of our absolute favourite dinners for piling ourselves in front of the TV with. The caviar in the title is an absolute misdirect too – there's nowt posh about this, and we very much doubt it's being served at fancy dinner parties before they bring out the cocaine and triple-stuffed-bird. Steady, steady, I'll do the jokes . . .

4 medium flour tortillas
6 tablespoons fat-free Greek yoghurt
1 small clove of garlic, crushed
1 avocado, halved, stone removed and sliced
50g (1¾oz) Cheddar cheese, grated
chilli sauce, to serve (optional)

For the cowboy caviar
2 × 400g (14oz) tins of black beans, drained
1 × 195g (7oz) tin of sweetcorn, drained
1 small red onion, finely chopped
1 red pepper, finely chopped
1 green pepper, finely chopped
2 tablespoons finely chopped jalapeño chillies, plus 2 tablespoons pickling juice

Preheat the oven to 200°C fan/425°F/gas mark 7.

Spray a couple of 18cm (7 inch) cake tins with spray oil. Put one tortilla into each tin, then cook in the oven for 15–20 minutes, or until crunchy. Repeat with the rest of the tortillas if you don't have enough tins to do this all at once.. You can do this in an air fryer in 5–8 minutes, if you have one. Set aside to cool.

Meanwhile, mix together the black beans, sweetcorn, red onion, red and green pepper, chopped jalapeños and the jalapeño pickling juice, with plenty of salt and pepper. Leave to stand.

Put the yoghurt into a bowl with the garlic and 2 tablespoons of water. Season with salt and pepper and mix until smooth.

Pile the black bean mixture into the crispy tortilla bowls, drizzle over the yoghurt sauce, top with sliced avocado and some grated cheese, and serve with chilli sauce if you like it spicy.

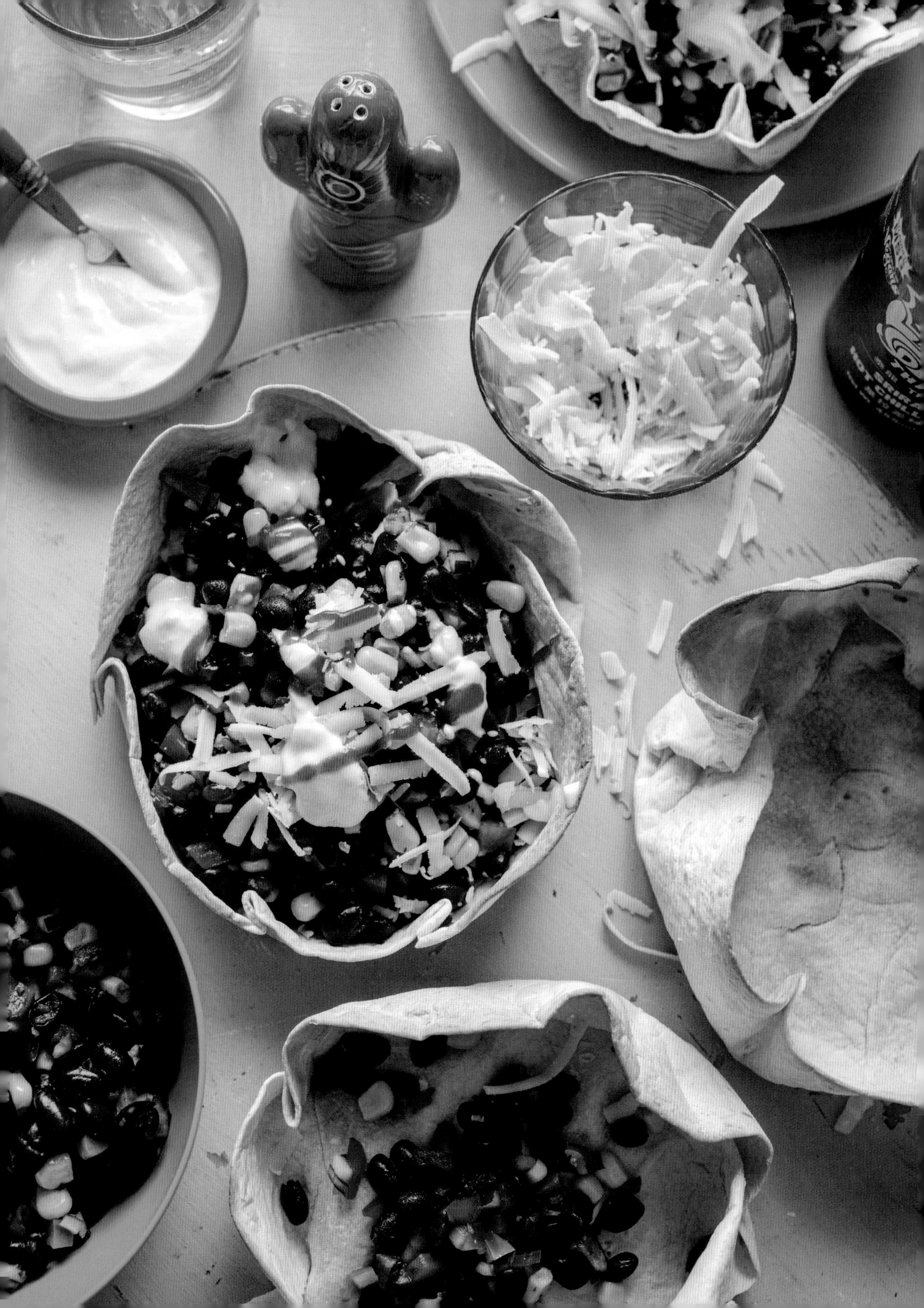

SERVES: 4
PREP: 15 MINS
COOK: 5 MINS
CALORIES: 275

SMOKY MUSHROOM TACOS

Here's a wonderful veggie dish in 'takeaway' form – tasty, smoky mushroom tacos. Nothing served stuffed into a shell can be a bad thing: unless it's a hermit crab, I guess, because it might bite your nose. Howdo – Paul here! James has insisted I do just one of these recipe intros, if only so I can understand what a terrible existence he has, bashing out 200 words every fifteen days while I go to work. It's little wonder he looks so haggard. I don't have a lot to say on mushrooms (not a single pun, ex*cept* that one), so I'll tell you two things about James that make me smile, as he has doubtless said something sweet elsewhere in the book in between jokes about my trousers. First, our nonsense communication: not a day will go by without one of us sending the other a video of a bin-lid closing with a scream or a lift door that looks shocked. We find hilarity in the mundanity. The second is his baffling belief in his singing ability: no matter the song, no matter the artists, and even when there's no lyrics to be found (he can't watch *The Chase* without caterwauling 'IT'S TIME FOR THE FINAL CHASE' as they walk down the stage), he'll be there, singing gaily away. It's like having a budgie you inherited from an endlessly drunk aunt. But boy, do we have fun.

- 8 large flat mushrooms, stalks removed
- 1 tablespoon butter
- 1 clove of garlic, crushed
- 2 tablespoons chipotle paste
- 4 tablespoons low-fat sour cream
- 4 tomatoes, chopped
- ½ red onion, finely chopped
- a handful of fresh coriander, finely chopped
- 1 lime: ½ juiced, ½ cut into wedges
- 8 small soft tacos

Heat a frying pan over a high heat. Once hot, spray the mushrooms with a little spray oil and cook for 3 minutes without disturbing them. Turn them over and continue to cook for 2 minutes, or until the mushrooms are juicy and soft. Turn off the heat.

Mix the butter, garlic and 1 tablespoon of the chipotle paste together and spread a little over the surface of each mushroom. Let it melt in the heat of the pan, turn the mushrooms in the butter, then slice the mushrooms like a steak.

Mix the remaining chipotle paste with the sour cream and set aside. Mix the tomatoes, onion and coriander with the lime juice and a pinch of salt.

Heat the tacos according to the instructions on the packet. Pile them with the sliced mushrooms and any resting juices, your tomato salsa, a dollop of smoky sour cream and a lime wedge for squeezing.

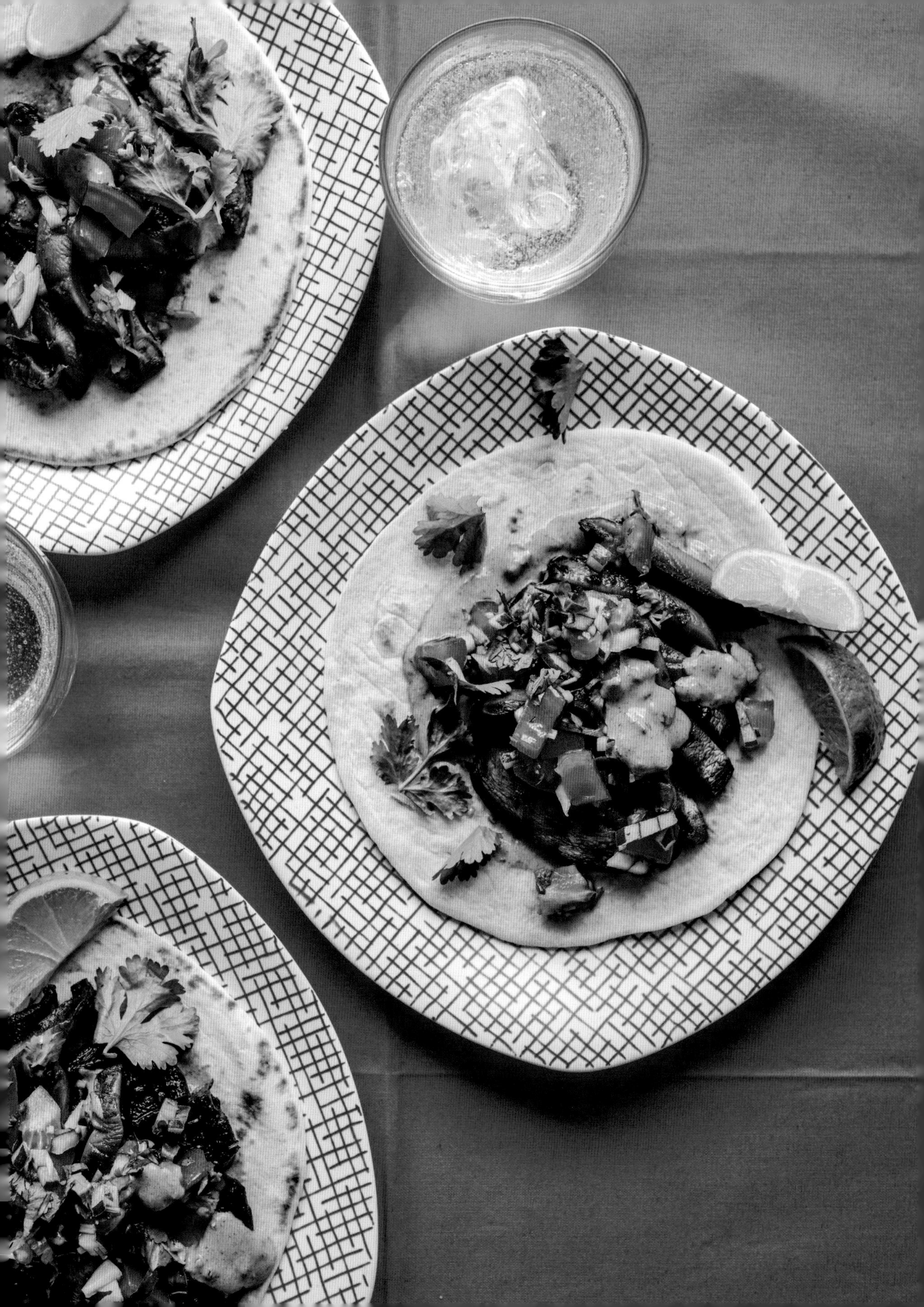

SERVES: 4
PREP: 10 MINS
COOK: 20 MINS
CALORIES: 492

30 mins | DF

DAN DAN NOODLES

I shall make you two promises here: this noodle dish is absolutely worth the effort with the ingredients (most of which you'll have in the house already), and I'll keep the recipe intro nice and short. I've just been reading a few reviews of our other books and there's an occasional mention of 'why is there always so much babble before the recipes'. It's a fair question, and here's why: it would be so unutterably boring to waffle on about the ripe tomatoes or the joyous blend of soy and sugar. We did try, promise, but I fell asleep about two sentences in. But let me take this opportunity to apologise to anyone who bought this book just for the recipes and has had to wade through all my treacle and nonsense. At least the food is delicious, and this recipe is a cracking example of that!

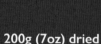

- 200g (7oz) dried egg noodles
- ½ teaspoon coriander seeds
- 400g (14oz) pork mince
- 4 cloves of garlic, crushed
- 4 spring onions, sliced
- 3 tablespoons sriracha
- 3 tablespoons soy sauce
- 2 tablespoons rice vinegar
- 1 tablespoon sugar
- ½ teaspoon black pepper
- 100ml (3½fl oz) chicken stock
- 40g (1½oz) dry roasted peanuts, roughly chopped
- 1 tablespoon sesame oil (optional)

Bring a large pan of water to the boil and cook the noodles for 3–5 minutes, until tender. Drain, rinse under cold water and set aside.

Spray a large pan with a little oil and place over a high heat. Add the coriander seeds and cook for 30 seconds, until fragrant. Add the pork mince and cook for 5–7 minutes, until browned, then remove from the pan and set aside.

Spray the pan with a little more oil, add the garlic and spring onions, and cook for 1–2 minutes. Add the sriracha, soy sauce, rice vinegar, sugar, black pepper and chicken stock and stir to combine.

Put the pork back into the pan, stir, then cook for 2–3 minutes until the sauce has thickened slightly.

Add the noodles and stir well to coat and warm through.

Divide between four bowls and top with the peanuts and a drizzle of sesame oil (if using).

Note: You can save some calories by skipping the peanuts and sesame oil, but you'll be doing yourself a disservice.

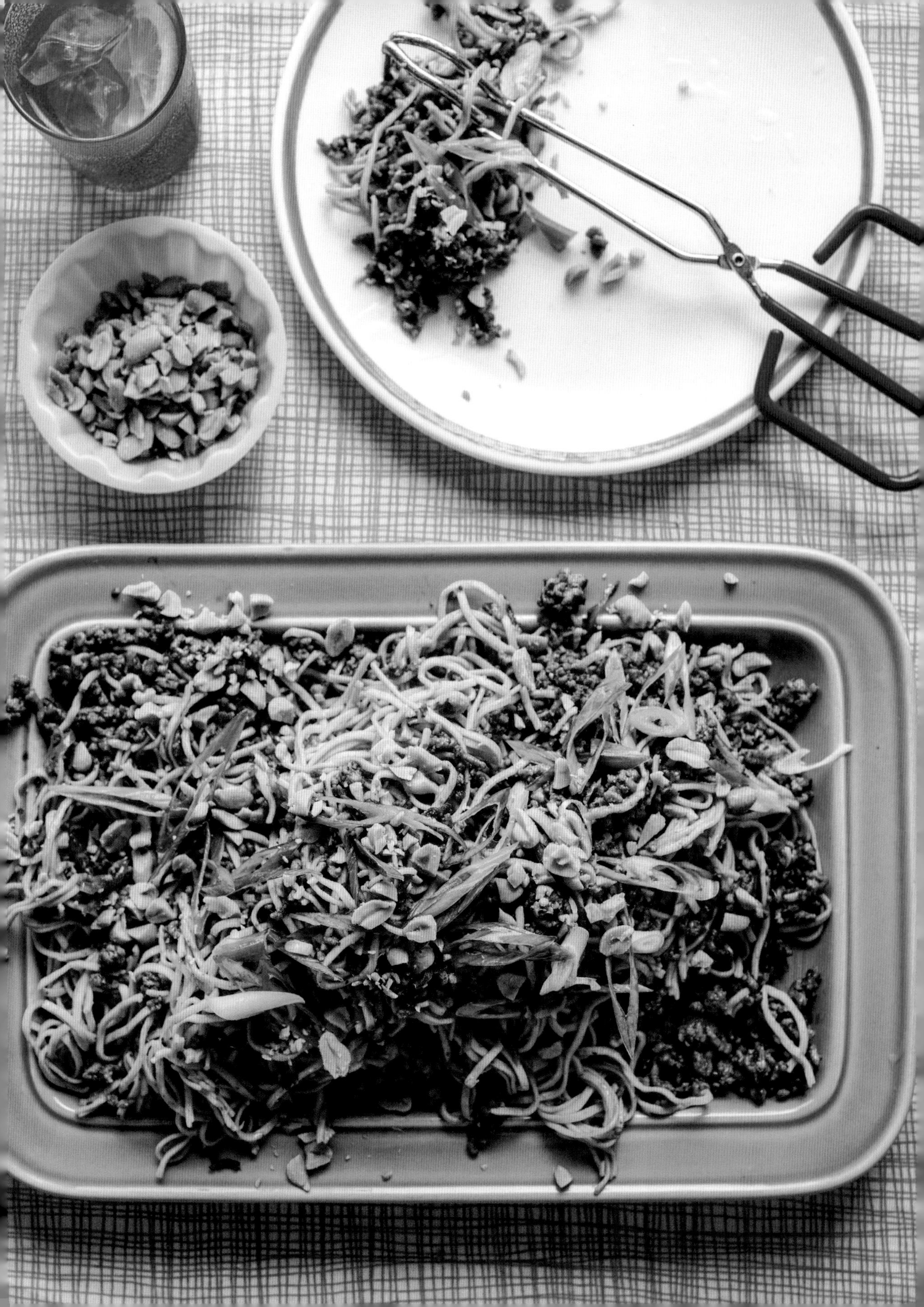

SERVES: 4
PREP: 10 MINS
COOK: 15 MINS
CALORIES: 314

30 mins DF

SPRING ROLL IN A BOWL

We adore spring rolls, especially the massive ones that come as part of a takeaway feast, all resplendent in their greasiness and ready to scatter shards all over your floor, no matter how primly you bite into them. Back in the infancy of twochubbycubs we tried to make healthy versions, knowing that no slimming club member would even consider a deep-fried version. I sourced some clear Vietnamese rice sheets, stuffed them with delicately sliced vegetables and made a wonderful dipping sauce. I remember being terribly excited with this healthy take on the spring roll and rushed out a blog entry to accompany them. The first comment? 'They look like someone stuffed a salad sandwich into a condom, no thanks.' Not saying the words stung, but we never made them again. However, this is a healthy compromise: all the good bits of a spring roll, but served bowl style. If you're missing the crunch of the roll itself, see Paul's notes.

- 500g (1lb 2oz) pork mince
- 1 clove of garlic, crushed
- 300g (10½oz) cabbage, thinly sliced
- 2 carrots, peeled and grated
- 4 tablespoons soy sauce
- 1 teaspoon ground ginger
- 1 egg
- 2 teaspoons sriracha
- 1 tablespoon sesame oil
- 3 spring onions, sliced

Spray a large pan with a little oil and place over a medium-high heat. Add the pork mince and cook until browned, then add the garlic and cook for another 30 seconds.

Add the cabbage, carrots, soy sauce and ginger and cook for 5–6 minutes, adding a splash of water it it's starting to get a little dry.

Reduce the heat to low. Make a well in the middle of the pan, add the egg, and gently scramble for 2 minutes.

Stir through the sriracha and sesame oil, and serve, sprinkled with the spring onions.

Note: For a bit of crunch you could bake some spring roll wrappers and crumble them on top, or some tortillas! Ooooh, he knows how to live, this one!

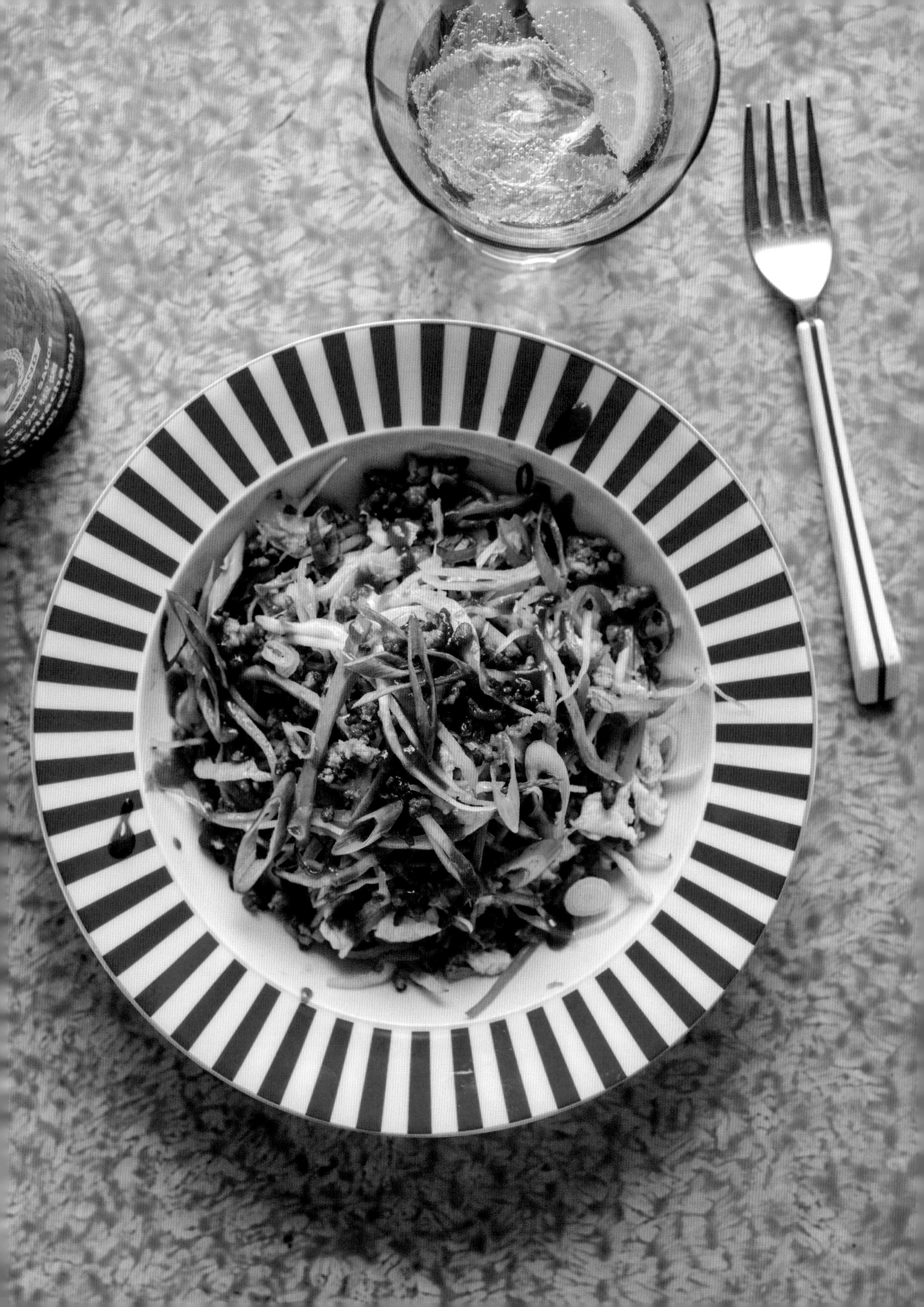

CHIMICHURRI BURGERS

SERVES: 4
PREP: 10 MINS
COOK: 15 MINS
CALORIES: 499

To steal from my father's vernacular: we will continue to include burger recipes in our slimming book for as long as I have a hole in my bum. I mean, those may not have been his exact words, granted, but certainly the spirit. See, to us, a burger epitomises that 'naughty' food when you're trying to lose weight. Anything that glistens and is covered in cheese is usually a terrible choice when dieting, but we refuse to bow to the idea that any food is naughty. Absolutely not, and this burger is a good example of that. The chimichurri sauce is a particular favourite that you may recognise from a previous recipe, but we're including it here because I want you to have a quick read of the notes. There's a wildcard addition you could make, see . . .

- 100g (3½oz) fresh parsley
- 50g (1¾oz) fresh coriander
- 3 cloves of garlic, crushed
- 2 tablespoons white wine vinegar
- 1 tablespoon lemon juice
- 1 teaspoon salt
- 6 sun-dried tomatoes
- 500g (1lb 2oz) lean beef mince
- 4 burger buns, sliced
- 4 handfuls of mixed lettuce leaves
- 4 slices of reduced-fat Cheddar cheese
- 2 tomatoes, sliced
- 1 red onion, sliced

Pulse the parsley, coriander, garlic, white wine vinegar, lemon juice and salt in a food processor, then pour into a bowl and set aside.

Rinse out the food processor bowl. Add the sun-dried tomatoes and pulse until they form a paste with a few chunks, then tip them into another bowl.

Add the mince to the sun-dried tomatoes and mix well, but be careful not to overmix.

Divide the mixture into 8 and roughly flatten into burgers (there's no need to be too neat, just smash them down!).

Spray a pan with a little oil and place over a medium-high heat. Add the burgers (in batches) and cook for a few minutes on each side until browned, then transfer to a plate.

Assemble the burgers by placing some lettuce on the base of each bun, followed by 2 burgers (with a slice of cheese in between), a dollop of chimichurri sauce, the tomato and onion slices, and finish with the top of the bun.

Notes: Lean mince can be quite dry, so we add the sun-dried tomatoes to give it a bit more moisture. Having two thinner burgers also stops it being too dry. Don't worry that they'll be too thin, it works great!

A good friend of mine made a chimichurri sauce using the green leaves and stalks off the top of his fancy carrots, and it worked really, really well. Naturally we can't do this because Ocado and their fancy carrots don't deliver to our area in case they get their tyres stolen during a drop-off, but if the option is available to you, do it!

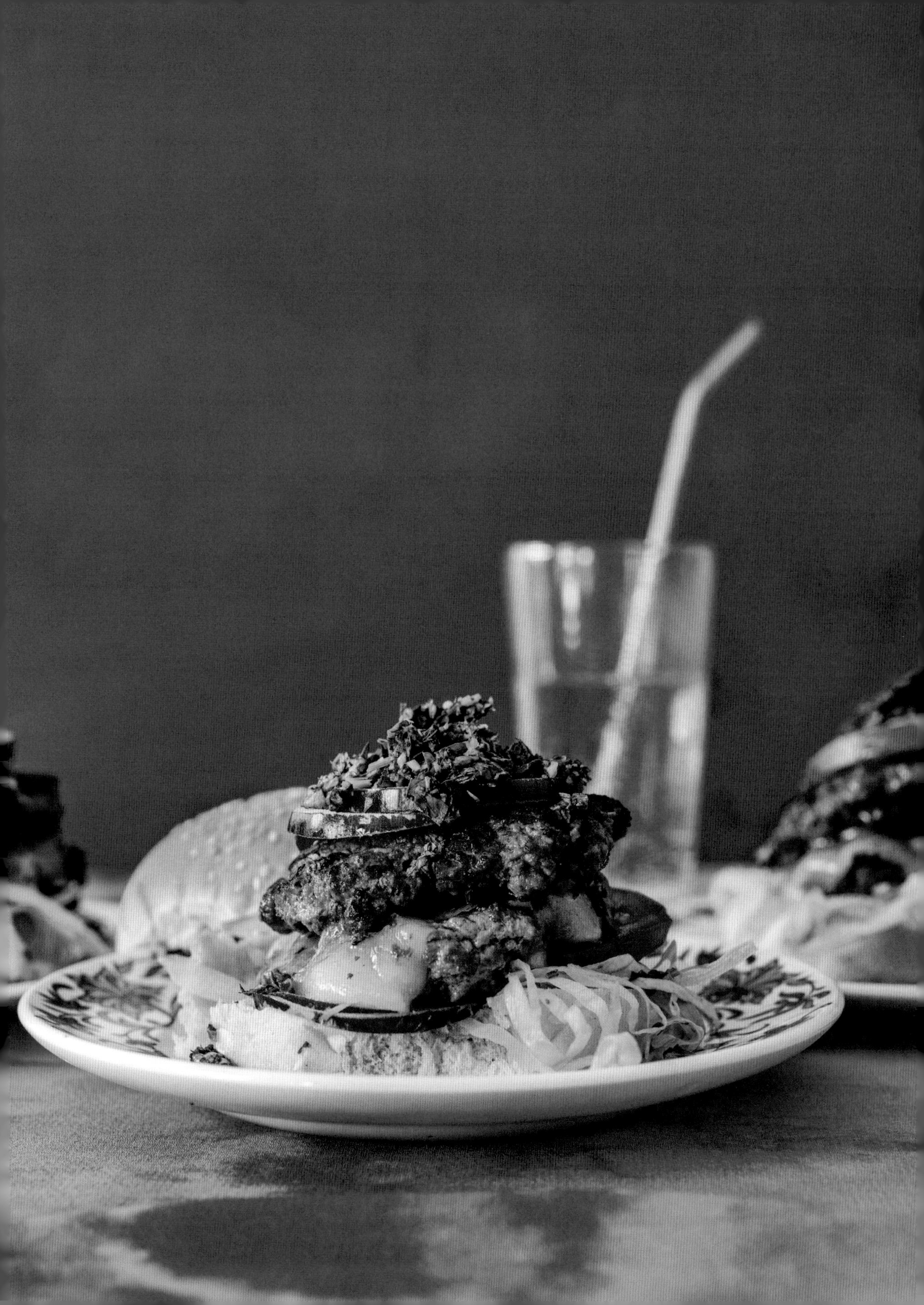

SERVES: 4
PREP: 5 MINS
COOK: 15 MINS
CALORIES: 481

EASY GARLIC NOODLES

This beautifully simple dish – noodles lifted with just garlic and spring onion – is a meal we cook often, and we consider it the next step up from the cacio e pepe in our previous book, *Dinner Time*. It's very much a light lunch sort of affair, and gets two thumbs up from one of our regular visitors, Emma. A past, how to say this politely, holiday conquest of ours once told us over dinner that people enter your life 'for a reason, a season or a lifetime'. It stuck with us, not least because it makes us dry-heave to remember it. It's very cheesy, no? But see, Emma's someone I used to work with over ten years ago and, on paper, we're an unlikely pairing: I'm a cynical, sarcastic soul and she is the most endlessly cheery person you could ever hope to meet. Being jaded takes no effort, but to be constantly smiling and laughing is a skill we could all use. We're talking about someone who still falls into genuine paroxysms of laughter about the time I sellotaped a pickle under her office chair or when she managed to convince me to ring the Mr Kipling factory and ask to speak to Mr Kipling himself under the guise of returning a missed client call. We meet twice a month for lunch, this noodle dish being one of her favourites, and I can say with a hand on my bitter, blackened heart that it is always a highlight of the week. In a world where we can all be awful, be more Emma.

- 350g (12oz) flat rice noodles (see notes)
- 5 tablespoons cooking oil
- 8 cloves of garlic, crushed
- 2 tablespoons sweet paprika
- 2 tablespoons toasted sesame seeds
- 4 spring onions, sliced
- 1½ teaspoons salt
- ½ teaspoon dried chilli flakes
- a handful of fresh coriander, chopped

Cook the noodles (or the pasta if using) according to the instructions on the packet, then drain, rinse with cold water, and return to the pan for later.

Heat the oil in a large pan over a medium-low heat, and add the garlic. Cook for 2 minutes, until it's got a little bit of colour, then add the paprika and sesame seeds and cook for another minute.

Add the noodles (or pasta) to the pan along with most of the spring onions (save a few of them for later) and the salt, and cook for 2 minutes, stirring continuously, until well coated. Sprinkle over the chilli flakes.

Serve in bowls, topped with the rest of the spring onions and the coriander.

Notes: We like to use flat rice noodles, but any noodles or pasta will work. Tagliatelle is a great alternative, but really, do feel free to use whatever you have in.

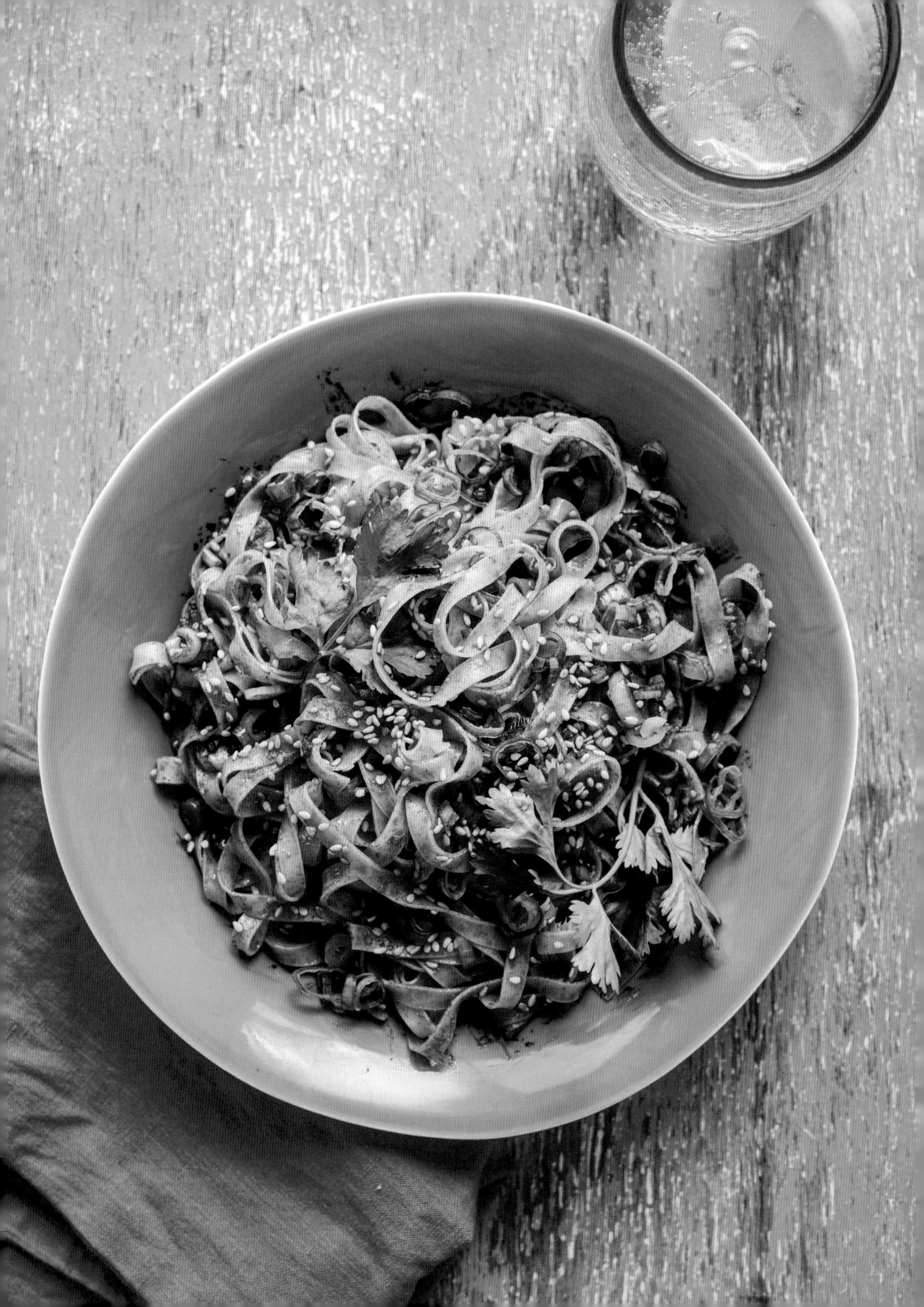

SERVES: 4
PREP: 5 MINS
COOK: 15 MINS
CALORIES: 498

LAMB 'N' MINT BURGERS

We're all aware that burgers have had quite the makeover in the last few years: smash burgers, giant burgers, burgers served inside a brioche bun. Whoever invented the latter deserves shooting into the sun, because a brioche bun is too sweet and too spongy for a burger, and that's a fact because I said so. Of course, we're fairly certain that we've done our own brioche-bunned-burger recipes ourselves, but that's fine, because we're cool. With the above in mind, we're keeping these lamb and mint burgers as simple as possible. Quite right, because a well-seasoned burger is a thing of joy, and you don't need it dripping in cheese and other unctuous additions to enjoy it. Oh, one final note: we're using mint sauce here purely for convenience: if you have access to fresh mint, get it chopped up and use that instead. Stick the rest of the plant in its own separate pot in the garden and you'll never be short of mint again.

- 500g (1lb 2oz) lean lamb mince
- 2 tablespoons mint sauce
- 4 tablespoons natural yoghurt
- 4 burger buns, sliced
- 1 red onion, sliced
- ½ iceberg lettuce, sliced

Preheat the grill to high.

Ridiculously easy, this one – mix together the lamb mince and half the mint sauce (wet hands is best), then divide into 4. Roll the mixture into balls and squash each one down into a burger shape.

Cook under the grill (or, even better – on a barbecue) for about 5–6 minutes each side (or until cooked to your liking).

Meanwhile, mix together the yoghurt and the remaining mint sauce with a pinch of salt and pepper.

To assemble, lay the lettuce on the base of the buns, top with the cooked burgers and a dollop of the mint yoghurt, add some sliced onion, and close with the top of the bun.

Notes: Don't get us wrong: there's occasionally a time and a place for a two-foot-tall burger served up by someone who spent more on his beard oil last year than we did on our mortgage, but this isn't it.

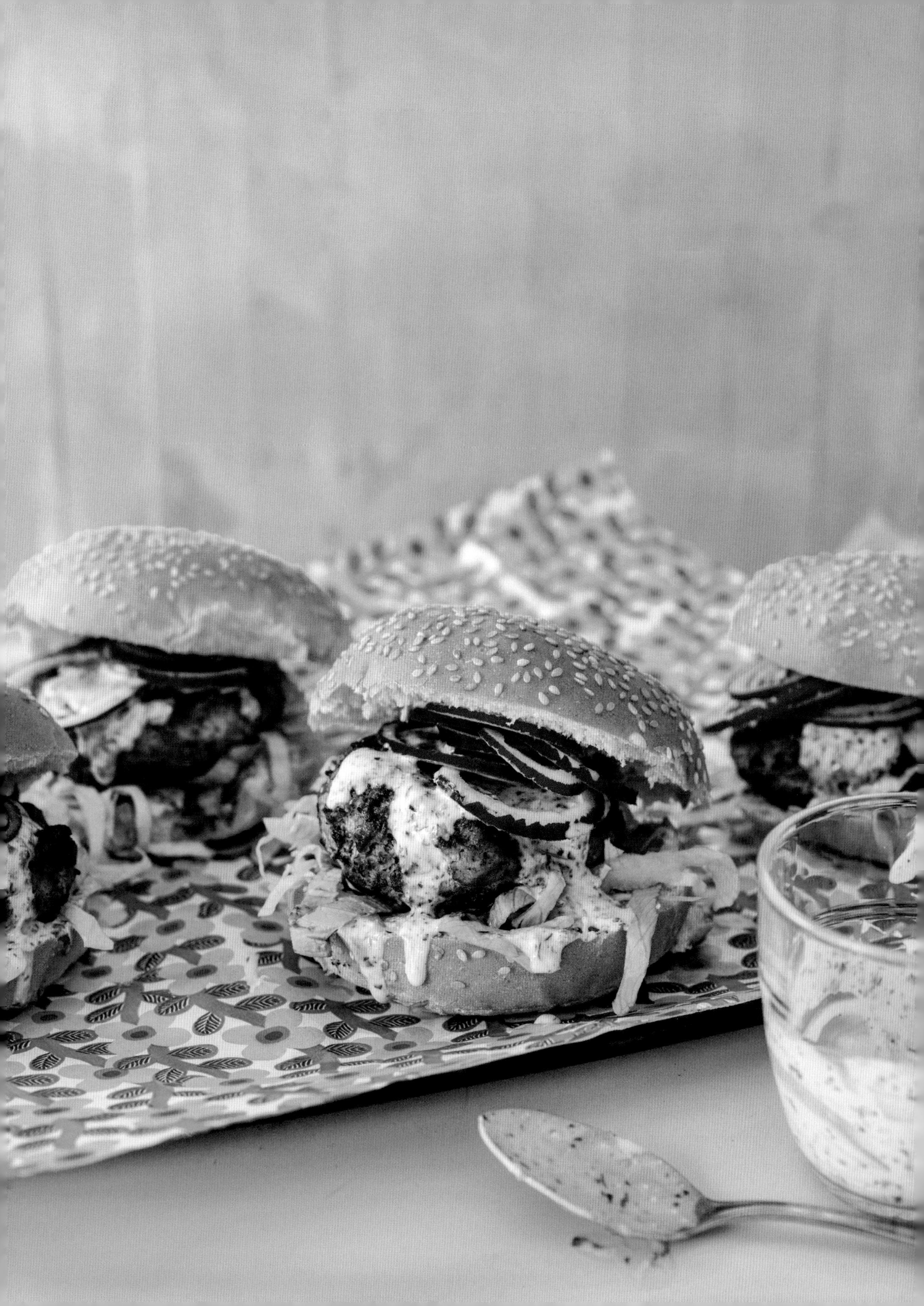

SERVES: 4
PREP: 10 MINS
COOK: 20 MINS
CALORIES: 495

- 1 × 120g (4oz) pouch of golden vegetable rice (see notes)
- 500g (1lb 2oz) lean beef mince
- 2 tablespoons taco seasoning
- 4 flour tortillas
- 125g (4½oz) reduced-fat soft cheese
- 70g (2½oz) reduced-fat Cheddar cheese, grated
- 125g (4½oz) tomato salsa
- 50g (1¾oz) reduced-fat crème fraîche
- a handful of tortilla chips
- 1 tablespoon butter

BOSTIN' BURRITO

Paul reliably informs me that 'bostin' means excellent in a Brummie dialect and as a result, this is an 'excellent burrito'. I'm inclined to agree, having tasted it, although questions are raised as to why he's suddenly cutting about talking like Jasper Carrott. Mind, I will say this: I prefer his tip and a wink to the Birmingham dialect far more than the occasional relapse into Estuary English (he's from Peterborough, remember) he will sometimes suffer. Nothing makes my eye twitch more than him replying 'I were there' instead of 'I was there' or 'He were hung like a church mouse.' It's really very distressing, isn't it? Luckily, you've got this deliciously cheesy, meaty burrito to take your mind off things.

Cook the rice according to the instructions on the packet and set aside.

Spray a large pan with a little oil and place over a medium heat. Add the mince and cook for 6–8 minutes, until browned. Add the taco seasoning along with 90ml (3fl oz) of water, stir, and cook for 2–3 minutes, until slightly thickened.

Meanwhile, microwave the tortillas for about 30 seconds, until softened.

Heat the soft cheese in the microwave for about 20 seconds, then stir in 25g (1oz) of the grated Cheddar.

Spoon equal amounts of mince, rice, cheese sauce, salsa, crème fraîche and tortilla chips into the tortilla wraps, fold up the sides towards the centre, then roll up tightly.

Heat the butter in the microwave in 10-second bursts, until melted.

Put the frying pan back over a medium heat. Brush the melted butter over the top of the burritos and sprinkle over half the remaining Cheddar, pushing it down to make sure it sticks.

Place the burritos in the pan, cheese side down, for about 1 minute, and as they cook, turn them over, brush the other side with the butter, sprinkle with the rest of the cheese, and do the same again.

Serve!

Note: We use golden vegetable rice for ease, but any is fine.

Fun fact: Paul's misspeaking is known as talking in the third-person singular zero. I say fun fact, I actually slipped into a coma researching that.

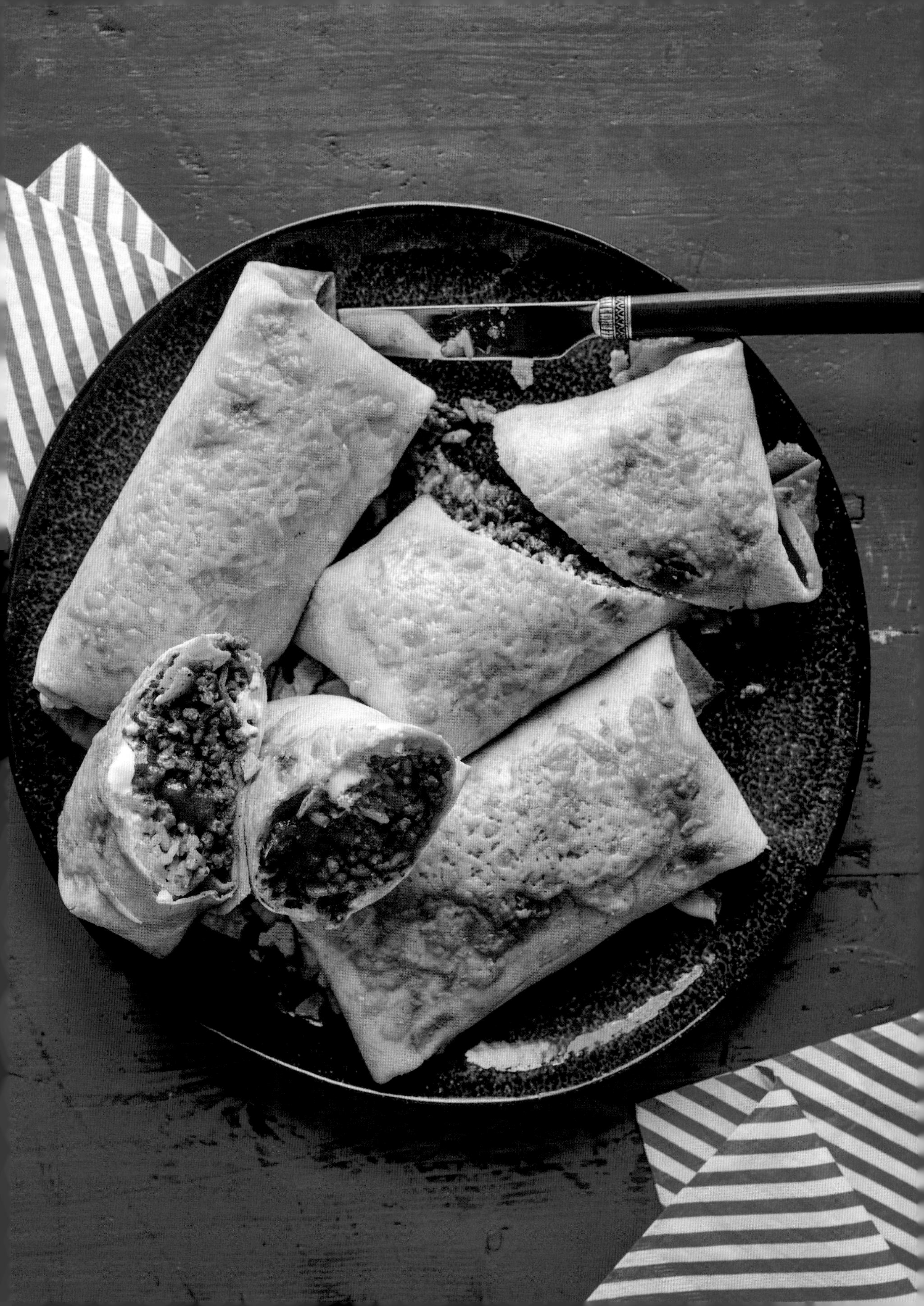

SERVES: 4
PREP: 20 MINS
COOK: 10 MINS
CALORIES: 371

30 mins V DF

- 150g (5½oz) rice vermicelli noodles
- 1 tablespoon sesame seeds
- ½ teaspoon chilli powder
- 280g (10oz) extra firm tofu, diced into 2cm (¾ inch) pieces
- 2 large carrots, coarsely grated
- ½ cucumber, halved lengthways and sliced
- 1 red pepper, thinly sliced
- 100g (3½oz) radishes, thinly sliced
- 150g (5½oz) frozen edamame, defrosted
- chilli sauce, to serve

For the dressing

- 3cm (1¼ inch) piece of ginger, grated
- 2 cloves of garlic, grated
- 3 tablespoons soy sauce
- 3 tablespoons rice vinegar
- 2 teaspoons honey
- juice of 1 lime

RICE NOODLE SALAD WITH CRISPY VEG & FRIED TOFU

We're using rice vermicelli noodles here because the thinness leaves far more room for the stars of the show: the crunchy and crispy vegetables paired with the tasty, slightly boingy tofu. Since publishing our first book what feels like eighty-seven years ago, we have tried with each new publication to improve and increase our vegetarian recipes. It's not always easy: we are confirmed meat-eaters, but the more vegetarian recipes you build into your diet, the less you miss meat. We encourage you to try. We get asked a lot to do a purely vegetarian recipe book and the idea is inviting, but as it stands at the moment we're still learning. All in good time, eh? In the meantime, please accept another one of our vegetarian wonders, and we hope you enjoy it as much as we do!

Put the noodles into a big bowl and cover with boiling water. Leave to stand for 10 minutes, then drain, refresh under cold water and drain again. Put back into the bowl and set aside.

Put the sesame seeds on a plate with the chilli powder and a pinch of salt. Roll the tofu in the mixture, pressing the sesame seeds into the surface.

Heat a non-stick frying pan, spray with a little oil, and cook the tofu cubes on all sides until crisp, golden and hot.

Throw the carrots, cucumber, red pepper, radishes and edamame on top of the rice noodles, then mix up the dressing ingredients and pour over. Use a couple of forks to toss it all together.

Divide the salad between plates and serve with the fried tofu on top and extra soy sauce and chilli sauce if you like.

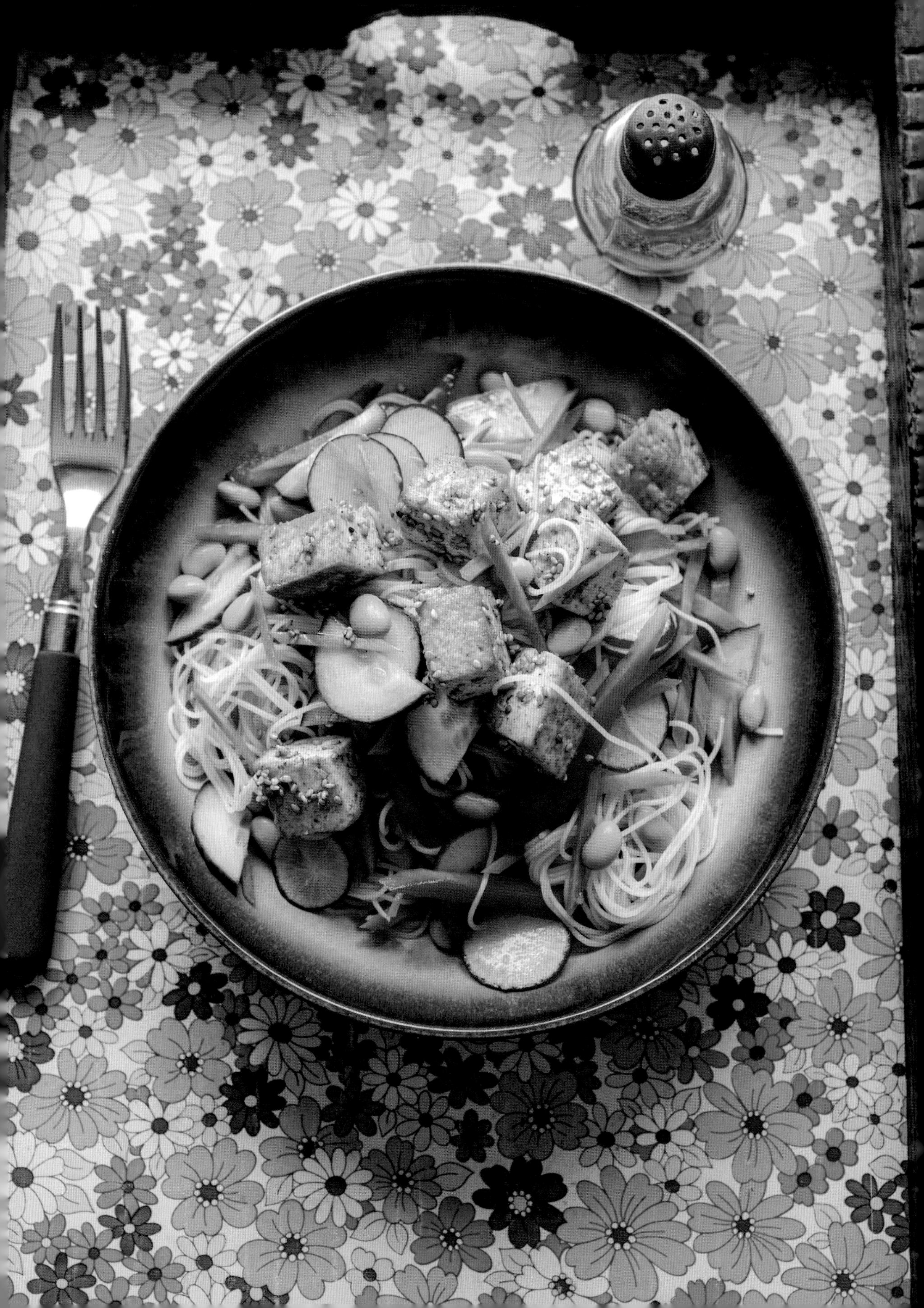

SERVES: 4
PREP: 15 MINS
COOK: 35 MINS
CALORIES: 397

SAUSAGE TART

Readers who have been with us since the early days of the blogs and books (and the planner too, but we don't talk about that: it's like the child you send away to boarding school because he keeps starting fires and whispering about Satan) will know that we have a somewhat eclectic range of neighbours around us. For the most part wonderful, but there's a few whose house I'm surprised hasn't burst into flame from the friction of the curtains twitching across the windowsill all day. But we absolutely must give a shout out to Colin and Pat and Wilf and Wilma, who are perfect neighbours indeed. Colin and Pat, clearly tiring of seeing me lumbering about trying to mow the lawn and then giving up when I realise such a task is tantamount to manual labour, have adopted our garden. They now spend merry afternoons making it beautiful while simultaneously shielding their eyes from my shimmering nakedness as I forget they're in the garden and blunder about on the other side of our open blinds in just a towel. Wilf and Wilma live opposite and keep us in fruit and vegetables from their allotment all year round, probably incentivised by Paul walking to the car with his rickets on show. They're always there for a chat, to take in my lovehoney purchases (a feat in itself, given they turn up on a flat-bed lorry and require a two-man installation and an electric point) and to keep us abreast of neighbourhood developments. As a quartet, they're wonderful, and I bring them up now not only to make them smile but also because this dish was the one we took over to Colin and Pat's anniversary party. See? We do give back!

- 2 red onions, finely sliced
- 1 tablespoon balsamic vinegar
- 4 reduced-fat sausages
- plain flour, for dusting
- 1 × 320g (11oz) sheet of light puff pastry
- 2 teaspoons wholegrain mustard
- 100g (3½oz) reduced-fat soft cheese

Preheat the oven to 200°C fan/425°F/gas mark 7.

Spray a large pan with a little oil and place it over a medium heat. Add the onions and cook for 10 minutes, stirring occasionally, until softened, then add the balsamic vinegar and cook for another 2–3 minutes.

While the onions are cooking, score the sausages with a knife and remove the casings, then gently break the sausage meat into chunks.

Sprinkle a little flour on your worktop. Lay out the pastry and score a 1cm (½ inch) border around the edge, then place it on a lined baking sheet.

Mix together the mustard and the soft cheese and spread it over the pastry, making sure not to go beyond the scored edges, then gently top with the caramelised onions and the chunks of sausage meat.

Bake in the oven for 15–20 minutes, until golden.

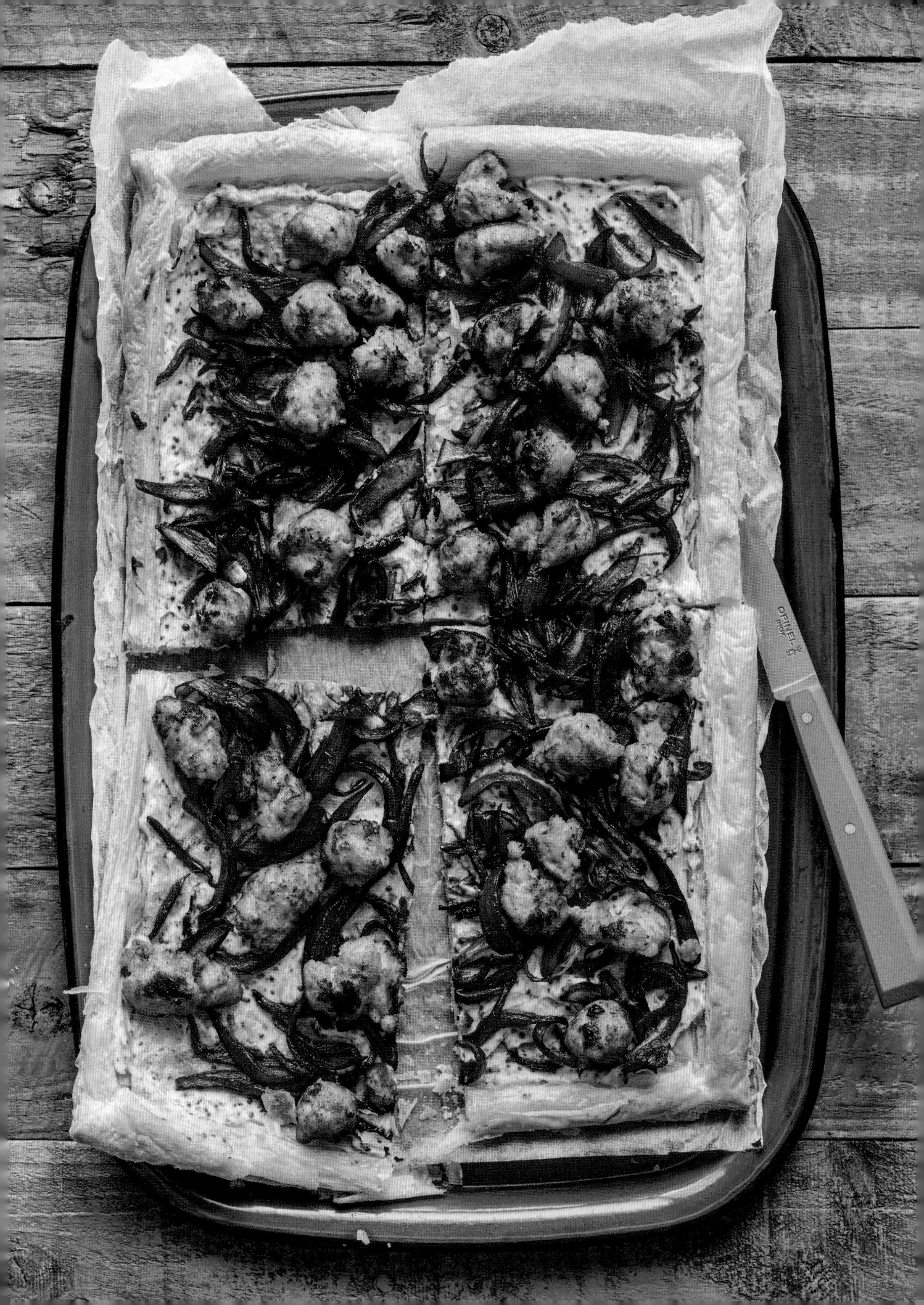
OPINEL
INOX

SERVES: 4
PREP: 10 MINS
COOK: 20 MINS
CALORIES: 452

30 mins · DF

ZINGY BASIL CHICKEN

This chicken dish is a doddle to cobble together and perfect if you're entertaining, and not in the way that requires you to throw your car keys into a bowl and get to know your neighbours better. Brr. I say perfect for entertaining, like Paul and I ever host people at ours for dinner. We would love to, honestly, but we're ever so busy and plus, can't bear having people in our personal space. Is that awful? Or normal? I always imagine when people come over that they're silently and icily judging our taste in decoration, or the state of the dog's ears (always full of sticky-jacks, thank you for asking), or even worse, the clip of our cooking. Even if we're having someone over to service the boiler – unusually, not a euphemism – I'll be polishing the kitchen cupboard doors and replacing the Bloo lest they think we're slatterns. And I mean, we are, but people don't need to know. Such reluctance to host is rendered even more silly given how much we love eating out at other people's homes. We always try to be the best guests too: offer to help with the washing, bring a good bottle of wine, keep the stealing of their scented candles to a minimum. But visit Chubby Towers? Absolutely not!

- 280g (10oz) long-grain rice
- 2 teaspoons soy sauce
- 1¼ teaspoons sriracha
- ½ tablespoon fish sauce
- 1 teaspoon cornflour
- 1 teaspoon dried chilli flakes
- 1 small brown onion, diced
- 3 cloves of garlic, crushed
- 4 chicken breasts, diced
- a handful of fresh basil leaves, chopped

Cook the rice according to the instructions on the packet, then drain and return to the pan to keep warm.

Meanwhile, in a small bowl, mix together the soy sauce, sriracha, fish sauce, cornflour and chilli flakes along with 1 teaspoon of water, and set aside.

Spray a large pan with a little oil and place over a medium-high heat. Add the onion and garlic and cook for 30 seconds, then add the chicken and cook for 8–10 minutes, until cooked through.

Add the sauce to the pan and cook for an extra minute, stirring well so the chicken is well coated.

Remove from the heat and stir through the basil.

Serve with the rice.

Note: Paul suggests rice and that's all well and good, but we've also tried it with those thick noodles you can buy that look utterly grim when you slide them out of the packet, but taste delicious when all saucy.

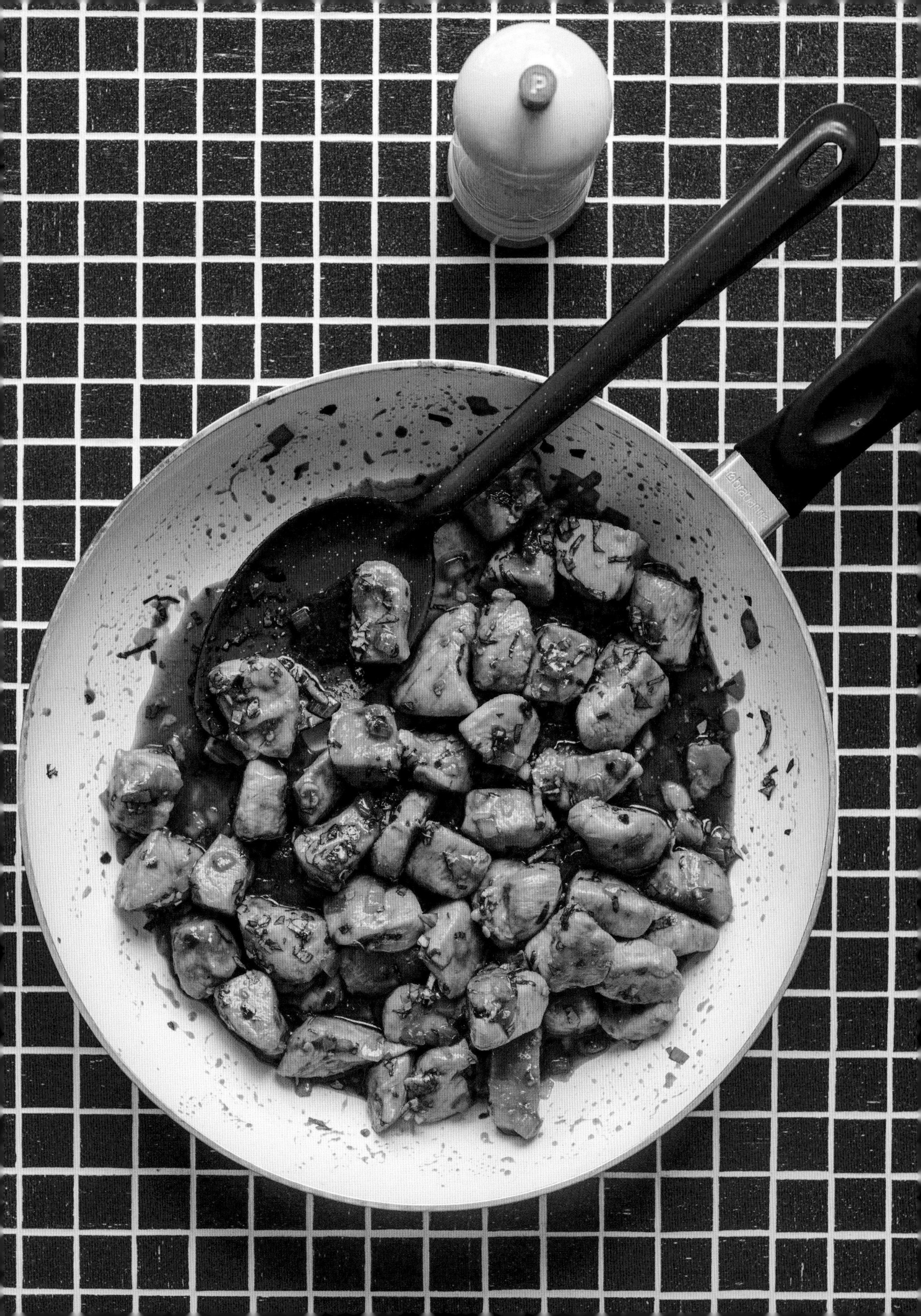
P
brabantia

SERVES: 4
PREP: 10 MINS
COOK: 30 MINS
CALORIES: 269

30 mins · GF · DF

- 1 onion, diced
- 1 green pepper, deseeded and diced
- 3 cloves of garlic, crushed
- 500g (1lb 2oz) lean beef mince
- 1 × 400g (14oz) tin of chopped tomatoes
- 80g (3oz) raisins
- 75g (2¾oz) pitted green olives, halved
- 1 teaspoon ground cumin
- 1 teaspoon dried oregano

PICADILLO

Four books and countless blog posts and we have never done a picadillo recipe – we ought to be ashamed. We have had a few variants over the years, and certainly we make absolutely no claim that this is in any way an authentic take on the Cuban classic. Actually, that goes for all the recipes in this book – we've learned our lesson since claiming the 'parmo' originated in Newcastle. We were gently persuaded via an avalanche of foaming instant messages on that one, and lordy-loo we'll never repeat that mistake again. All recipes are very much in the spirit of the dish, not the 'definitive' version. That's for the experts! With that little qualification in play, we should turn to this recipe anew: it's a delicious, beefy, fruity dish that tastes even better when you have it as leftovers the next day. I know, me neither.

Spray a large pan with a little oil and place over a medium heat. Add the onions, green pepper and garlic and cook for about 5 minutes.

Add the mince and cook until browned, stirring occasionally.

Add the tomatoes, raisins, olives, cumin and oregano and stir well. Reduce the heat to low and simmer for 10–15 minutes, until thickened.

Serve!

Note: This is perfect with plain, simple, unfussy white rice. But to each their own.

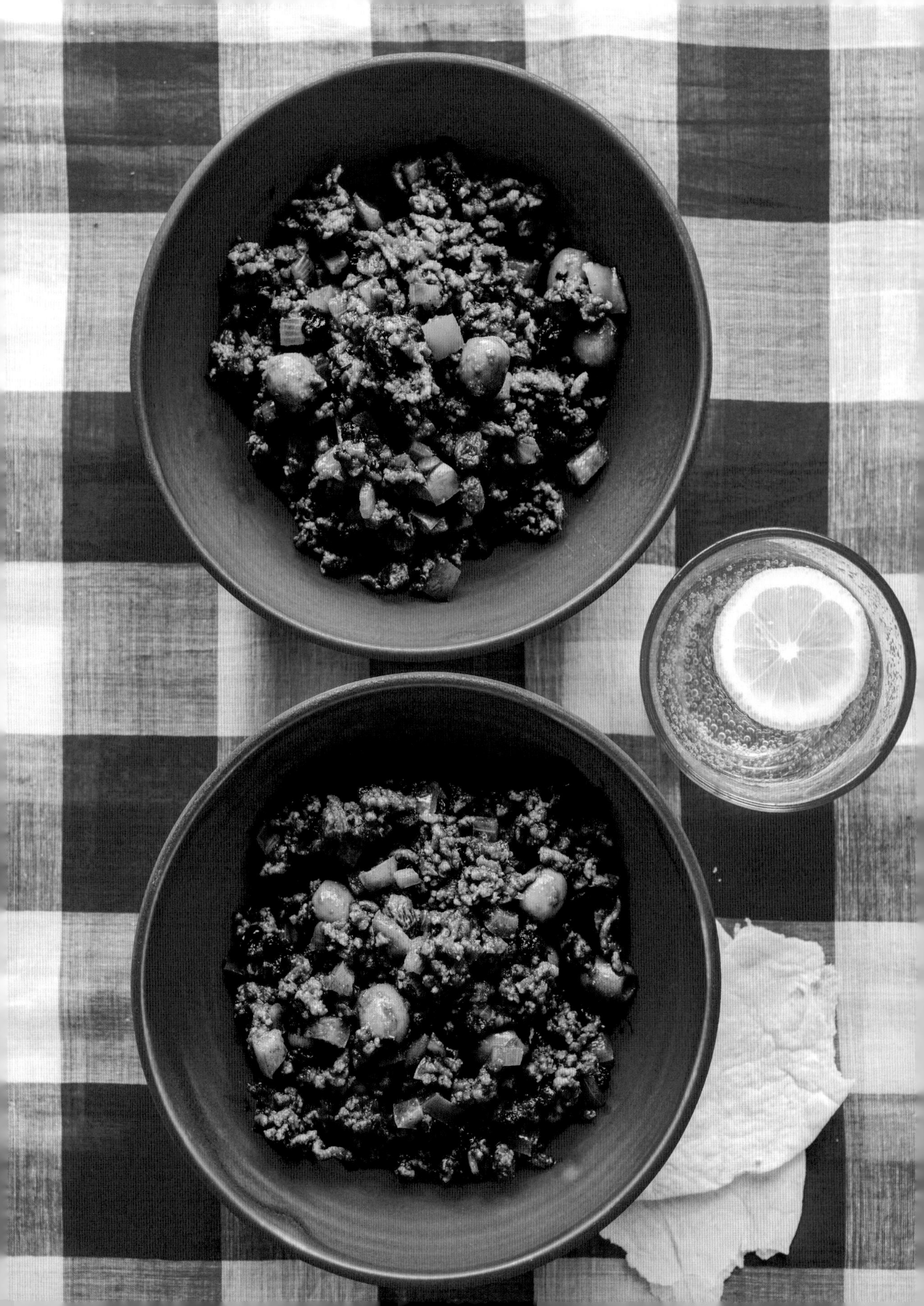

SERVES: 4
PREP: 15 MINS
COOK: 5 MINS
CALORIES: 269

30 mins · 10 · GF · DF

THE MOST RETRO PRAWN COCKTAIL

Take a deep breath, folks! We had a proper retro prawn cocktail *Somewhere* on a recent trip to Liverpool, where, would you believe, after sixteen years *Forever In Love*, we went to our first ever concert. I mean, *It's a Sin*, I know. And WHAT a concert: the Pet Shop Boys! They live *Rent* free in my *Heart* and certainly *Always on My Mind* and indeed, I've been *Dreaming of the Queen(s)* for years, so it was a no-brainer. We had to *Go West* to Liverpool because *It Couldn't Happen Here* in Newcastle, as we couldn't get tickets. *Se a vida é* indeed. However, a good *Sexy Northerner* friend of ours shocked us with his bi-annual moment of kindness (*It Always Comes as a Surprise*) and gave us his spare tickets, so before Paul could say *I Don't Wanna* and *Do I Have To?* and *I Wouldn't Normally Do This Kind of Thing*, we snatched them up. We were right at the front in the good seats with our *Delusions of Grandeur, One of the Crowd* in total *Pandemonium*. It was the *Single* best gig I've ever been to – *Absolutely Fabulous*, you might say, and clearly I'm a *Positive Role Model* because we were soon back to *The Way It Used to Be*, with Paul singing and *Domino Dancing* with me. 'Twas *The Night I Fell in Love* all over again.

- 1kg (2lb 4oz) peeled raw prawns, cleaned and deveined
- 4 tablespoons light mayonnaise
- 1 tablespoon tomato ketchup
- 1 teaspoon Worcestershire sauce
- 1 iceberg lettuce
- 1 cucumber
- 1 avocado
- 1 lemon
- ¼ teaspoon paprika

Bring a large pan of water to the boil. Add the prawns and poach for 2–3 minutes, until they turn pink, then drain and leave to cool.

In a bowl, mix together the mayonnaise, tomato ketchup, Worcestershire sauce, and a pinch of salt and pepper.

Chop the lettuce and cucumber into small pieces and place in serving glasses or bowls.

Slice the avocado and remove the stone, then gently scoop out the flesh and dice into small pieces. Add to the serving bowls.

Add the prawns to the bowls and squeeze over the lemon juice.

Finally, spoon over the sauce and chill for at least 30 minutes. Serve with the paprika sprinkled on top.

Note: Be very glad indeed I didn't try and work in The Truck Driver and His Mate, Love Comes Quickly, Did You See Me Coming? *or* Your Funny Uncle – *that was* So Hard! A Man Could Get Arrested!

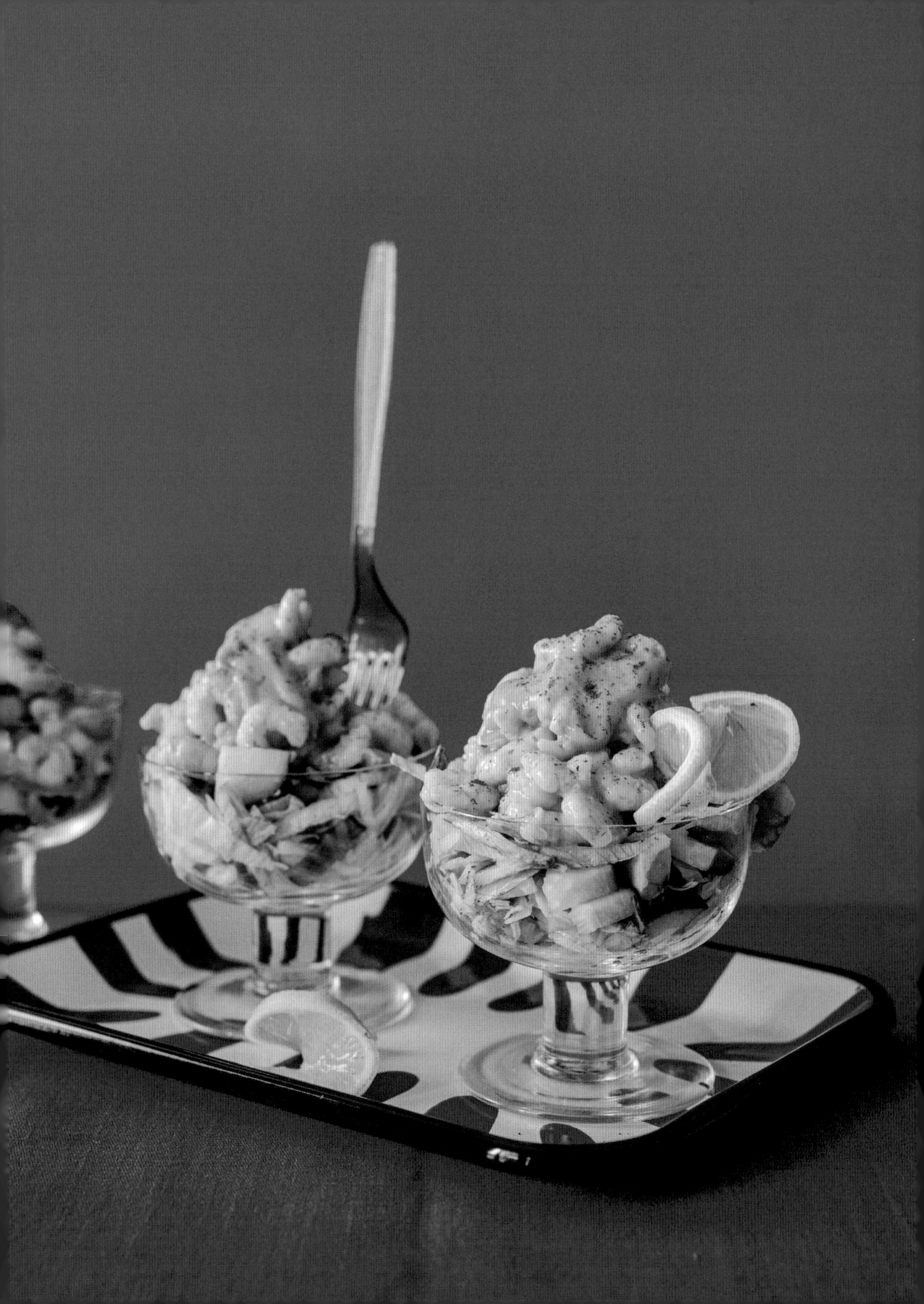

DA

D

ZLING

ISHES

PORK & SWEET POTATO CHILLI

SERVES: 4
PREP: 15 MINS
COOK: 1 HR 10 MINS
CALORIES: 498

We've done several takes on the traditional chilli over the years but the addition of sweet potato here was revelatory: it breaks down and adds a sweetness and a starchiness to what is usually quite a heavy dish. While I have your eyes on me, can we all agree now that sweet potato fries can get in the bin? They always cost more than normal chips when you order them as a side, and places never get them right. The only acceptable sweet potato fry is one that has been deep-fried and is crunchy on the outside and soft in the middle. Slicing up raw sweet potatoes and putting them in the oven for an hour does not make sweet potato fries: it makes sadness. So stop it.

- 320g (11oz) low-fat pork sausages, casings removed
- 1 brown onion, diced
- 1 green pepper, deseeded and sliced
- 300g (10½oz) sweet potatoes, peeled and chopped into bite-size chunks
- 1 tablespoon hot chilli powder
- 2 teaspoons smoked paprika
- 2 tablespoons tomato purée
- 2 bay leaves
- 1.2 litres (2 pints) chicken stock
- 1 × 400g (14oz) tin of kidney beans, drained
- 180g (6oz) basmati rice
- 2 tablespoons fat-free natural yoghurt

For the coleslaw

- 4 tablespoons cider vinegar
- 2 teaspoons sugar
- ¼ red cabbage, thinly sliced
- 1 green chilli, deseeded and thinly sliced
- a handful of fresh coriander, finely chopped

Spray a large pan with a little oil and place over a medium-high heat. Add the sausage meat, breaking it up with a wooden spoon, and cook for 6–8 minutes, until browned. Scoop out of the pan and set aside.

Add the onion and green peppers to the pan and cook for 5–6 minutes, until starting to soften. Add the sweet potatoes and cook for a further 5–6 minutes.

Add the hot chilli powder and paprika, stir and cook for 1 minute, then add the tomato purée and the bay leaves and cook for another 3–4 minutes.

Pour on the chicken stock, add the beans, then return the sausage to the pan and stir well. Bring to the boil, then reduce the heat, cover with a lid, and simmer for 30–40 minutes.

Meanwhile, put the cider vinegar and sugar into a bowl and heat in the microwave for 30 seconds, until the sugar has dissolved. Add the red cabbage, green chilli and coriander to the bowl along with a pinch of salt, toss, and keep in the fridge.

Cook the rice according to the instructions on the packet, then drain and keep warm.

Serve the chilli with the basmati rice and a dollop of yoghurt, with the coleslaw alongside.

Notes: Coleslaw may seem like an odd addition to this meal, but take our hand and trust us.

If you have leftovers, you can make some delicious wraps for lunch the next day. Chilli always tastes so much better the next day for sitting quietly in a pot.

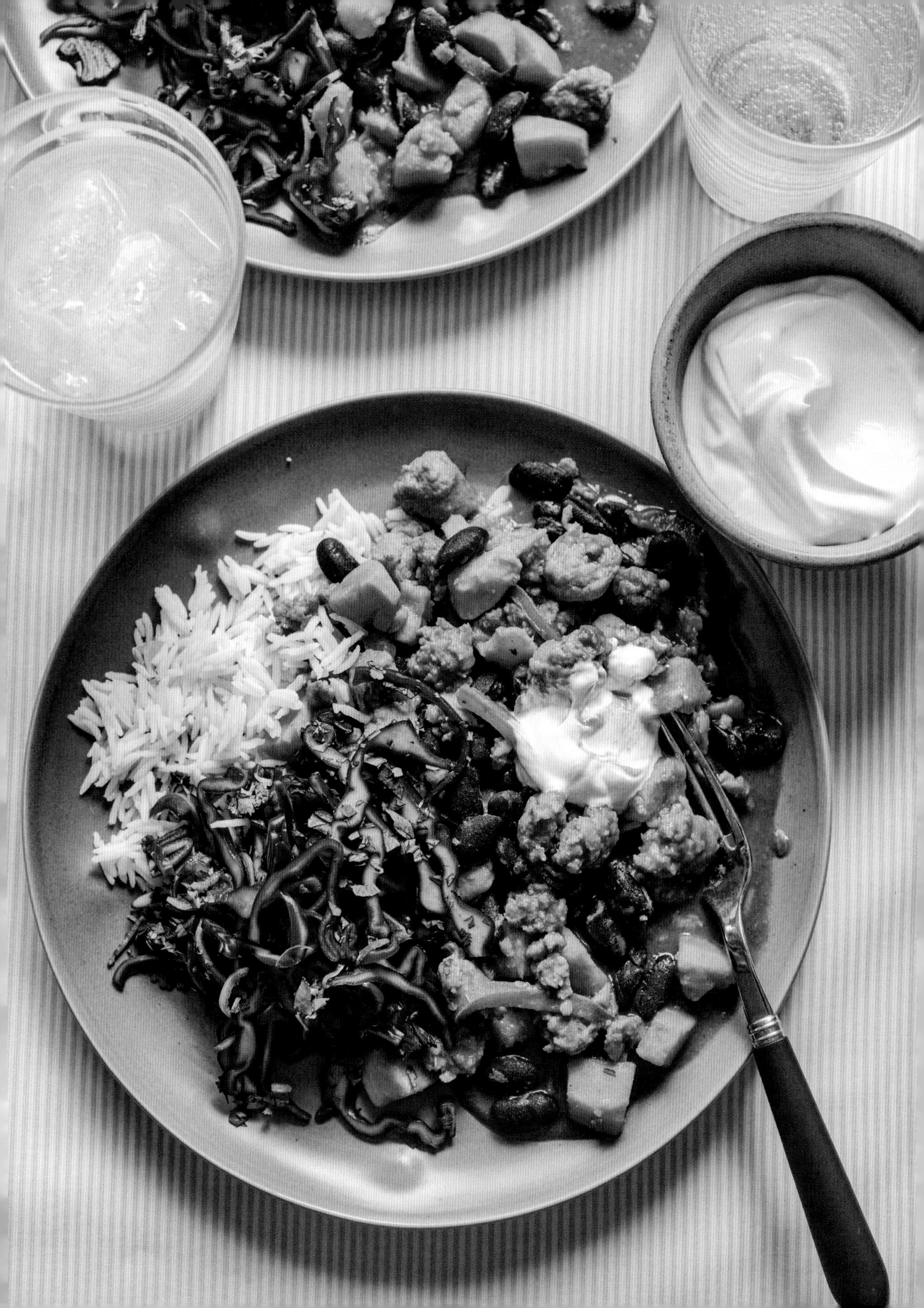

SERVES: 4
PREP: 10 MINS
COOK: 55 MINS
CALORIES: 489

- 8 boneless skinless chicken thighs
- 1 brown onion, sliced
- 1 red pepper, deseeded and diced
- 4 cloves of garlic, crushed
- ¼ teaspoon dried chilli flakes
- 1 tablespoon tomato purée
- 2 tablespoons plain flour
- 500ml (18fl oz) chicken stock
- 3 tablespoons paprika
- 1 × 400g (14oz) tin of chopped tomatoes
- 5 tablespoons natural yoghurt
- ¼ teaspoon salt
- a handful of fresh parsley, chopped

CHICKEN PAPRIKASH

It's a big surprise to me that we haven't managed a paprikash recipe yet, either in the books or online. Although traditionally a Hungarian dish, we first tried it in Ukraine back in 2020. It seems so far away, that holiday. Part of the reason it has stayed with us is it came just at the point when COVID started looming over the world – we travelled back through the airports seeing people in masks and still thought it was just a cold and would be over in a few weeks. We all know how that turned out. And now, the thought of going back to Kyiv, seeing that beautiful city once more, seems like an impossibility. It remains high on our 'must go back' list, though, and we recommend that you do the same. To the paprikash then, with a nod to its Hungarian origin.

Spray a large pan with a little oil and place over a medium heat. Add the chicken and cook for 10 minutes, turning halfway through, until browned, then remove from the pan. Do this in batches if you need to!

Add the onion and pepper to the pan and cook over a medium-high heat for about 5–6 minutes, until the onion has softened. Add the garlic, chilli flakes and tomato purée and cook for 1 minute.

Add the flour and stir continuously for 1 minute, then add the chicken stock, paprika and tinned tomatoes and stir well.

Add the chicken and bring to the boil, then cover the pan, reduce the heat to medium-low, and cook for 30 minutes, turning the chicken halfway through.

Mix together the natural yoghurt with the salt, and set aside.

Once the chicken is cooked, remove from the heat and leave to cool for about 5–10 minutes, then gently stir in the yoghurt until well combined.

Serve in bowls, sprinkled with the parsley.

Notes: Don't be tempted to use fat-free yoghurt in this, it'll probably split if you do!

We love this with mash, but it also works brilliantly with tagliatelle!

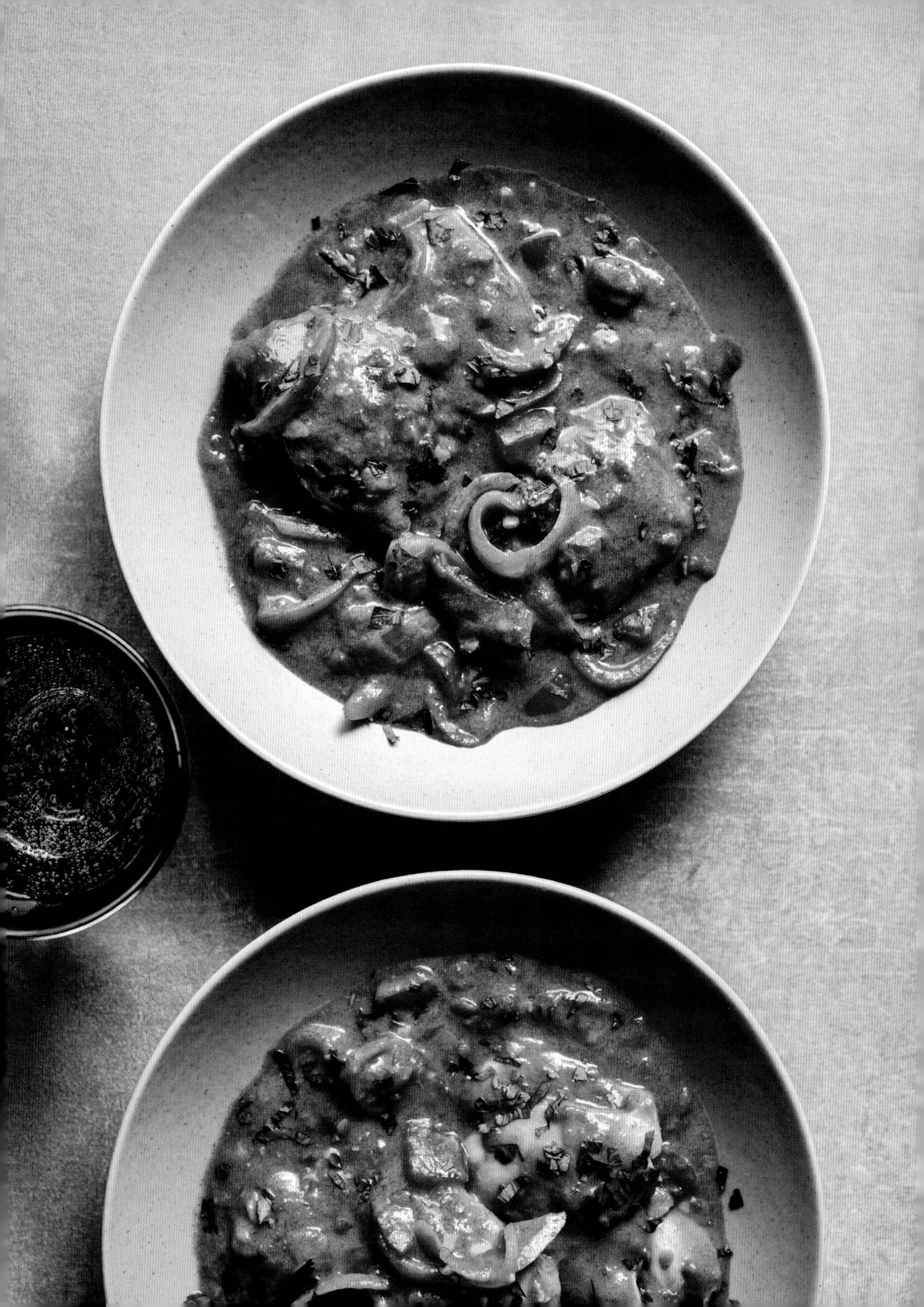

SERVES: 4
PREP: 10 MINS
COOK: 55 MINS
CALORIES: 491

CHICKEN & STUFFING BAKE

This is a pure guilty pleasure dinner, designed to be devoured in big steamy bowlfuls in front of some trashy television. It reminds me of Christmas, purely because of the stuffing, which we only tend to have during festive festivities – more's the pity. I'll get Paul on that right away. My nana used to make the most amazing stuffing, which looks nothing like what you get today, and in fact, sounds awful when I put it into words, but think of a thick sage and onion soup and you are almost there. We have tried replicating it several times over the years but never got it right, so we stopped trying. If she ever bursts forth from the afterlife in shimmering ethereality, I'll be sure to ask her. Now you may look at this and go that's a lot of packet and frozen food and indeed it is, but the key with this recipe is that it uses up all sorts of odds-and-sods you have kicking around and takes minimal effort to throw together. If you're not a fan of frozen veg, feel free to chuck in whatever you want, although we have come to love our freezer foraging. Vegetables especially have come a long way since the days of the 'pea, carrot and sweetcorn' mixes that were always such flavourless follies. I spent a good proportion of my school lunches stowing that in the pockets of whoever I used to be sitting near on the day. I wouldn't have been such a scoundrel had the school served this up though, so bear that in mind before you skip past.

- 170g (6oz) dried stuffing mix
- 1 brown onion, peeled and finely diced
- 2 cloves of garlic, crushed
- 30g (1oz) plain flour
- 1 × 400g (14oz) tin of cream of chicken soup
- 400g (14oz) frozen mixed vegetables
- ½ teaspoon dried thyme
- ½ teaspoon dried rosemary
- ½ teaspoon salt
- ½ teaspoon black pepper
- 400g (14oz) cooked chicken, diced

Preheat the oven to 200°C fan/425°F/gas mark 7.

Make the stuffing according to the instructions on the packet, and set aside.

Spray a large pan with a little oil and place over a medium heat. Add the onions and cook for 4–5 minutes, then add the garlic and cook for another minute.

Add the flour and stir to combine, then cook for about 2 minutes, stirring occasionally. Stir in the soup and keep stirring until no lumps remain.

Increase the heat to medium-high and add the mixed veg, thyme, rosemary, salt and pepper and simmer for 4–5 minutes.

Tip the mixture into an ovenproof dish along with the chicken and spread the stuffing mixture over the top (wet hands is best for this!). Place the dish in the oven and bake for 25–30 minutes.

Note: I'm going to let you into a terrible secret here: we occasionally use those packs of frozen cooked chicken you can buy in the Land of Ice.

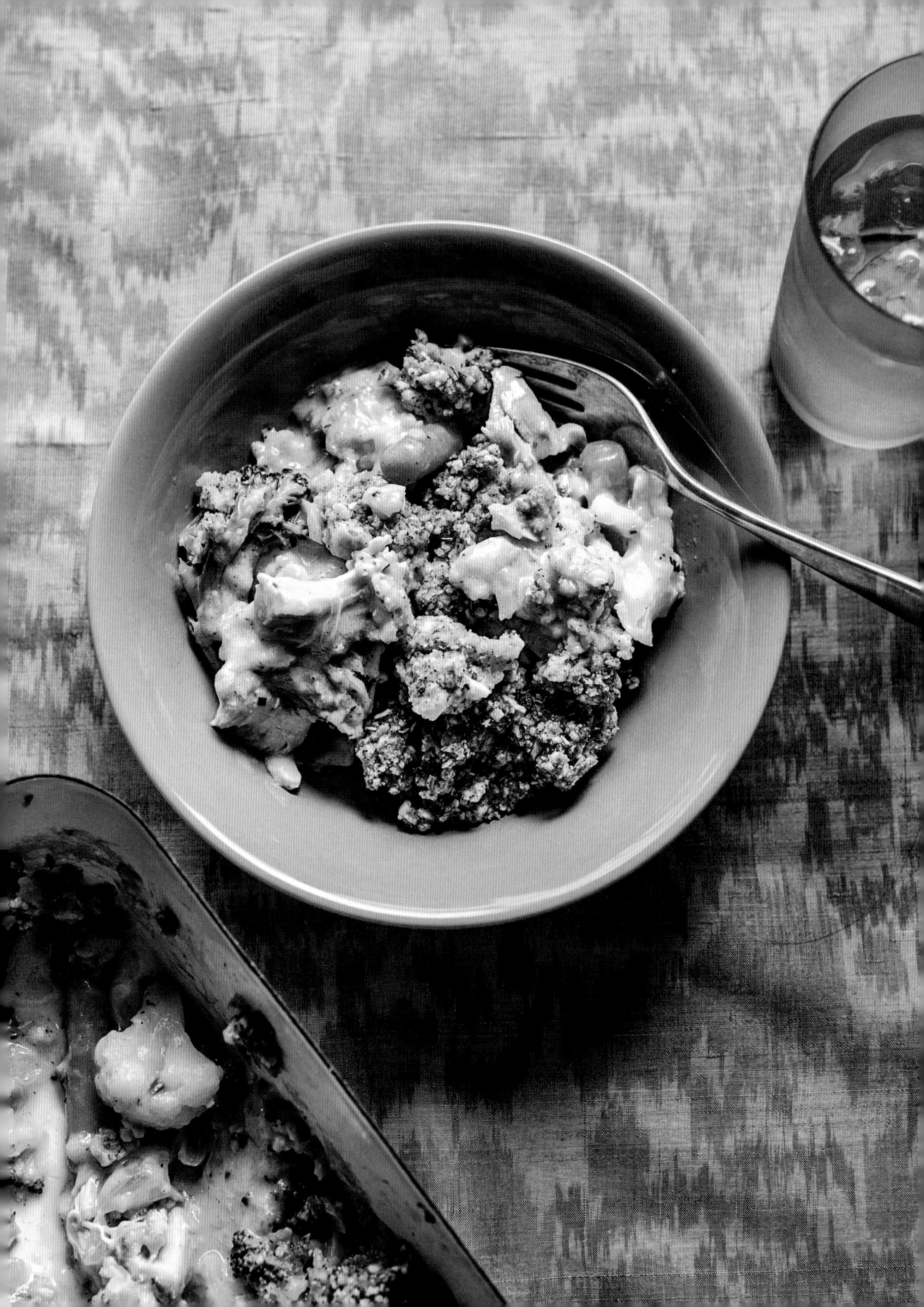

SERVES: 4
PREP: 15 MINS
COOK: 1 HR 20 MINS
CALORIES: 338

30 mins · GF · DF

- 500g (1lb 2oz) pork mince
- 100g (3½oz) brown rice, cooked and cooled
- 1 brown onion, finely diced
- 1 red pepper, deseeded and finely diced
- 30g (1oz) fresh coriander, chopped
- 1 teaspoon ground cumin
- 1 teaspoon smoked paprika
- ½ teaspoon salt
- ¼ teaspoon black pepper
- 1 egg
- 1 × 400g (14oz) tin of chopped tomatoes
- 500ml (18fl oz) beef stock
- 1 carrot, peeled and diced
- 2 celery stalks, diced

ALBONDIGAS

This is a *delicious* dish – meatball dishes always are, but it's the simmering sauce that makes this one shine. Veteran readers will remember our surprise trip to Benidorm a few years ago: literally a surprise, as we only found out at the airport where we were going. If I hadn't paid for a week's worth of long-stay car-parking I'd have backed out, and what a bloody fool I'd have been. It was a hoot. I mean, yes, you don't go there for outdoor performances of *Titus Andronicus* and braying laughter over a cheeky bottle of Teso La Monja: you go for pure fun and picking your dinner off a wipe-clean menu. It was here that Paul managed to order exactly one 'tapa' for our table, but even that one disc of bread with 'meat' on it was wonderful. Luckily, we found somewhere else to eat without embarrassment just a few doors down, and that's where we tried this. A few tweaks to make it a bit healthier, and it's yours to enjoy.

In a bowl, mix together the mince, rice, onion, red pepper, coriander, cumin, paprika, salt, pepper and egg, then roll the mix into 16 meatballs.

Spray a large pan with a little oil and place over a medium heat. Add the meatballs and brown on all sides (do this in batches if necessary).

In another large pan, stir together the tomatoes, stock, carrot and celery and bring to the boil.

Add the meatballs to the pan, then reduce the heat and simmer for 1 hour.

Serve!

Notes: This is perfect over lovingly cooked rice. Or indeed, poorly cooked rice. Or even chips. It always comes down to chips with us.

Freeze the meatballs and sauce separately.

I did spend a lot of time wincing at the poor tattoo choices, but that entitled snobbery is entirely on me.

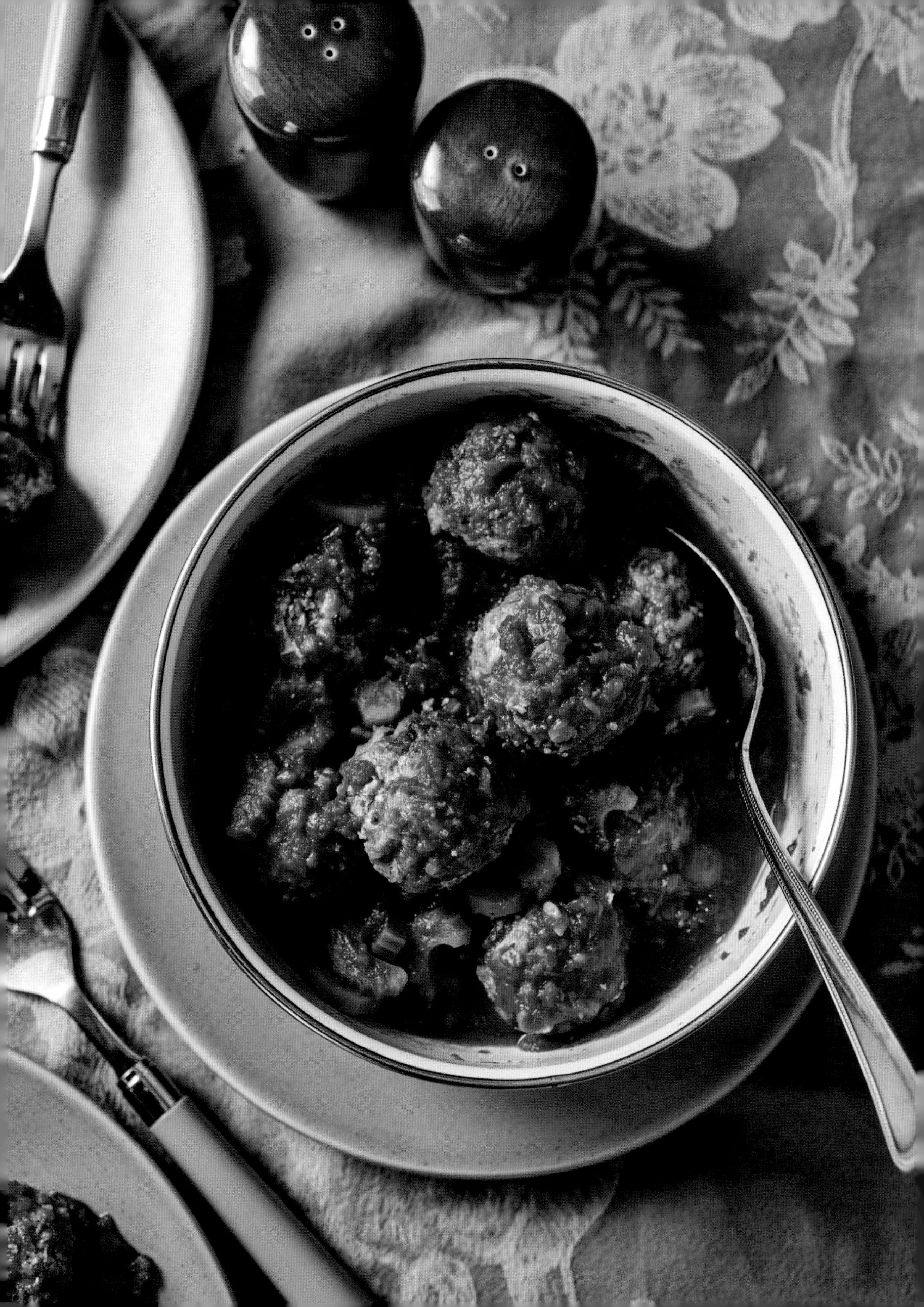

CHICKEN FRICASSÉE

SERVES: 4
PREP: 10 MINS
COOK: 1 HR 40 MINS
CALORIES: 324

↑30 mins ❄ GF

- 4 chicken breasts
- 1 brown onion, diced
- 2 cloves of garlic, crushed
- 1 carrot, peeled and diced
- 1 celery stalk, diced
- 1 bay leaf
- 1 sprig of fresh thyme
- 125ml (4fl oz) chicken stock
- 125ml (4fl oz) white wine
- 125ml (4fl oz) semi-skimmed milk
- 1 tablespoon cornflour

I'm going to be honest here: I have typed out an intro describing this chicken fricassée a couple of times, and although the dish is sublime, I'm yet to make the intro in any way interesting. So, because fricassée sounds like frisbee ... In the sixteen years Paul and I have been together, he's only ever caused me one direct injury: with a frisbee. On our very first holiday we took ourselves away to the seaside and, buoyed with the excitement that only dodging poos in the sea can bring you, we set about playing beach frisbee. I didn't know at this early point in the relationship that Paul can't throw, let alone frisbee, otherwise I'd have stood well back. As it was, he pitched back his arm, swung, and forgot to let go at the apex of the swing, instead electing to release about four foot from my face. The frisbee stotted (see notes) off my face, splitting open my eyebrow. I was hoping I'd be left with a sexy eyebrow scar but no, everything healed, bar perhaps Paul's self-esteem, as since then I won't let him throw a single thing without reminding him of the time he battered me with a beach frisbee. It's no life, is it?

Preheat the oven to 190°C fan/400°F/gas mark 6.

Spray a large ovenproof pan with a little oil and place over a medium-high heat. Add the chicken breasts and cook for 5–6 minutes on each side, then remove from the pan and set aside.

Add the onion, garlic, carrot and celery to the pan and cook for about 5–7 minutes, until softened. Add the bay leaf and thyme and cook for another minute.

Return the chicken to the pan, along with the stock and wine. Bring to the boil, then reduce the heat and simmer for 30 minutes.

Remove the chicken from the pan and keep aside, and discard the bay leaf and thyme sprig.

In a small jug, whisk together the milk and cornflour. Add to the pan and stir until the sauce thickens.

Return the chicken to the pan once again, then cover and bake in the oven for 30–40 minutes.

Notes: So, this is a filthy suggestion, but this served over steamy hot chips is absolutely the way forward. Purists say mash, but they can bore off.

'Stott' means 'throw' in Geordieland.

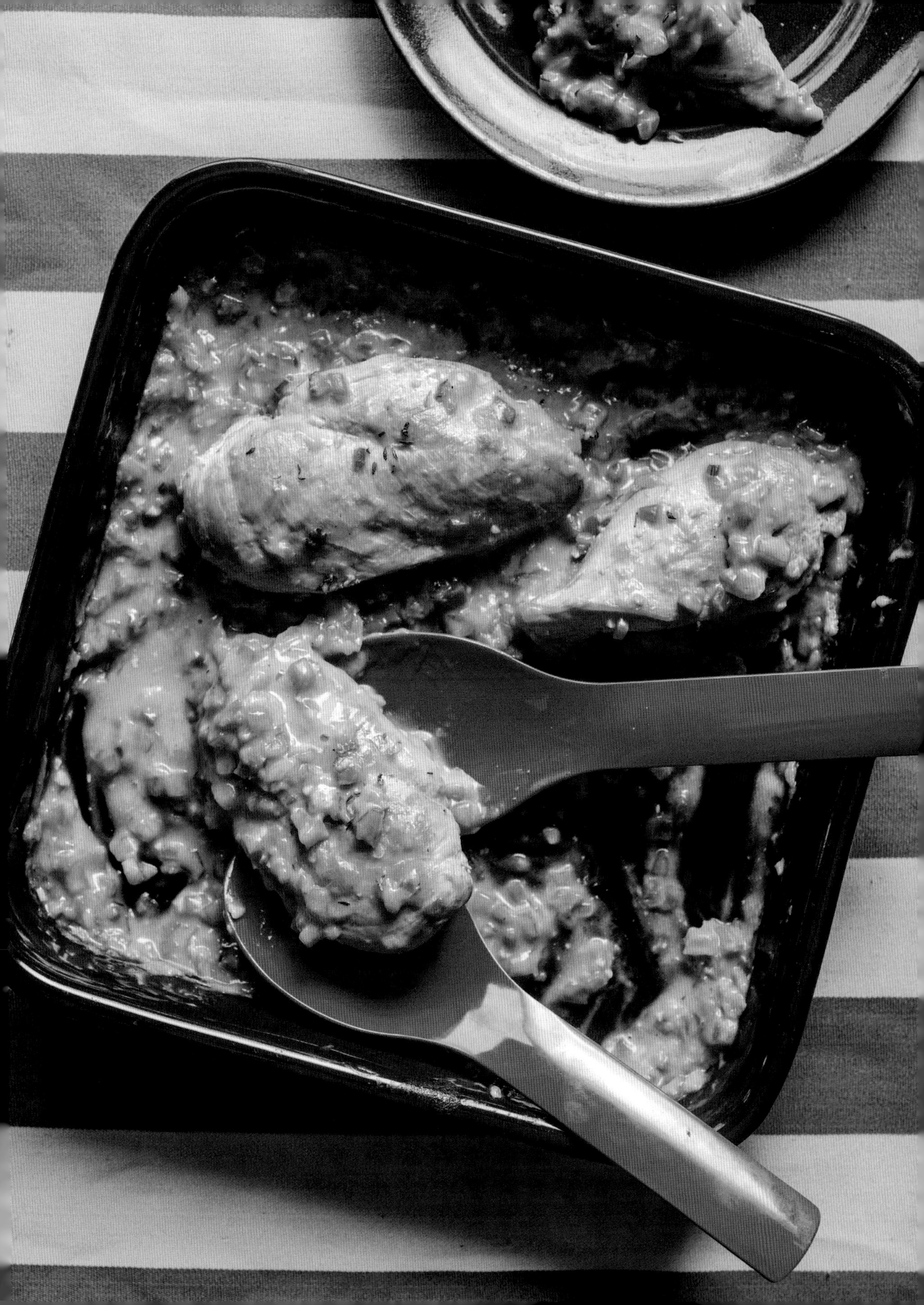

SERVES: 4
PREP: 10 MINS
COOK: 1 HR 20 MINS
CALORIES: 275

SPRING PIE

I'm not sure why Flossie (aka Paul) has called this spring pie: it could be that as a nice light dinner it'll put a spring in your step, but that seems oddly poetic for him. Maybe he knows that when spring comes, we're only a couple of months from every single person within a twenty-mile radius offering us spare courgettes? Who can say? Paul, presumably, but he's in another room and I'm just too lazy to ask. Just so we're all on the same page (very important, else how would you read the recipe), spring is, definitively, the second best season. Summer is all well and good, but I'm only ever two degrees from collapsing to the floor like Alex Mack (a reference that'll land with hardly any of you, but I'm keeping it in because I'm cool. Well, my best friend Ray thinks I'm cool). Winter I love, but I spend half the morning anxiously waiting to make sure Paul got into work – his Smart car can barely drive on a normal road, let alone an icy one. Spring is pleasant enough, but autumn, when the leaves start to turn and the air gets that fresh, chilly smell? That's my happy place.

- 3 courgettes, sliced
- 1 red onion, diced
- ½ teaspoon garlic granules
- ½ teaspoon onion granules
- 150g (5½oz) reduced-fat feta cheese
- 3 eggs, beaten
- 40g (1½oz) Parmesan cheese (or vegetarian alternative), grated
- 20g (¾oz) panko breadcrumbs
- ½ teaspoon dried mixed herbs
- 80g (3oz) mozzarella

Preheat the oven to 200°C fan/425°F/gas mark 7.

Put the courgettes and onion into a bowl with the garlic and onion granules. Spray with oil and toss until well coated.

Line a baking tray with baking paper. Spread the courgettes and onion on the tray, and bake for 20–22 minutes.

Meanwhile, mix together the feta, eggs, Parmesan, panko and mixed herbs. Gently stir in the cooked courgettes and onions, then tip the mixture into a greased ovenproof dish.

Tear up the mozzarella and spread across the top, then bake for 50 minutes.

Notes: Paul just chimed in with 'I love summer, but of course, I'm skinny now' which I think has to be one of the most passive-aggressive comments he's managed in years.

This freezes perfectly, if you have any leftovers. Ever the optimist!

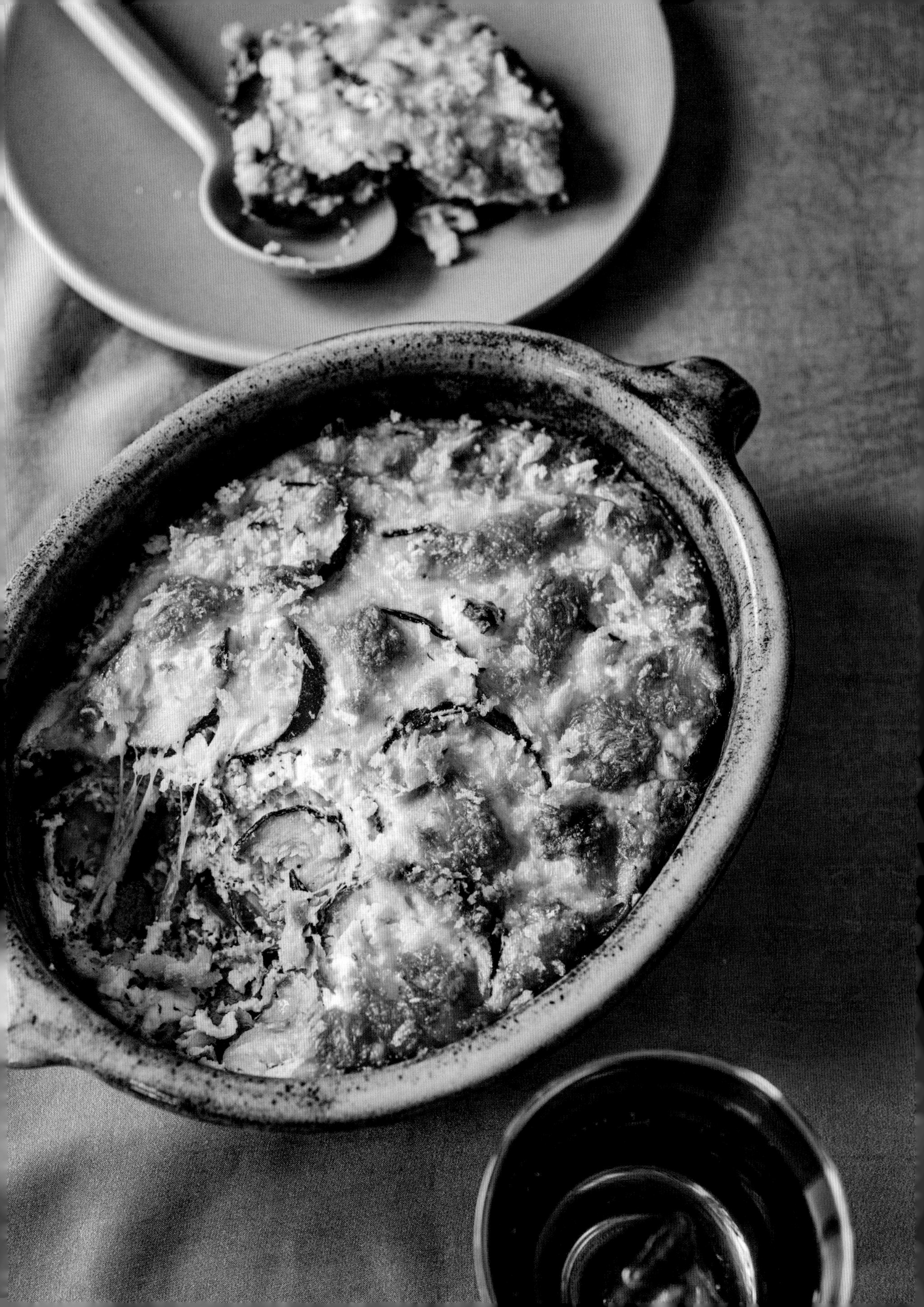

SERVES: 4
PREP: 10 MINS
COOK: 50 MINS
CALORIES: 494

30 mins, GF, DF

- 4 large peppers (any colour)
- 250ml (9fl oz) chicken stock
- 2 tablespoons tomato purée
- 180g (6oz) long-grain rice
- 500g (1lb 2oz) lamb mince
- 1 brown onion, finely diced
- 2 cloves of garlic, crushed
- 1 teaspoon ground cumin
- 1 teaspoon paprika
- ½ teaspoon ground cinnamon
- ½ teaspoon salt
- ¼ teaspoon black pepper

DELICIOUSLY DIFFERENT DOLMA

Dolmades, or stuffed vine leaves to give them their entirely non-fancy name, is easily one of our favourite dishes to find on a menu. However, finding vine leaves can be an absolute knacker, not least because Paul refuses to go into our local 'fancy' supermarket ever since one of the cashiers snootily assumed he wouldn't have a loyalty card. You can buy the leaves on Amazon, but as it goes against our 'cook with easy to find ingredients' ethos, we've swapped them out for peppers here. Trust us, it works beautifully. As a sidenote, I spotted in Paul's notes that he was struggling to find the right word for the 'foot' of a pepper, and that took me on a little bit of research because I adore learning new words. For reference, the word he is looking for is the 'apex' of the pepper.

Preheat the oven to 180°C fan/400°F/gas mark 6.

Slice the tops off the peppers, then carefully remove the seeds and scrape out the ribs from the inside with a teaspoon. Place them upright on a baking tray.

Put the chicken stock and tomato purée into a saucepan with 250ml (9fl oz) of water and bring to the boil, then add the rice. Reduce the heat and simmer for 18–20 minutes, until the rice is cooked, then drain and keep it warm in the pan.

Meanwhile, spray a large pan with a little oil. Add the mince and cook for 6–7 minutes, until browned.

Add the onion and garlic and cook for 5 more minutes, until the onion is translucent. Add the cumin, paprika, cinnamon, salt and pepper, stir, and cook for 2–3 minutes.

Add the cooked rice to the pan and stir well.

Spoon the mince mixture into the peppers (spoon any leftover mixture around the bottom of the peppers to get some lovely, crispy, nibbly bits), and bake in the oven for 30 minutes.

Notes: If you're struggling to keep the peppers standing up, slice the bottom nubs (not sure that's the correct word) to flatten them out.

We like to use lamb mince for this, but beef or vegetarian mince works just as well.

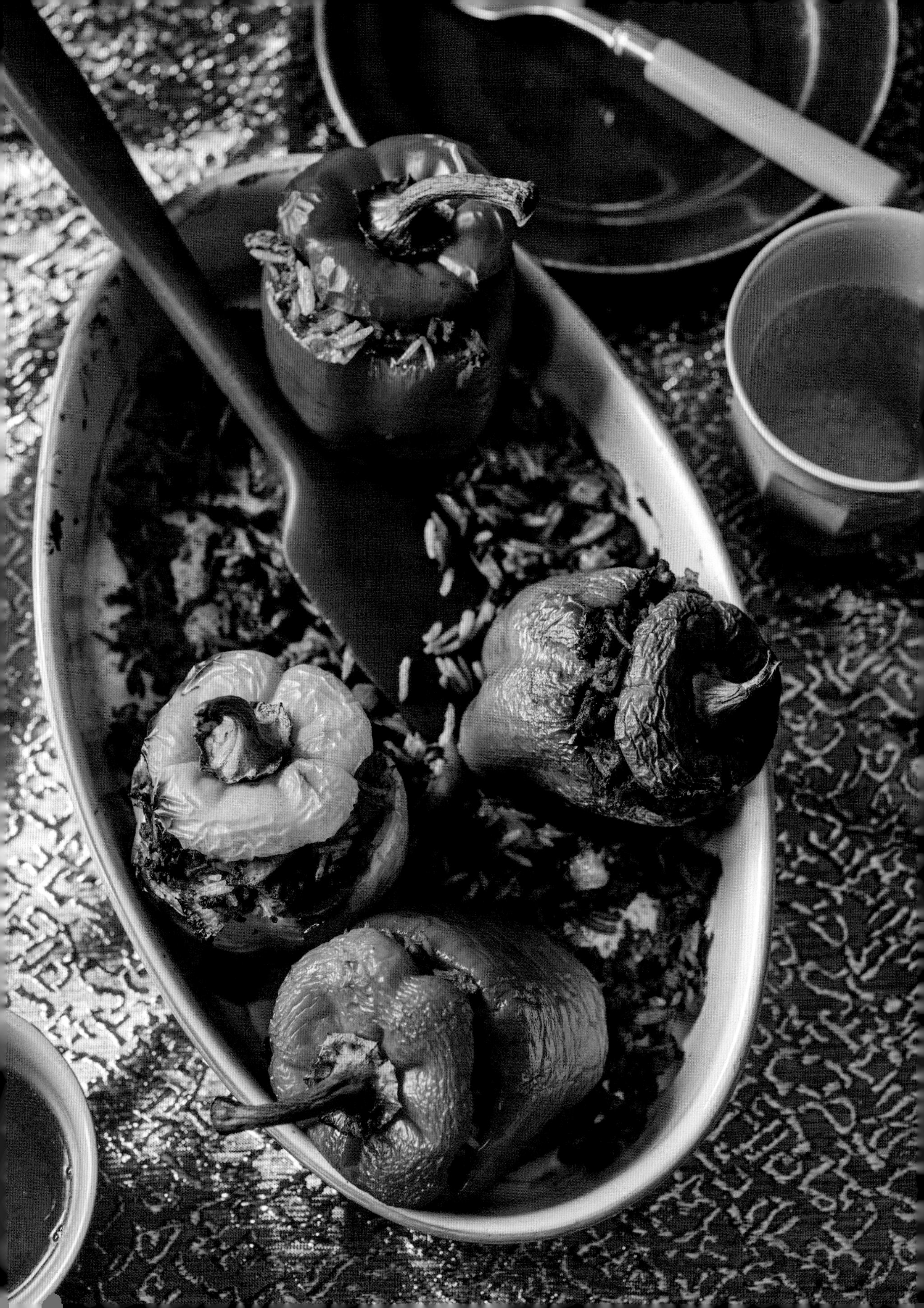

SERVES: 4
PREP: 10 MINS
COOK: 40 MINS
CALORIES: 207

30 mins, Family, V, GF, DF

PISTO

Since moving into Chubby Towers eleven years ago, I've had the grandest plans for our garden: we were to have a bountiful vegetable patch, lovely lawns and enough flowers to keep the bees bumbling all summer long. A life living like Barbara Good could have been mine, and would be perfect, as a boater is the only hat that will fit my jumbo noggin. However, last summer proved that this life was not for us. Take our vegetable patch: months of carefully tilling the soil and finding inventive ways of dispatching snails (in retrospect, the trebuchet was a mistake) yielded exactly four carrots. And we're not talking carrots that would make a judge at a village fête blush either, but more like the *Naked Attraction* studio if someone left the air-conditioner set to arctic. After a few months of looking at it furiously, and Goomba traipsing most of it into the house on his paws like he was in a reverse *Shawshank Redemption* remake, I took a huff and got rid. Of the vegetable patch, not Goomba – I'd miss his popcorn-smelling paws too much. I mention the garden only because we've finally come to a working arrangement that suits us all: the tomato hanging basket. My mum created a basket of tumbling toms, and as I write this in the middle of a long hot summer, we already have lovely little tomatoes ready for picking. Indeed, it is those that find themselves nestled in this recipe. Of course, like the proud parents we are, we must tell you how to raise your children: water regularly, tomato feed once every 2 weeks, and don't store them in the fridge. It's just common sense.

- 2 large onions, peeled
- 2 red peppers
- 2 green peppers
- 2 courgettes
- 4 large tomatoes or, as noted above, about 16 cherry tomatoes
- 4 cloves of garlic, finely diced
- 1 teaspoon salt
- 1 teaspoon black pepper
- 1 teaspoon smoked paprika
- 1 teaspoon honey
- 4 eggs

Chop all the vegetables into small pieces.

Spray a large pan with a little oil and place over a medium heat. Add the onions and garlic and cook for about 5 minutes, until the onions are translucent.

Add the peppers and courgettes and cook for a further 10 minutes, then add the tomatoes, salt, pepper, paprika and honey and cook for a further 20 minutes, stirring frequently.

Make four wells in the vegetable mixture and crack an egg into each one, then cover with a lid and cook for 3–4 minutes, until set to your liking.

Serve.

Note: You can use a tin of tomatoes instead of fresh if you prefer!

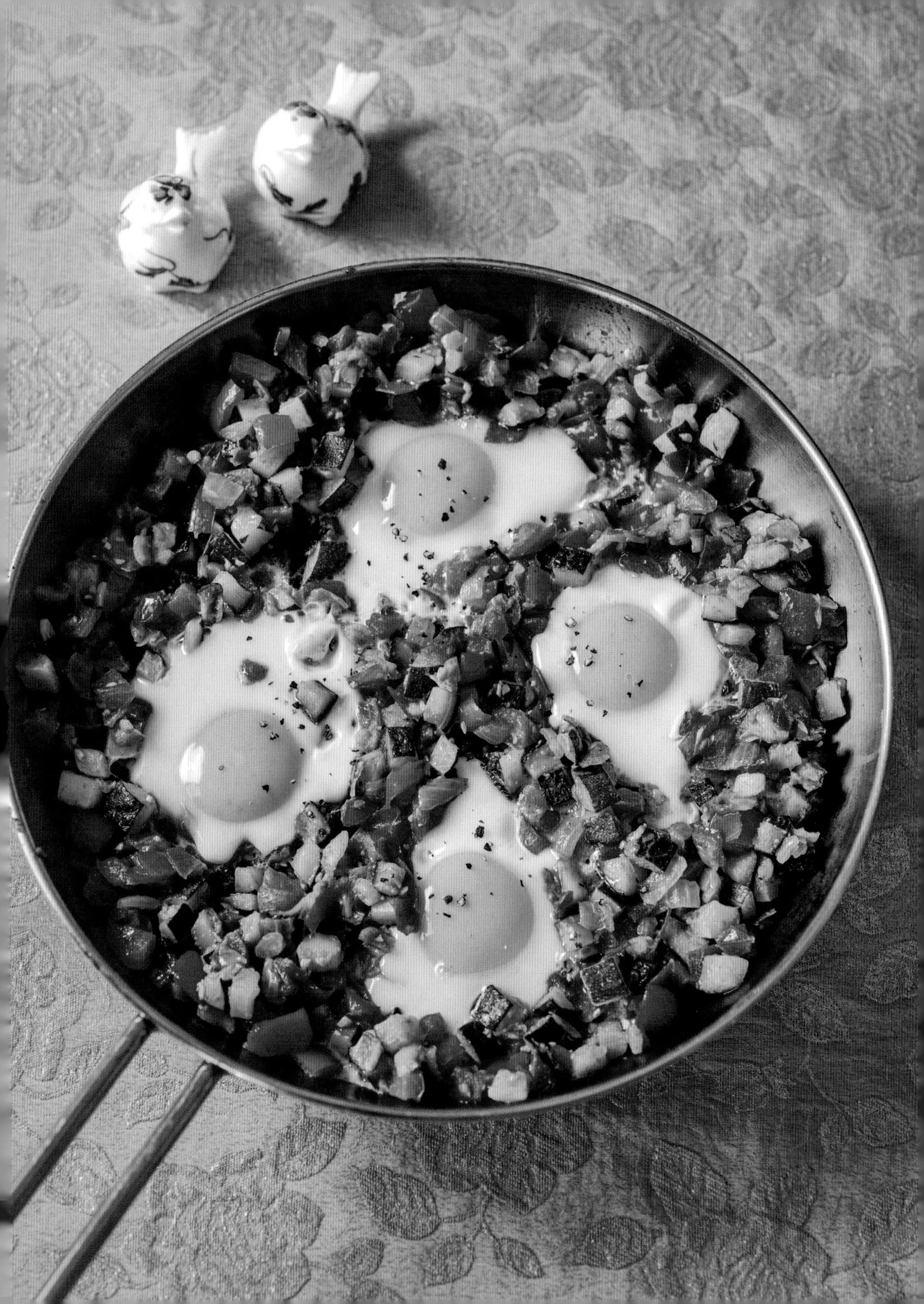

SERVES: 4
PREP: 15 MINS
COOK: 1 HR 50 MINS
CALORIES: 242

SPANISH CHICKEN & VEGETABLE STEW

A scrumptious dish that will whisk you to some sunny Spanish town without the need to get on a plane and spend three hours furiously staring at someone's hair while they drape it over the back of the seat in front. That's me exaggerating for effect, because I absolutely love flying. While I do indeed spend a good third of the flight imagining that we're only ever one loose bolt from plummeting to the ground, I've learned how to enjoy the rest of the time in the air. Have yourself a good meal, watch a couple of episodes of something you've been meaning to catch up on, then doze for the last hour or two with your eyes half-open lest you miss something from the trolley. Paul, on the other hand, always makes a friend. Because he's slender and unspeakably considerate, he always sits in the middle (which in turn allows me to gaze out of the window as though I'm leaving Walford in an *EastEnders* special) and, as a result, invariably ends up with a Chatty Cathy sat next to him. Paul hates small talk, but will end up gassing away and chortling for the entirety of the flight. If by a fluke you're one of the many folks who have become his best friend over the years, get in touch. We'll make you this chicken and vegetable stew by way of apology.

- 4 boneless chicken thighs
- 1 brown onion, diced
- 1 clove of garlic, crushed
- 1 red pepper, deseeded and sliced
- 1 yellow pepper, deseeded and sliced
- 1 courgette, sliced
- 1 × 400g (14oz) tin of chopped tomatoes
- 250ml (9fl oz) chicken stock
- 1 teaspoon smoked paprika
- 1 teaspoon ground cumin
- ½ teaspoon salt
- ¼ teaspoon black pepper

Spray a large pan with a little oil and place over a medium-high heat. Add the chicken and cook for 5 minutes on each side until nicely browned, then remove from the pan and set aside.

Add the onion and garlic to the pan and cook for 3 minutes. Add the peppers and courgettes and cook for 5 minutes, stirring occasionally, then add the tomatoes, stock, paprika, cumin, salt and pepper and stir well.

Put the chicken back into the pot and bring to a simmer. Reduce the heat to low, cover with a lid, and cook for 1 hour, stirring occasionally.

Remove the lid and cook for another 30 minutes.

Serve.

Notes: You'll see from the method that this is a very low-maintenance, low-prep dish. That extends to the ingredients: feel free to chuck in anything that looks vaguely healthy from your freezer. Case in point: a handful of frozen peas is never a bad addition.

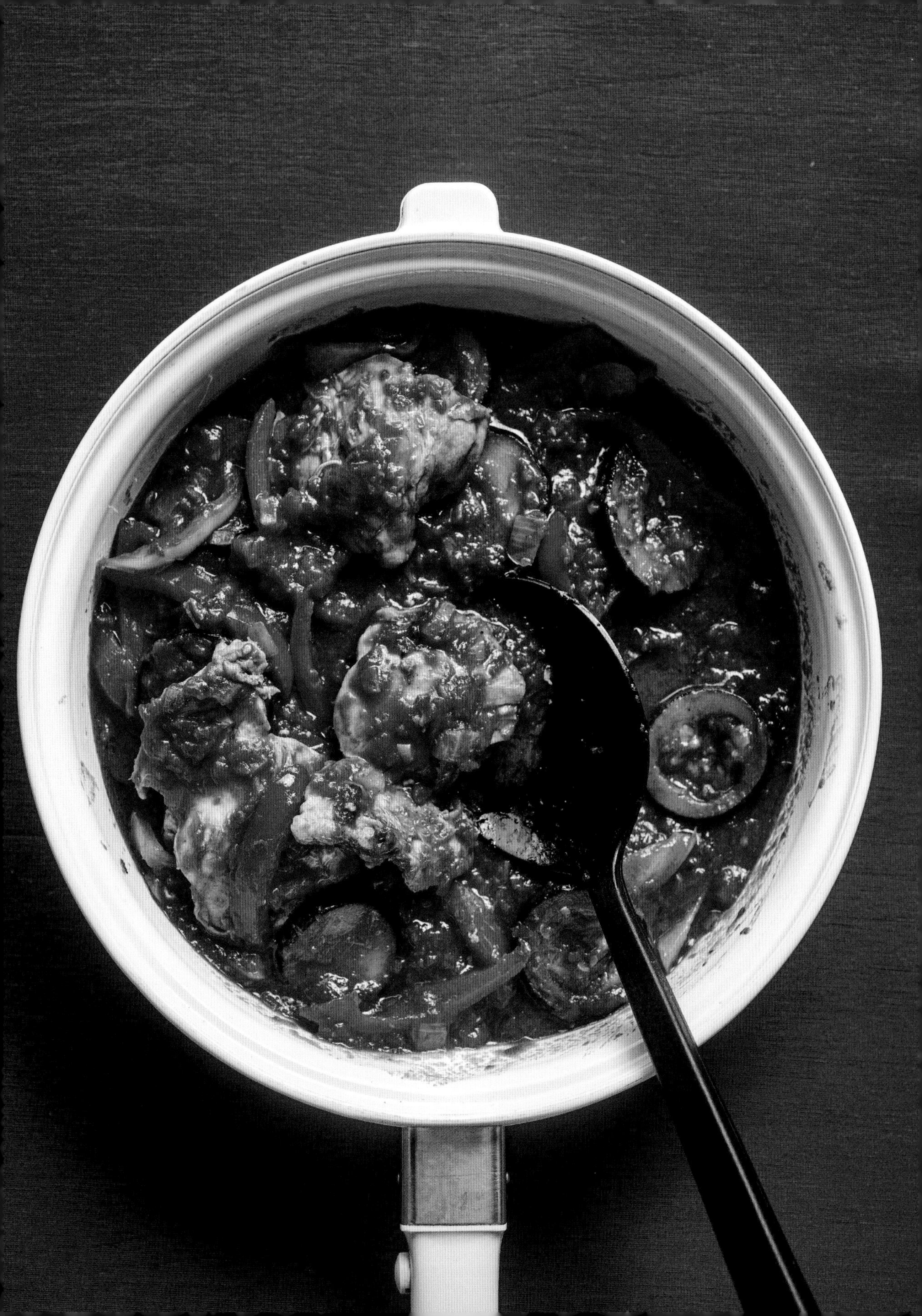

SERVES: 6
PREP: 10 MINS
COOK: 3 HRS 30 MINS
CALORIES: 500

30 mins 10 DF

- 30g (1oz) plain flour
- 1.4kg (3lb 2oz) beef roasting joint
- 2 brown onions, quartered
- 2 large carrots, peeled and sliced
- 4 cloves of garlic, crushed
- 500ml (18fl oz) beef stock
- 1 tablespoon fresh rosemary, chopped
- 2 bay leaves
- 440g (15½oz) potatoes, diced

LAZY ROAST BEEF

This is the sister recipe to the Lazy Roast Chicken recipe in our previous cookbook, *Dinner Time*: if only to give you an option for a Sunday when you're feeling especially languorous. There's always a time and a place for a lengthy roast dinner, served in a dazzling array of dishes while your face looks as though you've been staring into a nuclear explosion, but sometimes quicker is better. We would love to hear other variations on this recipe if you make them!

Preheat the oven to 150°C fan/325°F/gas mark 3.

Spray a large ovenproof pan with a little oil and place over a medium-high heat.

Sprinkle the flour on a plate and roll the beef in it until well coated. Put the beef into the pan and cook for 4–5 minutes per side, to brown, then remove and set aside.

Add the onions, carrots and garlic to the pan and cook for 3–4 minutes. Add the stock, stir to deglaze, bring to the boil, then stir in the rosemary, bay leaves and potatoes.

Put the beef back into the pan, reduce the heat to low and cover with a lid. Transfer the dish to the oven and cook for 3 hours.

Remove the beef from the pan and roughly tear with two forks, then return it to the pan and serve.

Notes: This makes a huge amount and is perfect with whatever you like – we particularly love it with mash and with a few other vegetables to make it into a roast dinner, but it's also great in sandwiches and wraps.

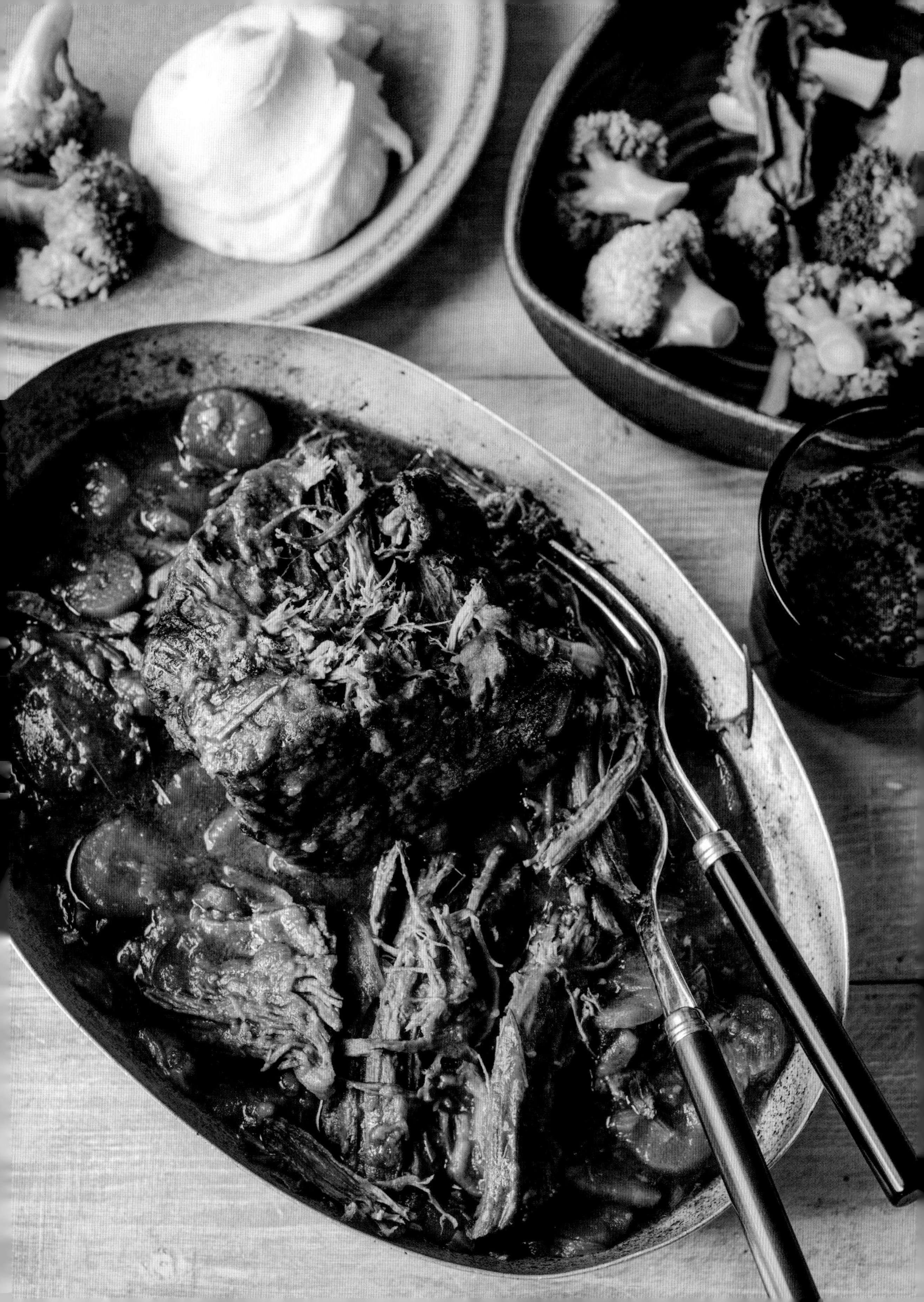

SERVES: 4
PREP: 10 MINS
COOK: 1 HR 30 MINS
CALORIES: 467

- 2 aubergines, sliced into 5mm (¼ inch) rounds
- 500g (1lb 2oz) lean lamb mince
- 1 brown onion, sliced
- 3 cloves of garlic, crushed
- 1 × 400g (14oz) tin of chopped tomatoes
- 1 tablespoon tomato purée
- 1 teaspoon ground cinnamon
- 1 teaspoon dried oregano
- ½ teaspoon salt
- ¼ teaspoon black pepper
- 2 tablespoons butter
- 2 tablespoons plain flour
- 250ml (9fl oz) semi-skimmed milk
- 40g (1½oz) Parmesan cheese, grated
- 1 egg

MOUSSAKA

As this is a lengthy recipe with a lot of steps (though you'll note, the actual preparation time is quite short and fragmented), we will keep the intro short. We used to make the sauce with blended-up tinned macaroni cheese thinned with milk, if you can believe. Clearly these days we know better, and we present you with a traditional, tasty and perfectly freezable dinner. Oh, though, such a dry intro with no obvious Greek puns? My Apollo-gies.

Preheat the oven to 190°C/400°F/gas mark 6.

Line a baking sheet with baking paper and spread out the slices of aubergine. Sprinkle them with a little salt and bake for 20 minutes, turning them halfway through.

Meanwhile, spray a pan with a little oil and place over a medium heat. Add the lamb mince, onion and garlic and cook until the lamb is browned.

Add the chopped tomatoes, tomato purée, cinnamon, oregano, salt and pepper and stir, then simmer for 10 minutes.

In a separate saucepan, melt the butter over a low heat, then add the flour and whisk until smooth. Increase the heat and slowly add the milk, whisking continuously, until the sauce thickens.

Remove from the heat and stir in the Parmesan and egg.

Layer half of the cooked aubergine slices in the bottom of a 28 × 21cm (11 × 8 inch) ovenproof dish. Top with the lamb, then layer with the remaining aubergine.

Pour the cheese sauce over the top and bake in the oven for 40–45 minutes.

Note: This also works well with beef mince.

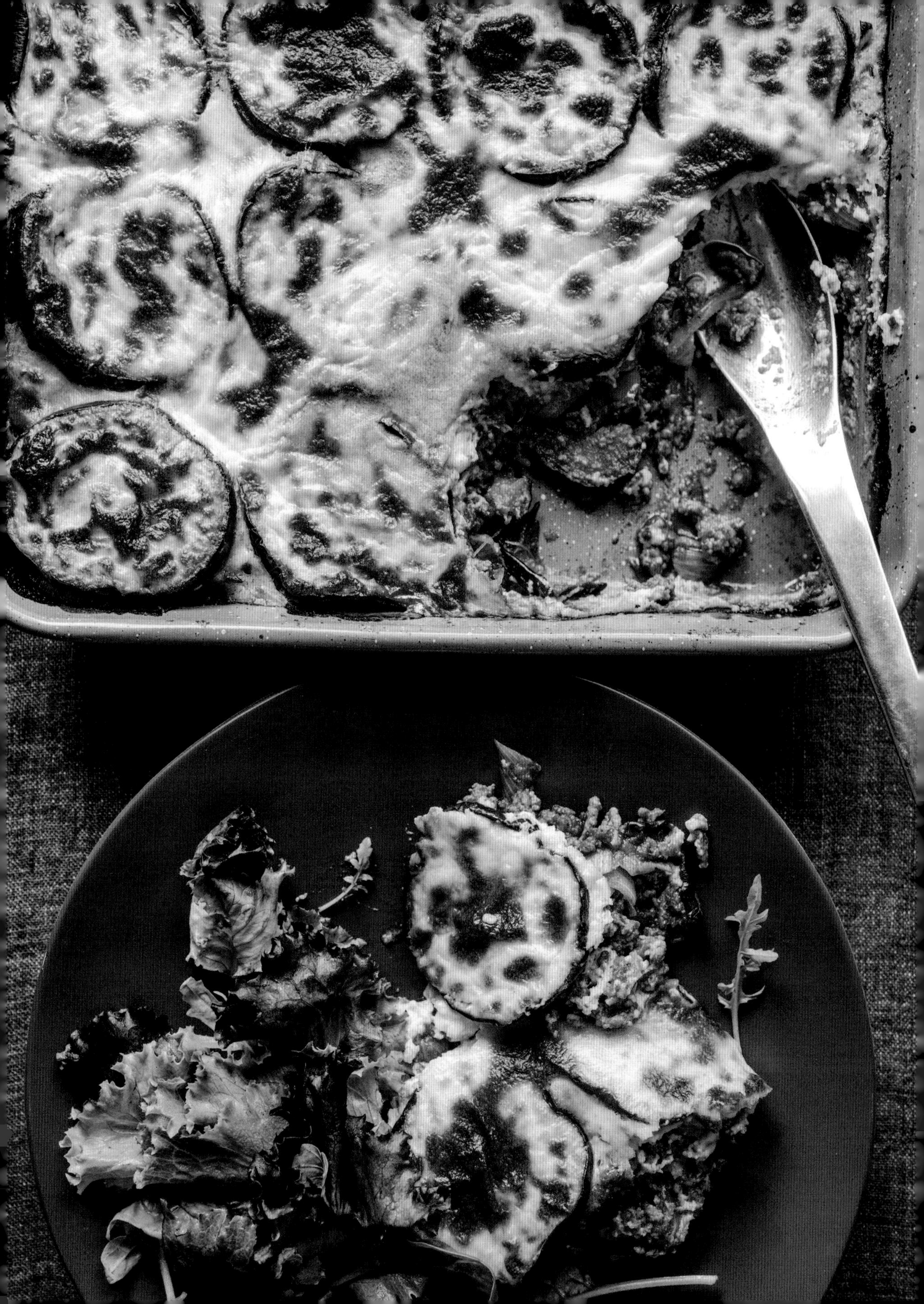

SERVES: 4
PREP: 10 MINS
COOK: 1 HR 30 MINS
CALORIES: 405

↑30 mins ❄ GF DF

- 100g (3½oz) chorizo, sliced
- 6 boneless chicken thighs
- 1 brown onion, diced
- 2 cloves of garlic, crushed
- 1 red pepper, deseeded and sliced
- 1 × 400g (14oz) tin of chopped tomatoes
- 1 teaspoon paprika
- 1 teaspoon dried oregano
- 1 bay leaf
- 400ml (14fl oz) chicken stock
- a handful of fresh parsley (optional)

CHICKEN & CHORIZO STEW

We've been cooking with chorizo for as many years as we have been together, and it was only a couple of months ago when I sat in the kitchen to keep Paul company / make sure I got my fair share that I realised you're supposed to peel off the casing. I had no idea! What followed was a full and frank discussion about how silly I was, and my, admittedly poor, defence, that life is too short to skin a chorizo. Well, good news: some internet research has pulled up that although it is recommended, you're not going to keel over and die. Luckily, if that does happen, you'll have had a wonderful final meal, assuming you chose this chicken and chorizo stew to go out with.

Place a large pan over a medium heat. Add the chorizo and cook for 2–3 minutes, then add the chicken and cook for 4–5 minutes on each side. Remove the chicken and chorizo from the pan and set aside.

Add the onion, garlic and red pepper to the pan and cook for 5–7 minutes.

Add the tinned tomatoes, paprika, oregano, bay leaf and stock and bring to a simmer.

Put the chicken and chorizo back into the pan and cover with the sauce, then simmer for 1 hour.

Serve topped with a handful of parsley (if using).

Note: Paul mocks, but I've received a text from him stating that I'm a 'pre-Madonna' – he maintains it was an error in dictation, but we both know. We know.

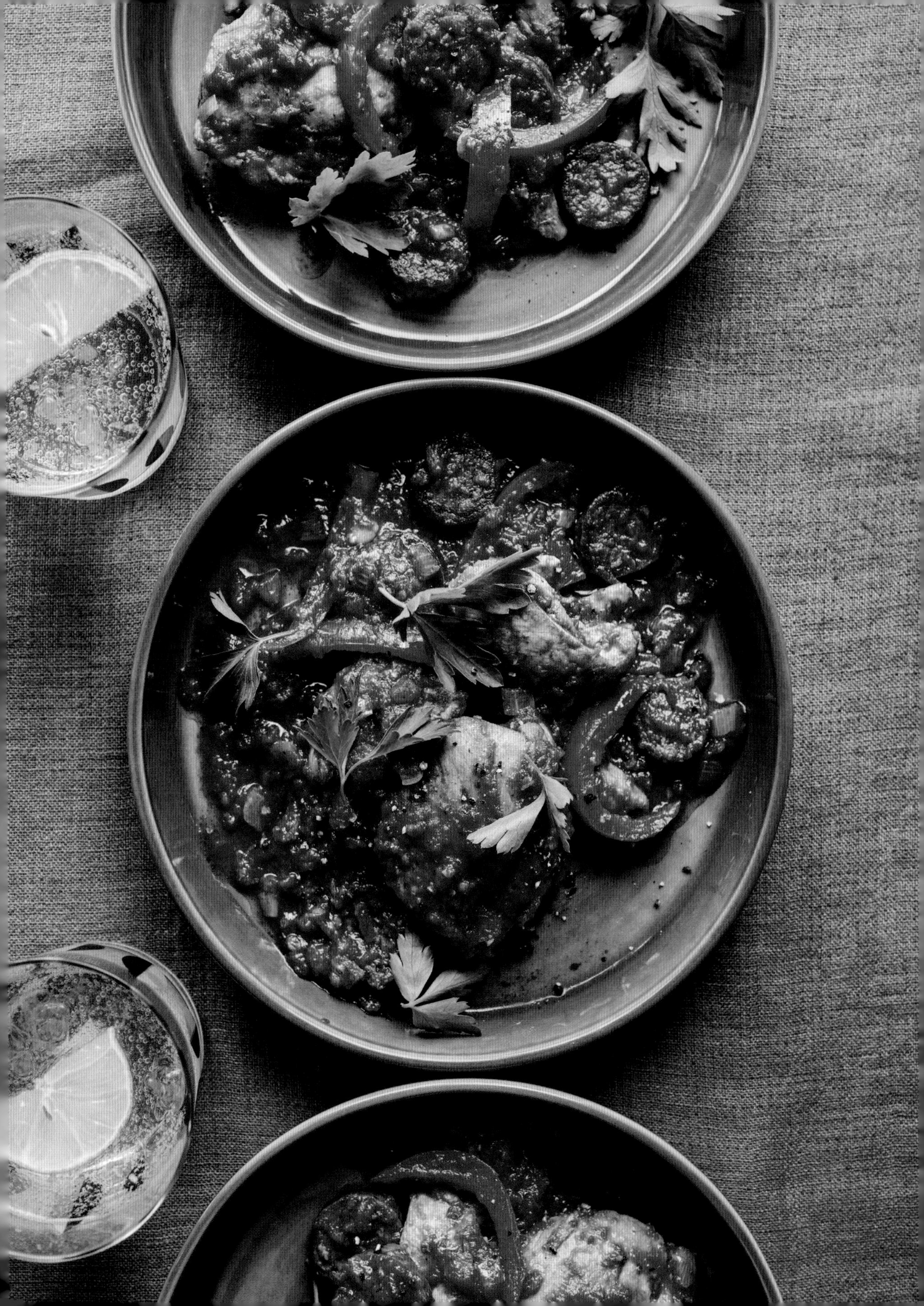

SERVES: 4
PREP: 15 MINS
COOK: 1 HR 10 MINS
CALORIES: 372

FANCY FISH FILL-UP

The word 'fancy' is doing a lot of heavy lifting here: as with all of our recipes, there's nothing fancy about it, but I'm a stupendously super sucker for alliteration, so we're running with it. I mean we sprinkle a packet of crisps on the top of it, for goodness' sake, we're aware of what we are. You could very easily turn this into a more substantial dish by mashing up some potatoes and spreading that on the top to turn it into more of a pie, but we like the simplicity of this as it is. It almost goes without saying that although we have given a recommended amount of cheese, we both expect and encourage you to double or triple the amount.

- 20g (¾oz) butter
- 1 small brown onion, finely chopped
- 2 cloves of garlic, crushed
- 2 tablespoons cornflour
- 1 tablespoon Dijon mustard
- 2 tablespoons dry white wine
- 320ml (10½fl oz) semi-skimmed milk
- 50g (1¾oz) Parmesan cheese, grated
- 60g (2oz) reduced-fat Cheddar cheese, grated
- 1 teaspoon dried thyme
- 600g (1lb 5oz) cod fillets (see notes), cut into 2.5cm (1 inch) chunks
- 1 bag of ready-salted crisps, crushed

Preheat the oven to 180°C fan/400°F/gas mark 6.

Place a saucepan over a medium heat and add the butter. Let it melt, then add the onion and garlic and cook for 3–4 minutes, until the onion is translucent.

Add the cornflour and whisk continuously for about a minute, then add the mustard and mix well. Add the wine (or water if you prefer) and whisk continuously, until smooth, for around 2 minutes, then add the milk and continue to whisk until the mixture starts to thicken.

Add half the Parmesan and a quarter of the Cheddar, along with the thyme, and stir until melted and smooth.

Spread the fish evenly in the bottom of a medium baking dish and pour over the cheese sauce mixture. Mix well, spread the mixture out evenly, then sprinkle over the rest of the Parmesan and Cheddar, and the crushed crisps.

Bake in the oven for 45–50 minutes.

Notes: As always, any white fish will do here – cod, pollock, haddock, basa – use whatever you have! If you're using frozen fish, make sure it's fully defrosted.

No wine? Sherry will do, but if you've none of that either, feel free to leave it out. We've had the same four bottles of sherry on the go for years now: when we moved in, we found all manner of hard liquor secreted around the place courtesy of the old dear who lived here before. Every time we think we're running low, we'll move an old suitcase in the garage and discover another one. It's marvellous!

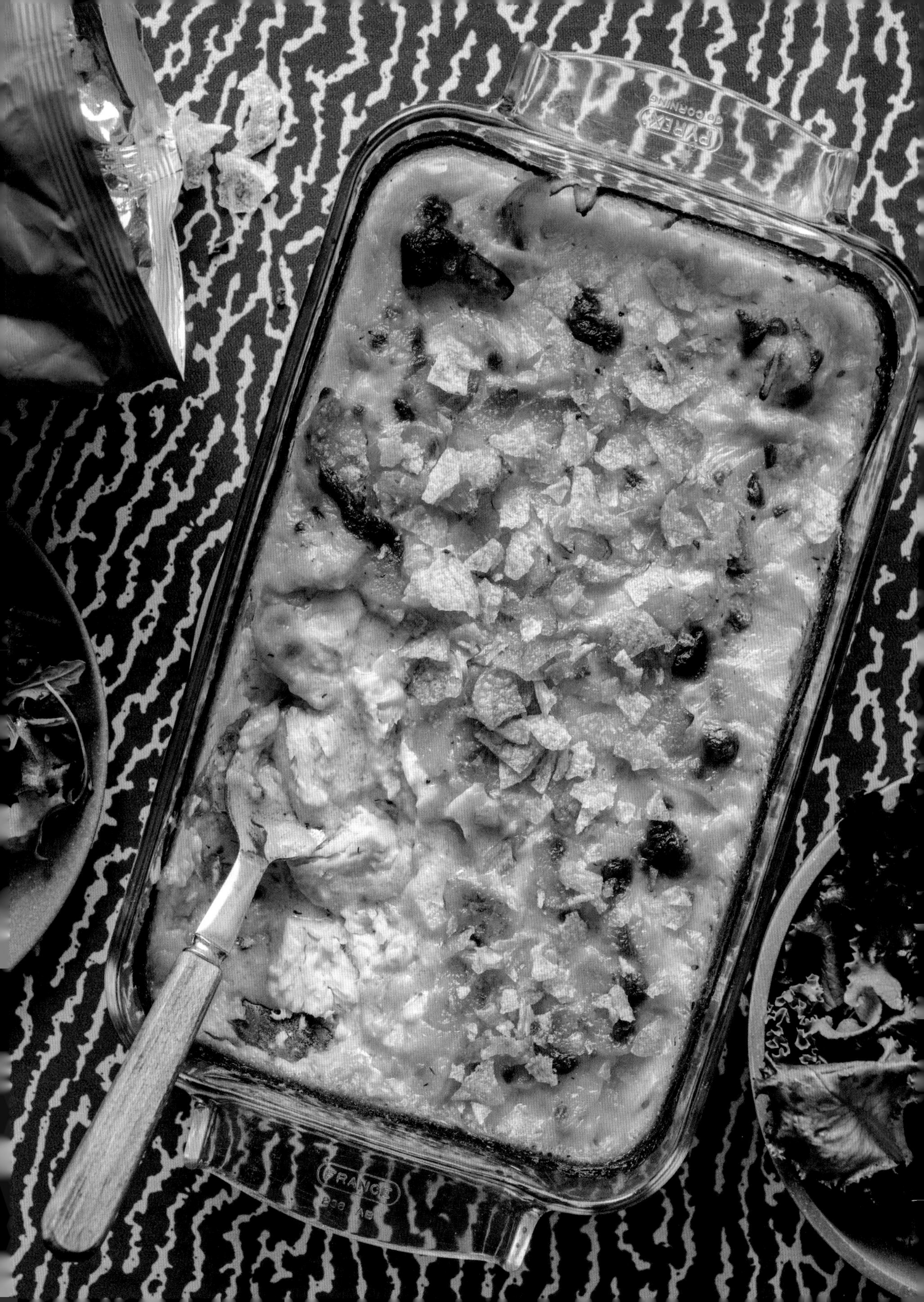
PYREX
FRANCE

LEMON & GARLIC CHICKEN STEW

SERVES: 4
PREP: 10 MINS
COOK: 25 MINS
CALORIES: 498

GF DF

2 onions, finely diced
750g (1lb 10oz) skinless, boneless chicken thighs
5 cloves of garlic, crushed
185ml (6½fl oz) chicken stock
1 teaspoon dried parsley
1 teaspoon salt
¼ teaspoon paprika
juice of 1 lemon
200g (7oz) long-grain rice
4 teaspoons cornflour

A pressure cooker recipe for this wonderfully saucy and simple stew, because we do love them so, though Paul has taken pains to explain how you could easily do it on the hob if you didn't have a hissing doom contraption to hand. I jest of course: your modern pressure cooker, assuming you haven't ordered it off a dodgy website and paid £4.87 for it, is a perfectly safe and very efficient way to cook food. People remain confused and befuddled by them and what they do, but the easiest explanation is: they're like an anti-slow cooker. If slow cooking is all about cooking for ages on a low heat, a pressure cooker is cooking for a vastly reduced time under high pressure. I mean, the clue is in the name. Pretty much anything you can do on the hob for a few hours can be thrown into a pressure cooker for twenty minutes or so, although always check the instructions. And, as we always find ourselves saying, they're safe. Gone are the days when a clattering tin-pot would be hissing and shrieking on the hob. Our pressure cooker even serves a dual purpose as an air fryer. Give it a year or two and it'll probably drive itself to the supermarket to pick up the ingredients.

Set your pressure cooker to 'sauté' and spray with a little oil. Add the onions and cook for 5–10 minutes.

Add everything else, apart from the rice and cornflour, and give it a good stir. Seal the cooker and cook under high pressure for 15 minutes, and when finished use 'quick release'.

Meanwhile, cook the rice according to the instructions on the packet.

When the chicken has cooked and the pressure has been released, scoop out about half a mugful of the cooking liquid and mix it with the cornflour, making sure there are no lumps.

Remove the chicken from the pan and set aside, then pour in the cornflour mix, stirring until the sauce has thickened slightly.

Serve the chicken on top of the rice, and ladle over the sauce.

Note: No pressure cooker? Nee worries pet, just cook everything (add an extra 50ml/2fl oz of stock) in a lidded casserole dish in the oven at 170°C fan/375°F/gas mark 5 for about 2 hours, following the same steps for the cornflour.

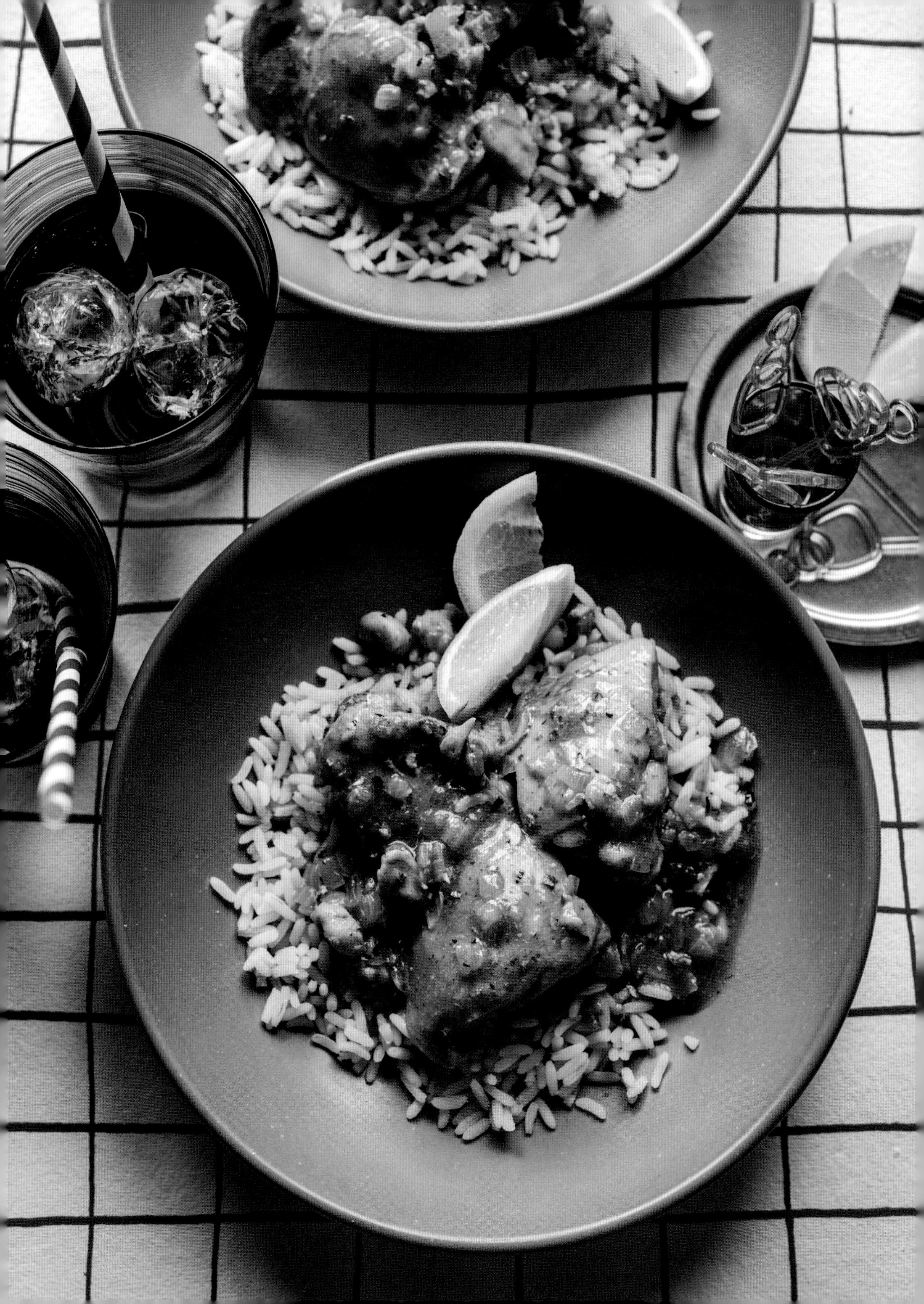

SERVES: 4
PREP: 10 MINS
COOK: 1 HR 10 MINS
CALORIES: 466

30 mins · DF

SAUSAGE COLCANNON BAKE

This is pure comfort, and the dish Paul will make for me if he knows I'm having a rough day. A bowl of this is just the thing for curling up and feeling sorry for yourself with. Now, in every book, I've used one of the intros to mix up my constant teasing of Paul and say something lovely, and I won't be breaking with tradition here. He is the real hero of our partnership. I come out with the funny words (occasionally, admittedly), but he's the one tinkering with recipes, cooking all the meals, going to work so I can do what I wish. He never grumbles, he never complains, just plods through life being Paul, the kindest, sweetest bloke you could ever hope to meet. He listens to my nonsense, calms my anxieties, and best of all, if I come to bed after him of an evening (happens quite a lot, as he needs to be up early), he will always shuffle over like a walrus in his sleep and grab hold of my little roll of belly-flab. People like me – sarcastic and teasing and endlessly anxious – are ten-a-penny, but Paul is an absolute diamond. Once this book is published and he's reading all my bits (he doesn't like to do so beforehand, he likes the surprise), he'll chastise me for this sentimentality, but you know what, he deserves it. Everyone, be more Paul!

- 8 reduced-fat sausages
- 6 medium potatoes, cut into large chunks (skins on)
- 80g (2¾oz) kale or spring greens
- 1 egg
- 1 large onion, sliced
- 2 tablespoons plain flour
- 500ml (18fl oz) beef stock
- 125g (4½oz) mushrooms, sliced
- 100g (3½oz) frozen peas
- 1 teaspoon Worcestershire sauce
- 1 bay leaf

Preheat the oven to 200°C fan/425°F/gas mark 7.

Put the sausages into an ovenproof dish and cook in the oven for 25–30 minutes, turning halfway. Set aside and reserve the dish for later.

Boil the potatoes in a large pan of water. Reduce the heat and simmer for 15 minutes, then drain and put back into the pan. Meanwhile, put the kale (or spring greens) into another pan and add a splash of water. Cook over a high heat for 3–4 minutes, until softened.

Crack the egg into the potatoes, then add the kale and a pinch of salt and pepper, mash together, and set aside.

Spray a large pan with a little oil and place over a medium-high heat. Add the onion and cook for about 10 minutes, until starting to caramelise. Add the flour and stir for about a minute, then slowly pour in the stock a little at a time, until thickened. Add the cooked sausages along with the mushrooms, peas, Worcestershire sauce and bay leaf, and mix well.

Tip the sausage mixture into the ovenproof dish and top with the mash, spreading it evenly across the top (drag a fork across the top to get those nice crispy bits). Bake in the oven for 20–25 minutes, and serve.

Note: Don't be too much like Paul, though: the world isn't ready for that many pastel-coloured canvas shorts.

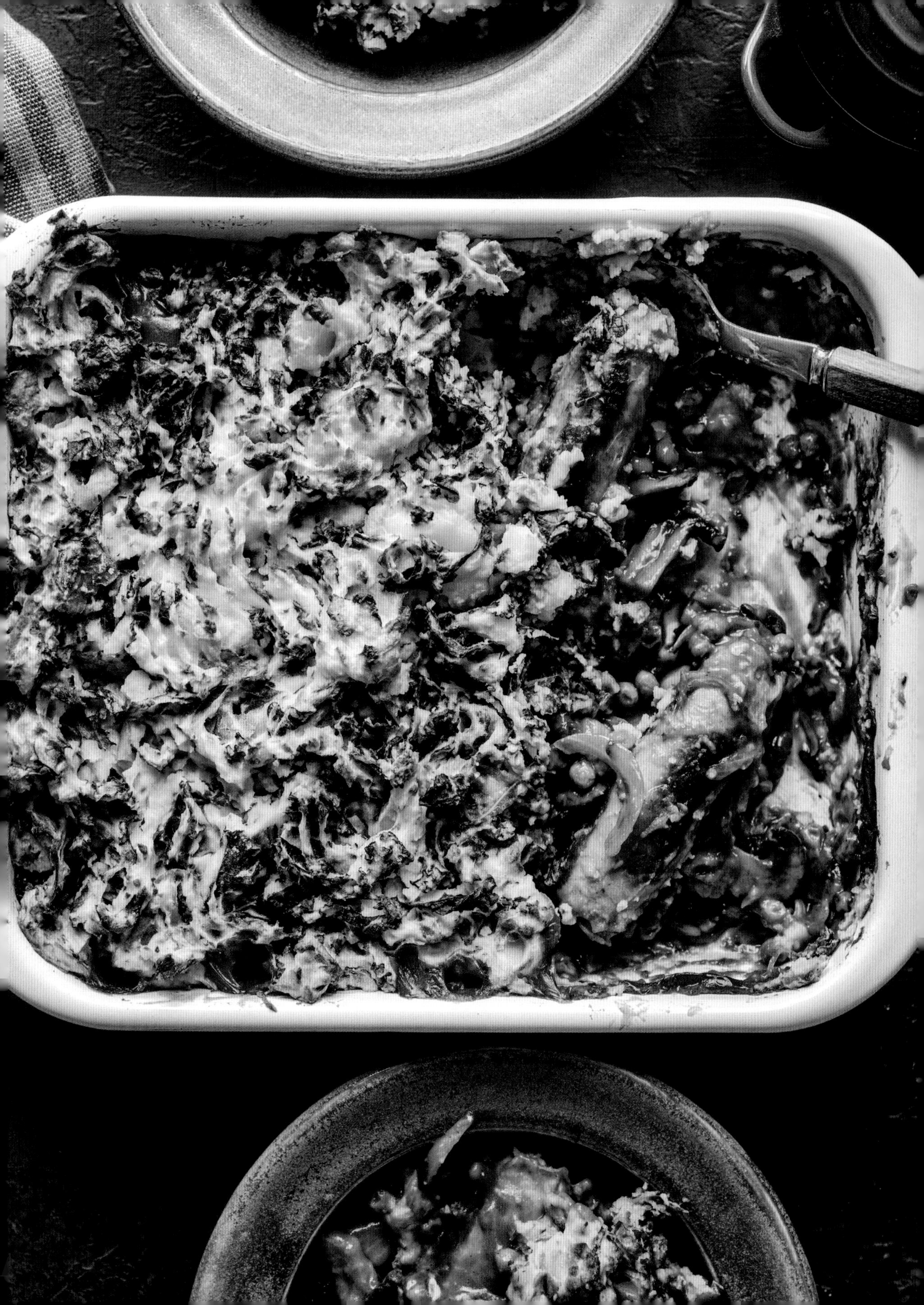

SERVES: 4
PREP: 10 MINS
COOK: 1 HR 20 MINS
CALORIES: 460

4 baking potatoes
4 reduced-fat sausages
1 brown onion, diced
1 clove of garlic, crushed
1 × 400g (14oz) tin of kidney beans in chilli sauce
1 × 400g (14oz) tin of chickpeas, drained
2 tablespoons Worcestershire sauce
200g (7oz) chopped tomatoes
1 red pepper, deseeded and sliced
½ teaspoon Marmite
1 tablespoon sriracha

ONE-POT SAUSAGE & BEANS

A jacket potato, served with a perfect topping, is a thing of wonder – and lord knows we don't have them enough in our house. If you're equally all about saving money, stick a load of jacket potatoes in the oven at once. It'll take a little longer, but once they're done, spare jacket potatoes freeze beautifully – just wrap them up in foil once they're cooled and then try to eat them within six months. Similarly, this bean and sausage mix works well if you scale up the ingredients, cook a big panful, and then freeze for later use. Oh, and a final tip! We used to buy our beans and peas from a well-known brand and pay through the nose for the privilege. No need: have a look in the world food aisle in your supermarket and you'll find giant tins of both, considerably cheaper.

Preheat the oven to 200°C fan/425°F/gas mark 7.

Prick the potatoes all over, spray them with a little oil and sprinkle them with salt. Put them into the oven and bake for 1 hour–1 hour 20 minutes.

Meanwhile, spray a large pan with a little oil and place it over a medium-high heat. Add the sausages and the onion and cook for 15–20 minutes, until cooked.

Remove the sausages from the pan and slice thinly, then set aside.

Add the garlic to the onion in the pan and cook for 30 seconds, then add the kidney beans, chickpeas, Worcestershire sauce, tomatoes, red pepper, Marmite and sriracha and give it all a good mix.

Put the sausages back into the pan, then reduce the heat to a low simmer and cook until the potatoes are ready.

Cut a cross in the top of each potato, open them up, and top with the sausage and bean mix.

Notes: Not a fan of chickpeas? A tin of baked beans works just as well!

Not a fan of Marmite? Then take yourself to the foot of the stairs and think about what you've done.

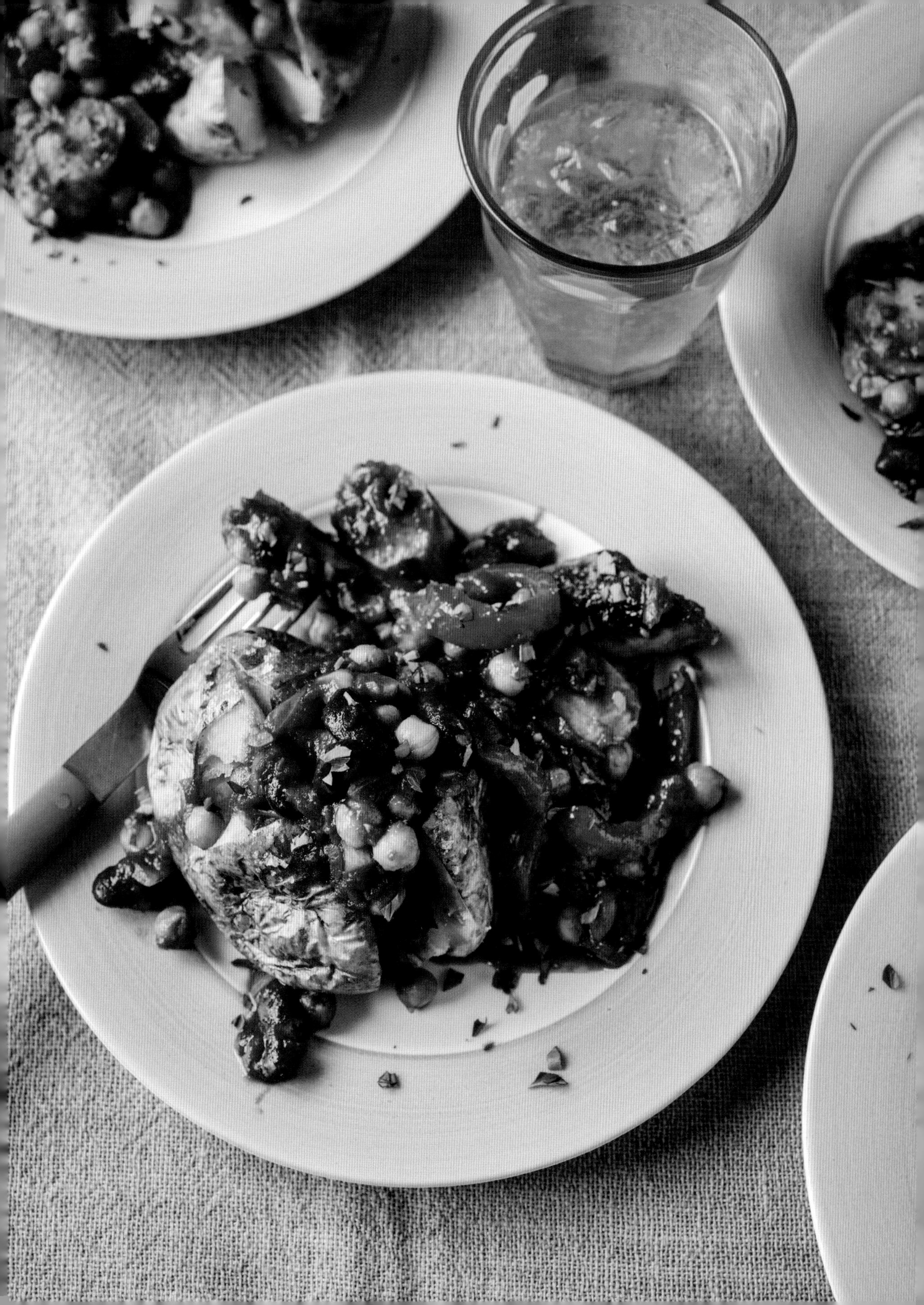

SERVES: 4
PREP: 15 MINS
COOK: 8 HRS
CALORIES: 498

PORK & APPLE STEW

Seeing as we included a pressure cooker recipe earlier, it makes sense to balance it out with a slow cooker recipe for this terrific pork and apple stew. A proper winter warmer, though don't restrict yourself to seasonal eating. If you don't have a slow cooker, fret not, just reduce the cooking time down to an hour or so and hubble-bubble it on the hob. Paul and I had the bright idea of getting up at insane-o'-clock and travelling to our local car-boot sale a few weeks ago (I mention this purely because I think it was the Actual Law to have a slow cooker on your selling table). We had no big purchases planned and just wanted to have a nosey and a burger that contained less meat than the grass we were standing on, but still, even with those lowest of expectations, managed to leave disappointed. We went expecting to find treasure, we came away realising that your average British household has four slow cookers, two toastie makers and a collection of DVDs that even the most remote petrol station wouldn't put up. Still, live and learn.

- 450g (1lb) diced pork
- 300g (10½oz) baby carrots
- 1 onion, diced
- 2 celery stalks, finely sliced
- 250ml (9fl oz) apple juice
- 150ml (5fl oz) chicken stock
- 3 green apples, peeled, cored and quartered
- 1 tablespoon wholegrain mustard
- 2 teaspoons dried thyme
- 2 tablespoons reduced-fat crème fraîche
- 2 teaspoons cornflour
- 2 sprigs of fresh sage (optional)

For the mash

- 800g (1lb 12oz) potatoes, peeled and cut into chunks
- 15g (½oz) butter
- 40ml (1.3fl oz) milk

Chuck everything except for the crème fraîche, cornflour and sage into a slow cooker and cook on low for 8 hours (or high for 4 hours).

When the stew is about half an hour away from being ready, bring a large pan of water to the boil and add the potatoes. Cook for 15–20 minutes, until tender, then drain and mash with the butter and milk.

When the stew is cooked, stir the cornflour into a little cold water until dissolved, then pour into the stew and stir until nicely thickened.

For an extra flourish, if you like, spray a frying pan with a little oil and place over a high heat. Add the sage leaves and cook for no more than 10–15 seconds, so they're nice and crispy.

Serve the stew with the mash and top with the sage leaves.

Notes: If you want to make this a little naughtier, swap the apple juice for cider.

The sage leaves are worth the effort, but feel free to leave them out if you don't have them to hand.

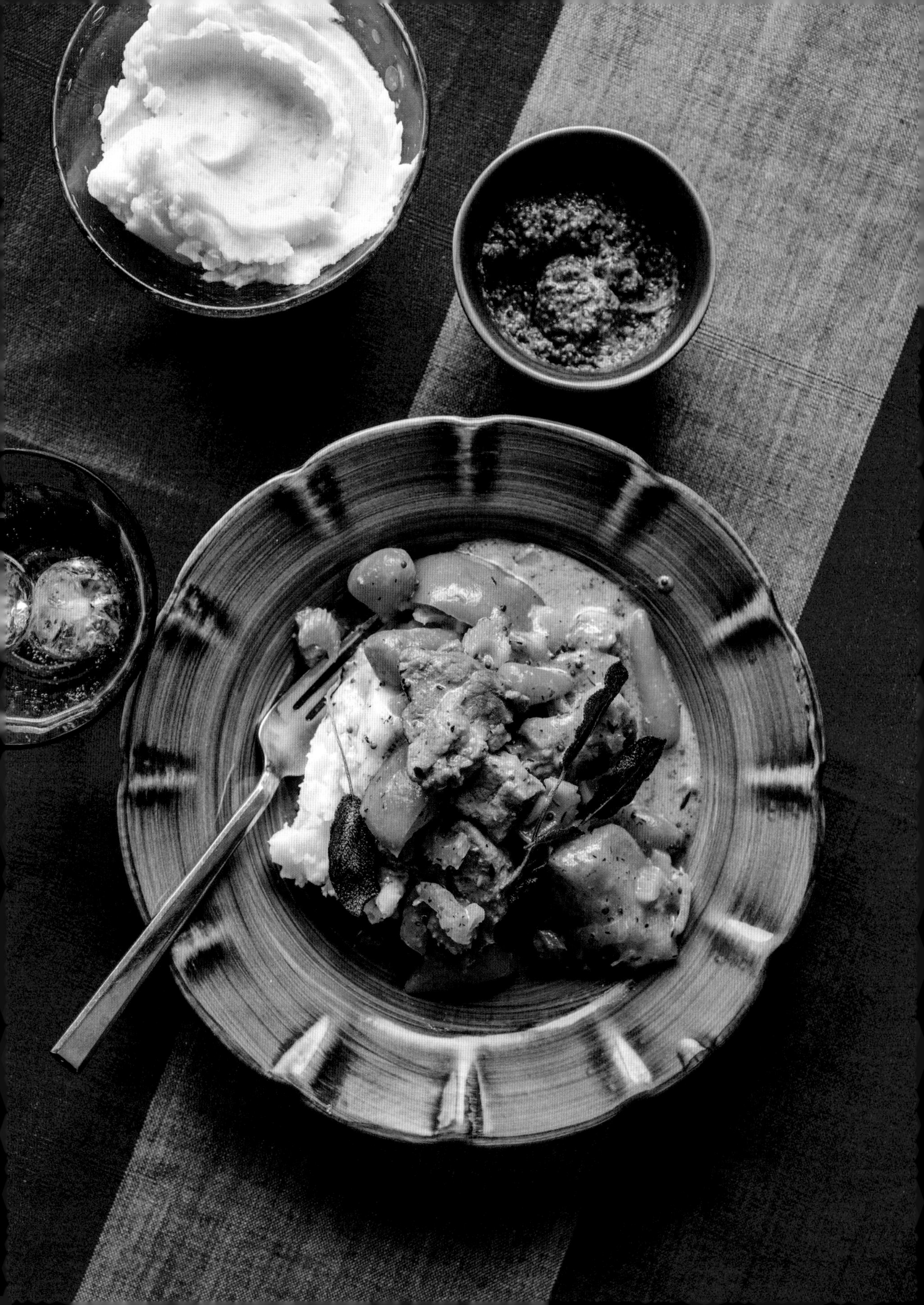

SERVES: 4
PREP: 15 MINS
COOK: 30 MINS
CALORIES: 420

30 mins · ❄ · GF

PIZZA-STUFFED MEATLOAF

You can't beat a simple, tasty meatloaf, can you? Although turns out you can if you cram a load of cheese, ham and basil into the middle, perfect for eating and then wondering why your right arm hurts at 3am in the morning. You know what we would love, though? Meatloaf and gravy served in one of those wonderful American diners you see in the movies, with red and white chequered floors, coffee served from a bottomless glass pitcher and all sorts of bleary-eyed chaps taking a break from falling asleep at the wheel of their 18-wheelers to choke down a burger. You can see the waitress, can't you? A lady called Flo or Val or Dolly or Marge who last took her make-up off in 1978 and who calls you darlin' with every enquiry. We want meatloaf in this roadside utopia, followed by a slab of cherry pie with the crisscrossing pastry on the top. Then we'd leave, sated and elated, and promptly get hit by one of those 18-wheelers I mentioned before. But what a way to go! Anyhoo, the meatloaf . . .

- 4 tablespoons tomato purée
- 1 tablespoon cider vinegar
- 1 teaspoon dried oregano
- 500g (1lb 2oz) beef mince
- a few slices of ham
- 70g (2½oz) reduced-fat mozzarella
- 30g (1oz) Parmesan cheese, grated
- a handful of fresh basil leaves

Preheat the oven to 190°C fan/400°F/gas mark 6.

In a small bowl, mix together the tomato purée, vinegar and oregano to make a paste – add more vinegar or water if you need to thin it a bit.

Lay out some baking paper and shape the mince into a rectangle shape, about 23 × 18cm (9 × 7 inches). Spread 2 tablespoons of the tomato mix over the mince, leaving about 1cm (½ inch) uncovered around the edge.

On one half of the mince rectangle, layer on a few slices of ham, half the grated mozzarella and half the Parmesan.

Use the baking paper to help you 'fold' over the uncovered half on top of the other half, and pinch together the seams to form a meatloaf. Carefully move it on to a baking sheet.

Spoon the rest of the tomato mix on top of the meatloaf and sprinkle over the remaining cheese and some salt and pepper.

Cook in the oven for about 30 minutes, then remove and top with the basil leaves to serve.

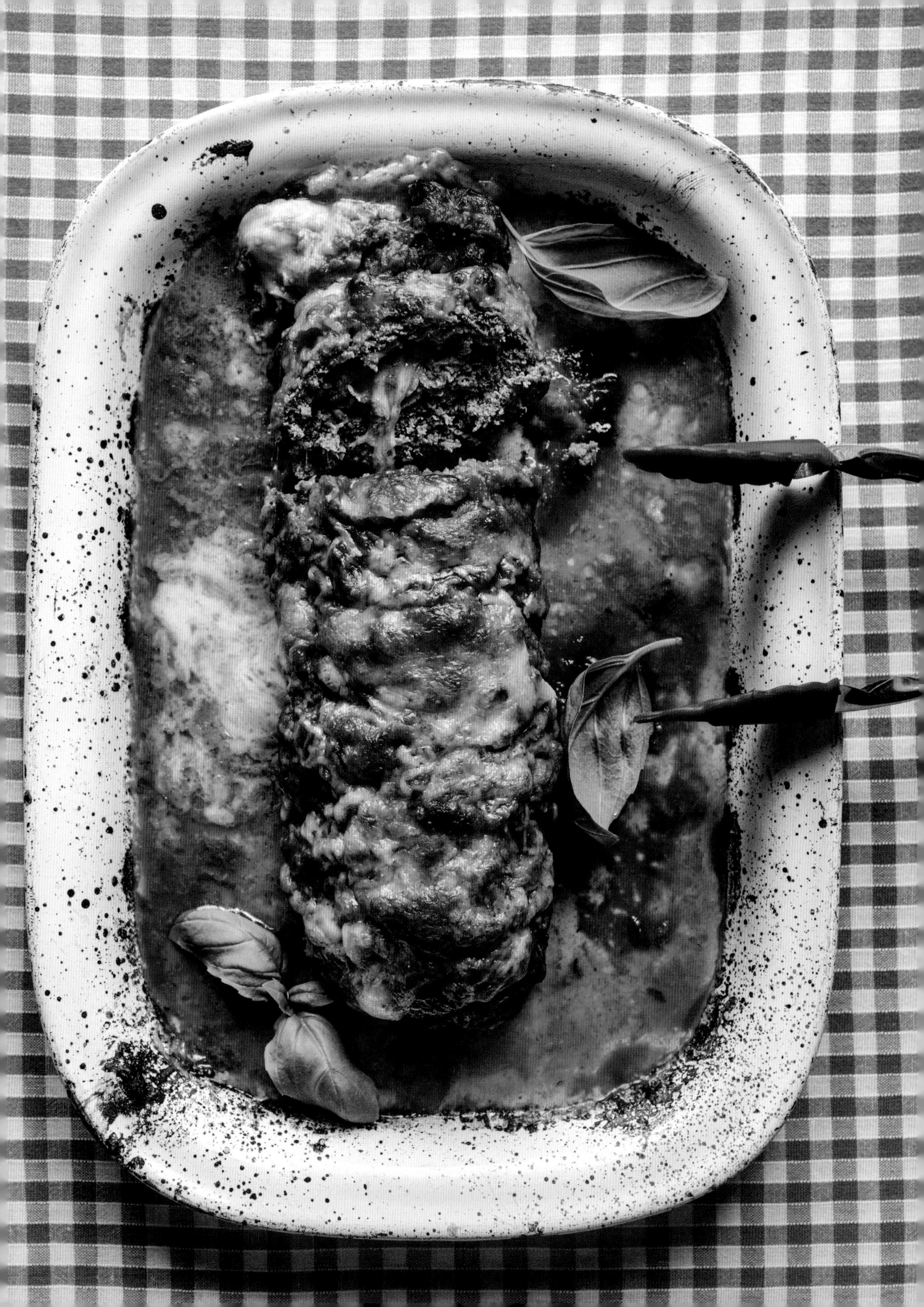

SERVES: 4
PREP: 5 MINS
COOK: 1 HR
CALORIES: 434

THICC CHICKEN

It seems like Paul is determined in each of our books to give our recipes titles that make me wince and demand an explanation for those of you not conversant with the modern vernacular. He certainly didn't learn his lesson with green eggs and fam from *Dinner Time*: I had to sit him down and explain that he's about as urban and street as a shopping spree around a Cotton Traders outlet store. Bless. But here he is again with 'thicc chicken' – to be fair to the little stinker, this recipe is indeed chicken in a very thick sauce, so he's halfway right. Thicc is just a way to passively-aggressively wind me up when I come to writing these introductions, because he knows I hate it. See, when people say thicc (and doubly so when they say '*thicccccccccc*', lisping those Cs like Sylvester the Cat trying to be seductive), they mean big and juicy. So you can perhaps imagine the conversations in which the word appears, and frankly I'm just too old for any of that nonsense. Not too old for this chicken dinner, though, because I promise you this: it's incredible – if this doesn't end up on your regular rotation, then we will never agree on anything.

- 15 cherry tomatoes, halved
- 4 chicken breasts
- 70g (2½oz) plain flour
- 4 cloves of garlic, crushed
- 150ml (5fl oz) vegetable stock
- 150g (5½oz) natural yoghurt
- 1 teaspoon tomato purée
- 1 tablespoon mixed herbs
- 1 teaspoon dried chilli flakes
- 100g (3½oz) sun-dried tomatoes, drained and chopped
- fresh basil leaves
- 30g (1oz) Parmesan cheese, grated

Preheat the oven to 140°C fan/325°F/gas mark 3.

Place the cherry tomatoes in a small baking tray, drizzle with a little olive oil, salt and pepper, and roast for 45 minutes.

Sprinkle the chicken breasts with a little salt and pepper and toss in the flour, then set aside.

Spray a large frying pan with a little oil and place over a medium-high heat. Add the chicken and cook for 4–5 minutes on each side, then remove to a plate.

Put the pan back over the heat. Add the garlic and cook for 1 minute, then add the vegetable stock, yoghurt, tomato purée, mixed herbs and chilli flakes, stir well, and simmer for 4–5 minutes.

Add the sun-dried tomatoes, put the chicken back into the pan, stir and cook for a few more minutes.

Serve, with the roasted cherry tomatoes, basil leaves and Parmesan scattered over.

Notes: Buy yourself a basil plant and once you have finished it, pop the plant on a saucer and water it regularly from the bottom – it'll last you all summer long. Or, buy a jar of pesto. Less maintenance!

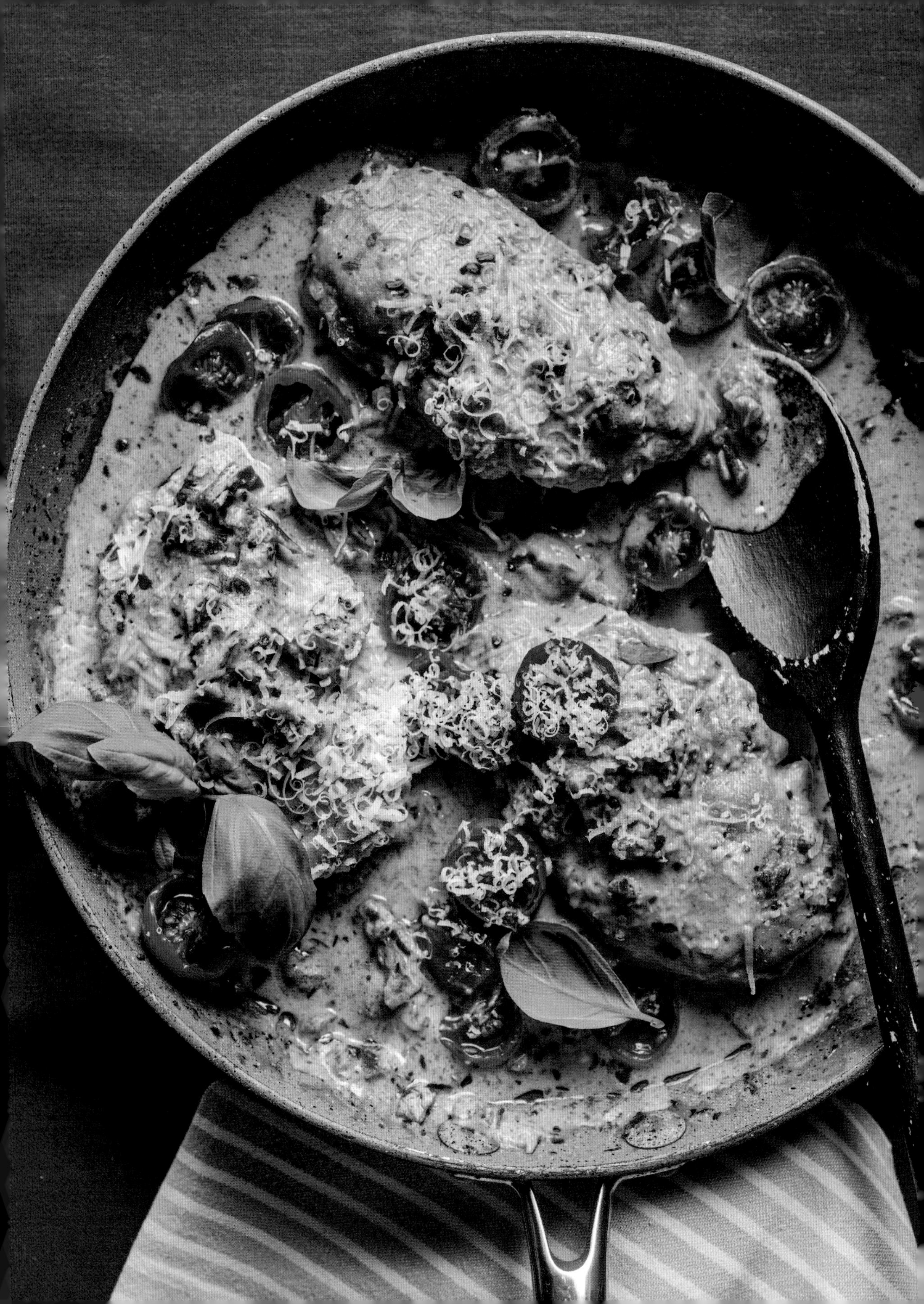

SERVES: 4
PREP: 15 MINS
COOK: 2 HRS 15 MINS
CALORIES: 500 (OURS), 338 (NAN'S)

30 mins · GF

ANN'S CORNED BEEF HASH

The second contender in the Battle of the Nanas (explained on page 52) comes from the Nan of the Queen of the Emotional Support Potatoes (book one), Paul Hawkins (46) (approx.). You can see her battle card for her official stats, and we need to keep this intro short to fit it all on the page so I'll say only this: we've included her traditional and delicious recipe *and* the gussied-up version if you're fancying something a little more decadent. I say decadent: it has crisps on it.

OUR WAY

- 700g (1lb 9oz) potatoes (we use Maris Piper)
- 1 egg and a splash of milk
- 2 large onions
- 1 × large tin of reduced-fat corned beef
- 200g (7oz) reduced-fat extra mature Cheddar cheese
- chilli sauce, as much as your arse can handle
- optional: one bag of Walkers Max Flame Grilled Steak Crisps

Make the mash by boiling chunks of potato (don't peel them) until soft and mashing them up with an egg and some milk, plus salt and pepper to taste.

While the mash is cooking, finely dice your onions and fry gently until golden and soft.

In a big bowl, mix the mash, corned beef and half the cheese together, seasoning to taste.

Slop into a baking dish and cover with the rest of the cheese and, if using, the crisps – but crunch the crisps up first so they go into wee tiny bits.

Pop into the oven on about 170°C fan/375°F/gas mark 5 for 30 minutes, covering the top with foil for the first 20 minutes so the crisps don't burn. Feel free to finish it off under the grill to make it super crispy.

Serve with beans if you like, but we prefer just old-fashioned chilli sauce.

NAN'S WAY

- 700g (1lb 9oz) potatoes (we use Maris Piper) – peel them!
- a good knob of butter and a splash of milk
- 1 × tin of reduced-fat corned beef
- 100g (3½oz) extra mature Cheddar cheese

Peel your potatoes and cut into chunks, then boil until softened. Add milk and butter until creamy. Mash in a tin of corned beef. Top with grated cheese and grill until crispy.

Notes: Serve with beans for the traditional, serve with beans and chilli sauce for the fancy version.

Paul kindly volunteered up his nan's recipe here: partly because he wants to keep her sweet for any inheritance dividends, partly because he forgot to put his own recipe in because there was something more interesting to consider on the internet for six whole months.

ANN "BRUISER" NETHERCOT

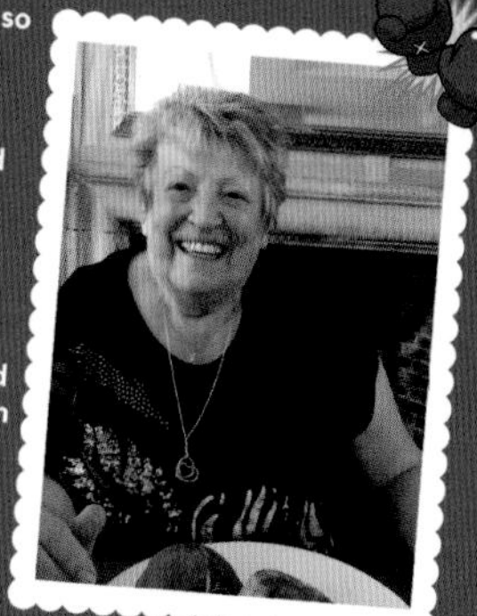

Ann to her friends, and so Mrs Nethercot to you, loves nothing more than being around family. As long as they're quiet and well-behaved, and they're out of the door before the Emmerdale theme tune kicks in.

Despite nearing the grand old age of [redacted], Ann remains a competent and definitely not terrifying force behind the wheel of her souped up motor, a go-faster silver Hyundai.

FIGHTER STATS

PREFERRED TITLE	NAN
HOLIDAY STYLE	INEBRIATED
WARS SURVIVED	WW2, FAMILY
COVID JABS	7 AND RISING
GRANDCHILDREN	10

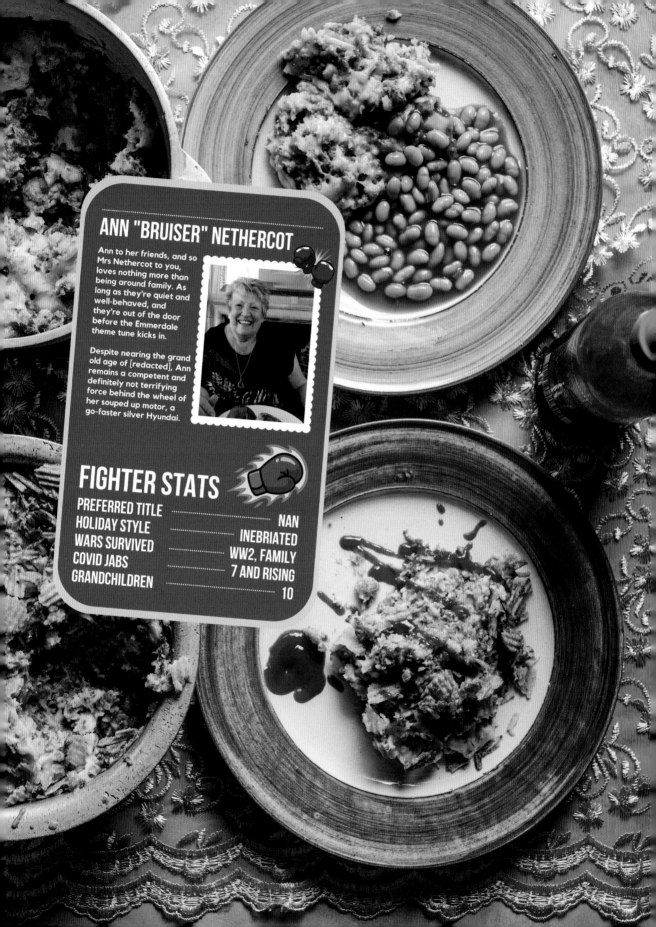

SERVES: 4
PREP: 15 MINS
COOK: 50 MINS
CALORIES: 361

- 150g (5½oz) cooked rice
- 50g (1¾oz) mushrooms, finely diced
- ½ brown onion, finely diced
- a handful of spinach leaves
- 50g (1¾oz) mozzarella, torn into small chunks
- 20g (¾oz) panko breadcrumbs
- 20g (¾oz) Parmesan cheese, grated
- 1 teaspoon salt
- ½ teaspoon black pepper
- 4 chicken breasts

CHICKEN ROLL-UPS

These tasty little chicken numbers are absolutely terrific – a personal favourite of ours if you're after a high-protein, simple enough to make dinner that you can serve with a simple salad – but boy howdy do they need a better name. Roll-ups make me think of two things: one I can't really describe in a family cookery book, the other smoking: neither of which scream good health. It baffles the both of us that we used to be such committed smokers: even when times were incredibly tight or we were poorly sick, resources would always be found to fund our habit. We've long since quit (although I've replaced one deleterious habit with another and can now be found entering rooms in a cloud of menthol mojito, as though I'm a minty magician), and the key thing we found was how much better everything tasted. It perhaps goes some way to explaining why some of the very early recipes on the blog were either incredibly bland or seasoned to the point they were almost sentient. If that isn't a reason to give up, what is? Perhaps you can think of a more charming name, then: if so, do let us know.

Preheat the oven to 190°C/400°F/gas mark 6.

In a bowl, mix together the cooked rice, mushrooms, onion, spinach, mozzarella, panko, Parmesan, salt, pepper and a drizzle of olive oil.

Lay the chicken breasts on a chopping board. Using a rolling pin (or the bottom of a heavy pan), bash them until they're around 5mm (¼ inch) thick. Alternatively, butterfly the breasts and then bash them.

Spoon some of the rice mixture on to each chicken breast and roll up tightly, securing with toothpicks if needed.

Place the chicken roll-ups in a baking dish and bake in the oven for 45–50 minutes, or until cooked through.

Notes: These are lovelier still cooled down and taken into work for a quick lunch the next day, we might add.

Forgive us for the gentle nag, but if you were thinking about giving up, we can't recommend Allen Carr's Easy Way to Stop Smoking *enough. Although we've both had little wobbles since, it made a frighteningly daunting task into nothing at all.*

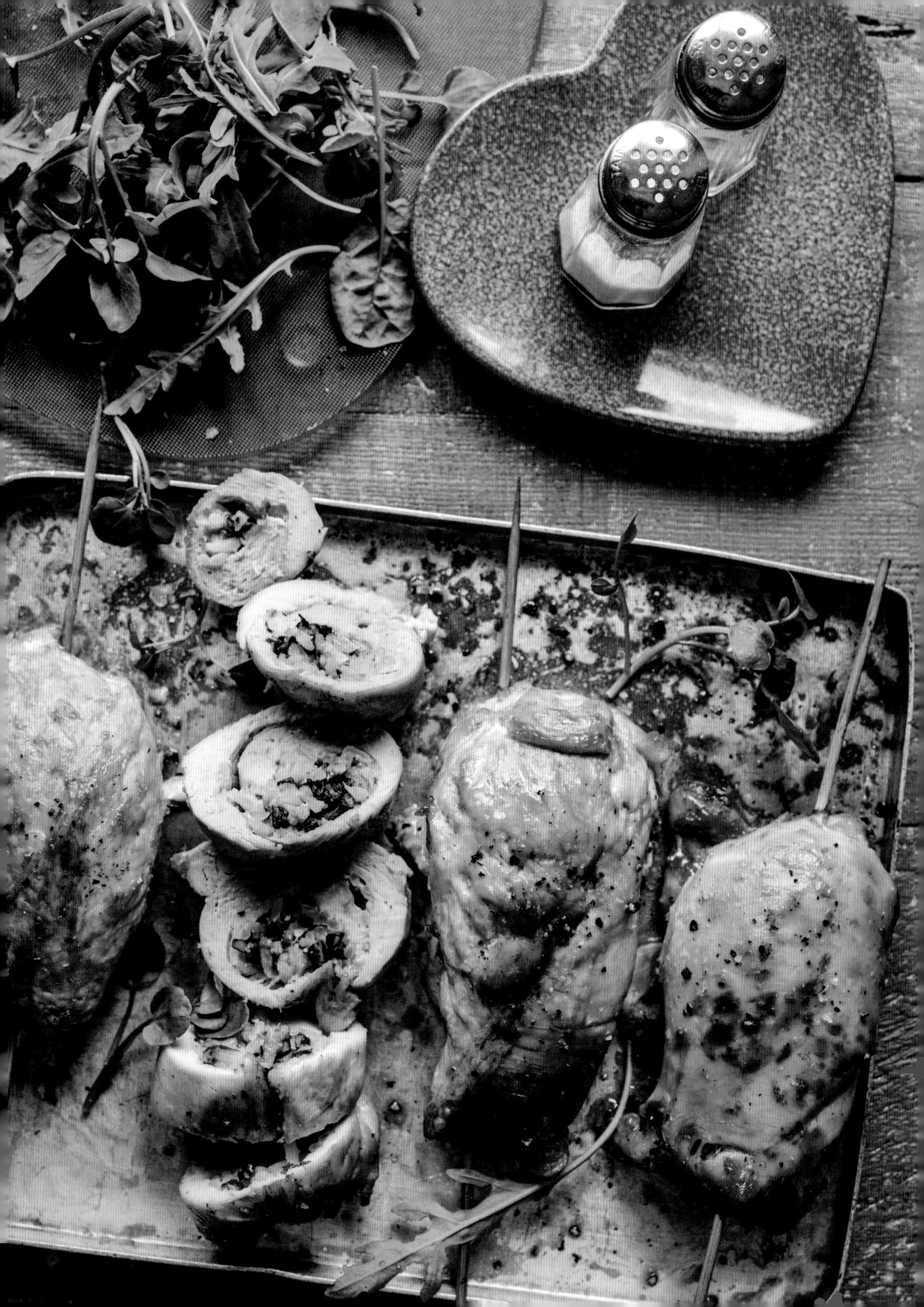

SERVES: 4
PREP: 10 MINS
COOK: 30 MINS
CALORIES: 455

- 4 frying steaks
- 250g (9oz) mushrooms, sliced
- ½ brown onion, diced
- 2 cloves of garlic, crushed
- 30g (1oz) plain flour
- 500ml (18fl oz) beef stock
- 60g (2¼oz) low-fat soft cheese

STEAK 'N' SHROOMS

Although Paul has gone for the somewhat non-descriptive description of 'frying steak' for this recipe, which could encompass everything from a strip of shoe-leather through to an expensive cut from a cow that enjoyed summers in Tuscany, he's right to keep it simple. See, we hate food snobbery here at Chubby Towers, and no more so than when it comes to people telling you how you should have your steak. You see it an awful lot with discussions around steak. Some folks will think your life isn't complete unless you've taken on their sage advice about how it should be cooked, others will tell you that if you haven't taken out a mortgage to pay for it, it's hardly worth having. All, and I say this with love and an eye to our PG rating, poppycock. Tastes are personal, and what works for you, works for you.

Spray a large pan with a little oil and place over a medium-high heat. Season the steaks on both sides with a little salt and pepper, add to the pan, and fry for 2–3 minutes per side. Remove from the pan and set aside.

Add the mushrooms, onion and garlic to the pan and cook for 5–7 minutes, stirring occasionally.

Sprinkle over the flour and stir well, then gradually pour in the stock, whisking continuously, and bring to a simmer. Cook for 5–7 minutes, until thickened.

Stir in the soft cheese and add a bit more salt and pepper to taste.

Return the steaks to the pan, then cover and simmer for 10 minutes.

Serve.

Notes: Regarding frying times: I like my steaks very rare indeed – very much a 'wipe its bum and serve it up' sort of approach, so a flash on each side. Paul prefers the middle ground, with a little bit of pink on show, so follow the timings above. My best friend, however, likes his steak to resemble a shoe you'd find discarded in the aftermath of a raging forest fire (cook for fourteen years on the surface of an exploding sun). Horses for courses (though stick to cows).

Serve with chips. Let's be realistic here.

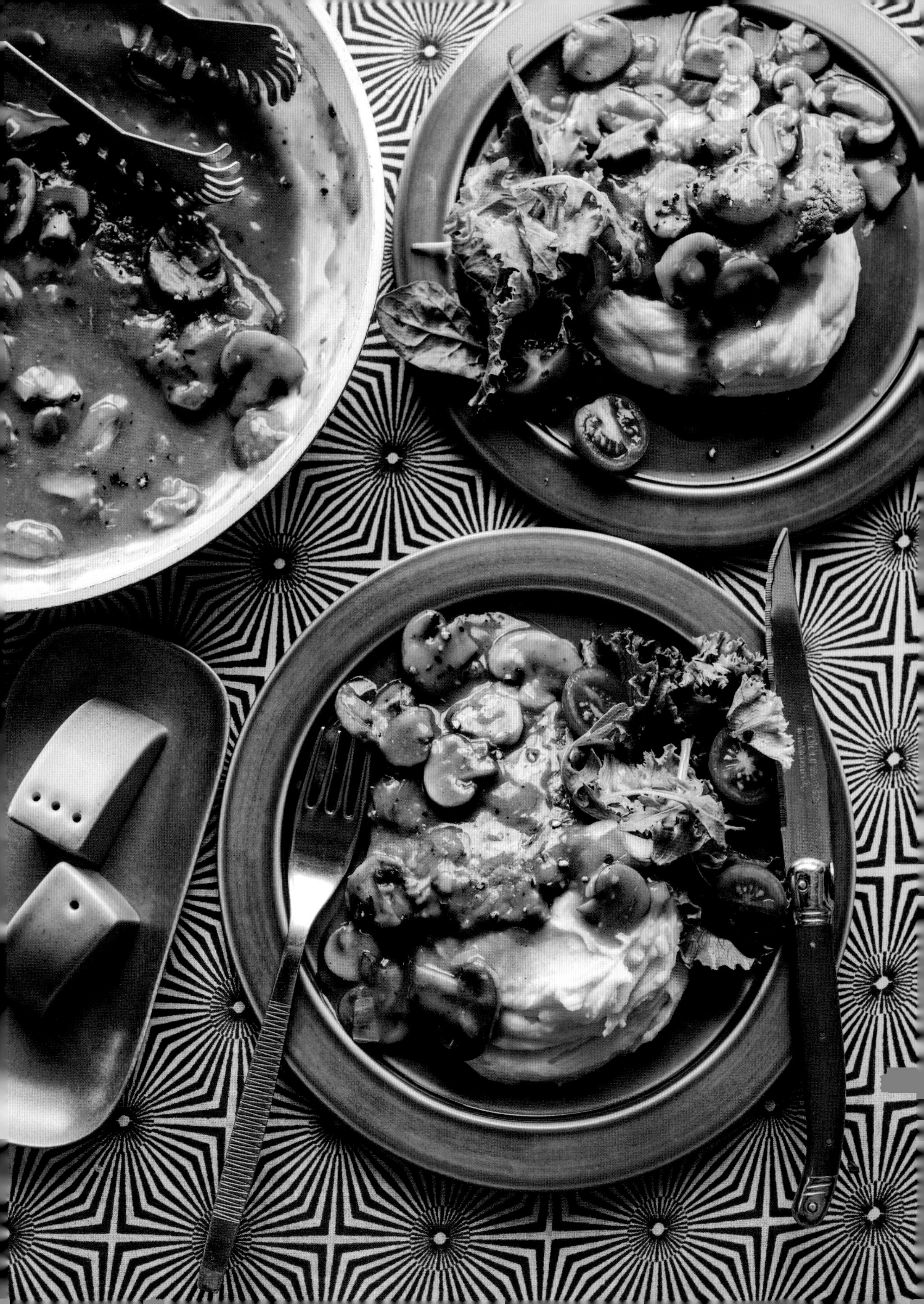

SERVES: 4
PREP: 10 MINS
COOK: 2HRS 20 MINS
CALORIES: 301

↑30 mins · DF

- 12 reduced-fat sausages
- 2 leeks, washed and sliced
- 2 cloves of garlic, crushed
- 1 teaspoon fennel seeds
- 1 teaspoon smoked paprika
- 1 bay leaf
- 500g (1lb 2oz) red cabbage, sliced
- 1 × 400g (14oz) tin of chopped tomatoes
- 500ml (18fl oz) beef stock
- ½ teaspoon salt
- ¼ teaspoon black pepper

SCABBAGE

Scabbage: like a muscly fireman called Percival, it's a tasty little dish with a terrible name. Now if you're called Percival, or indeed if you know of a loved one with this name, we of course give our immediate apologies. It can't be easy. Now we've got that creaky joke out of the way, we can turn to scabbage, a snappy little portmanteau of cabbage and sausage, if you're not quite keeping up at the back. Cabbage just doesn't get enough love (although we refer you to the cauliflower consequences on page 68), and considering how cheap it is, it really needs some time in the sun. Literally: it won't grow otherwise. I know, it's just bit after bit in this recipe! We're using reduced-fat sausages here because frankly the other ingredients more than make up for the reduction in taste (how often it is that when they remove fat, they remove flavour), but if you were feeling like a daring renegade, you could of course use full-fat sausages here. Simply cook them and serve with egg and chips, then make scabbage tomorrow.

Spray a large pan with a little oil and place over a medium heat. Add the sausages and cook for 10 minutes, until browned on all sides, then remove from the pan and set aside.

Add the leeks to the pan and cook for 6–7 minutes, until softened.

Add the garlic, fennel seeds, smoked paprika and bay leaf, and cook for 1–2 minutes.

Add the cabbage, tomatoes, stock and sausages, season with salt and pepper, bring to the boil, then simmer over a low heat for 1–2 hours.

Serve.

Note: Save money on expensive bay leaves by spotting that your neighbour has a bay tree growing in their garden and surreptitiously stealing a few every time you walk your dog past their house.

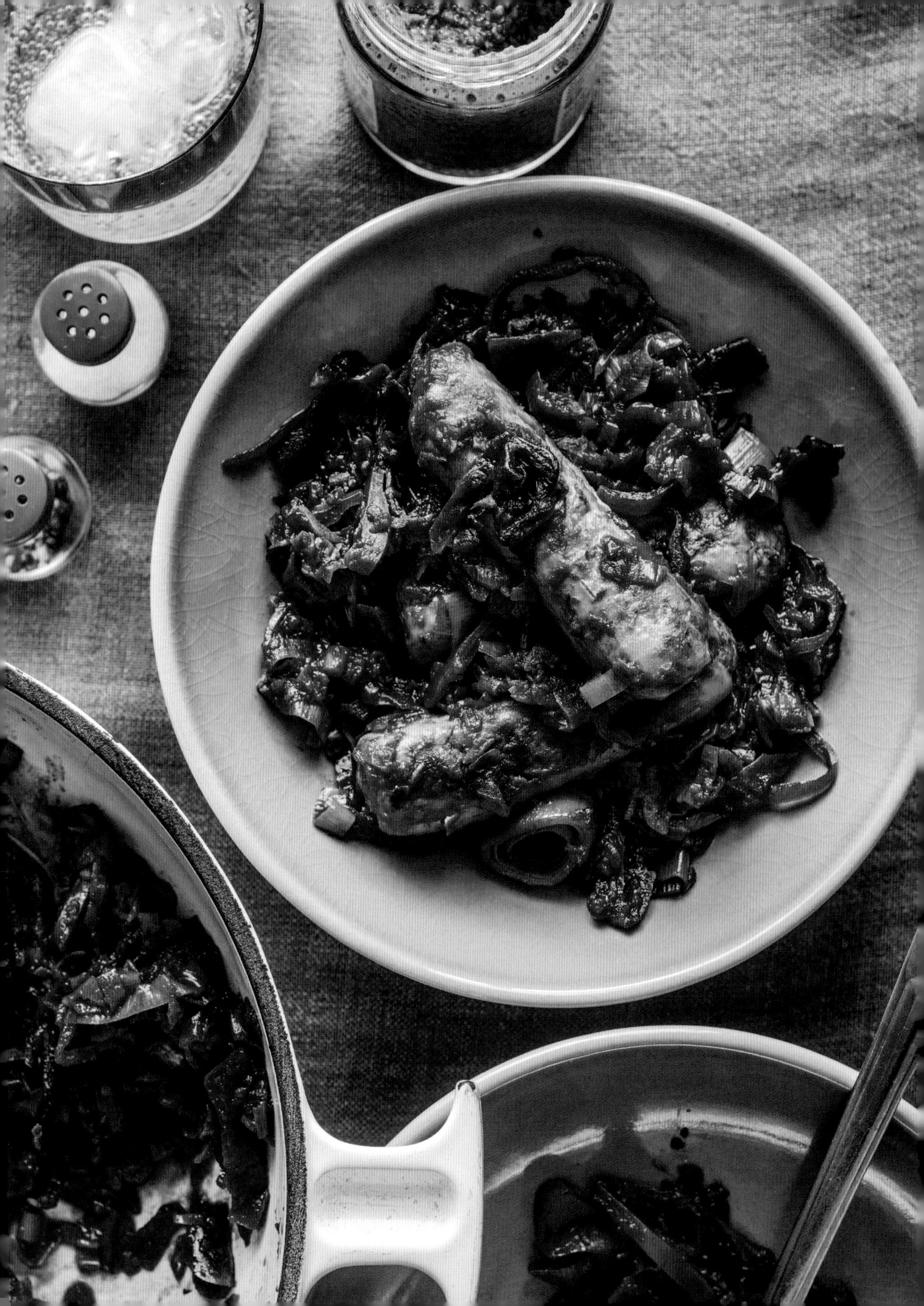

SERVES: 4
PREP: 15 MINS
COOK: 50 MINS
CALORIES: 261

- 1 tablespoon fennel seeds
- 200g (7oz) reduced-fat feta cheese
- 150g (5½oz) fat-free Greek yoghurt
- 1 egg
- 600g (1lb 5oz) potatoes

GREEK POTATO PIE

Paul calls this a pie, but as far as I'm concerned, a pie has to have pastry sides and a lid, and needs two hands on the fish-slice to hoik your serving on to the plate. However, in the spirit of having an easy life, we'll allow him this indiscretion. If anything, this is more of a cheesy hot-pot, but let's not open that argument up either. We're using reduced-fat feta and fat-free Greek yoghurt here, and it works, it truly does, but if you're feeling like throwing calorie caution to the wind, upgrade to the full-fat version. Plus, add some cheese on top. And more in the sauce. And have a biscuit while it cooks. It's what we do.

Preheat the oven to 200°C fan/425°F/gas mark 7. Line a 20cm (8 inch) sandwich tin with greaseproof paper.

Using a pestle and mortar (or the edge of a rolling pin), grind the fennel seeds.

Put the feta into a bowl with the yoghurt and mash with a fork, making sure they're well combined. Add the fennel seeds and egg, mix well, then set aside.

Scrub and peel the potatoes, then slice thinly. Spray the slices with a little oil on both sides.

Spread a layer of potatoes in the bottom of the prepared tin and add a layer of the cheese mix on top. Repeat the layers of potatoes and cheese twice more.

Cover the tin with foil and bake in the oven for 30 minutes, then remove the foil and bake for another 20 minutes.

Allow to cool, then serve.

Note: Hoik, of course, is a good Geordie term for lifting. For those of you who didn't pledge allegiance to Ant and/or Dec at birth, I apologise for the occasional slip into Geordie.

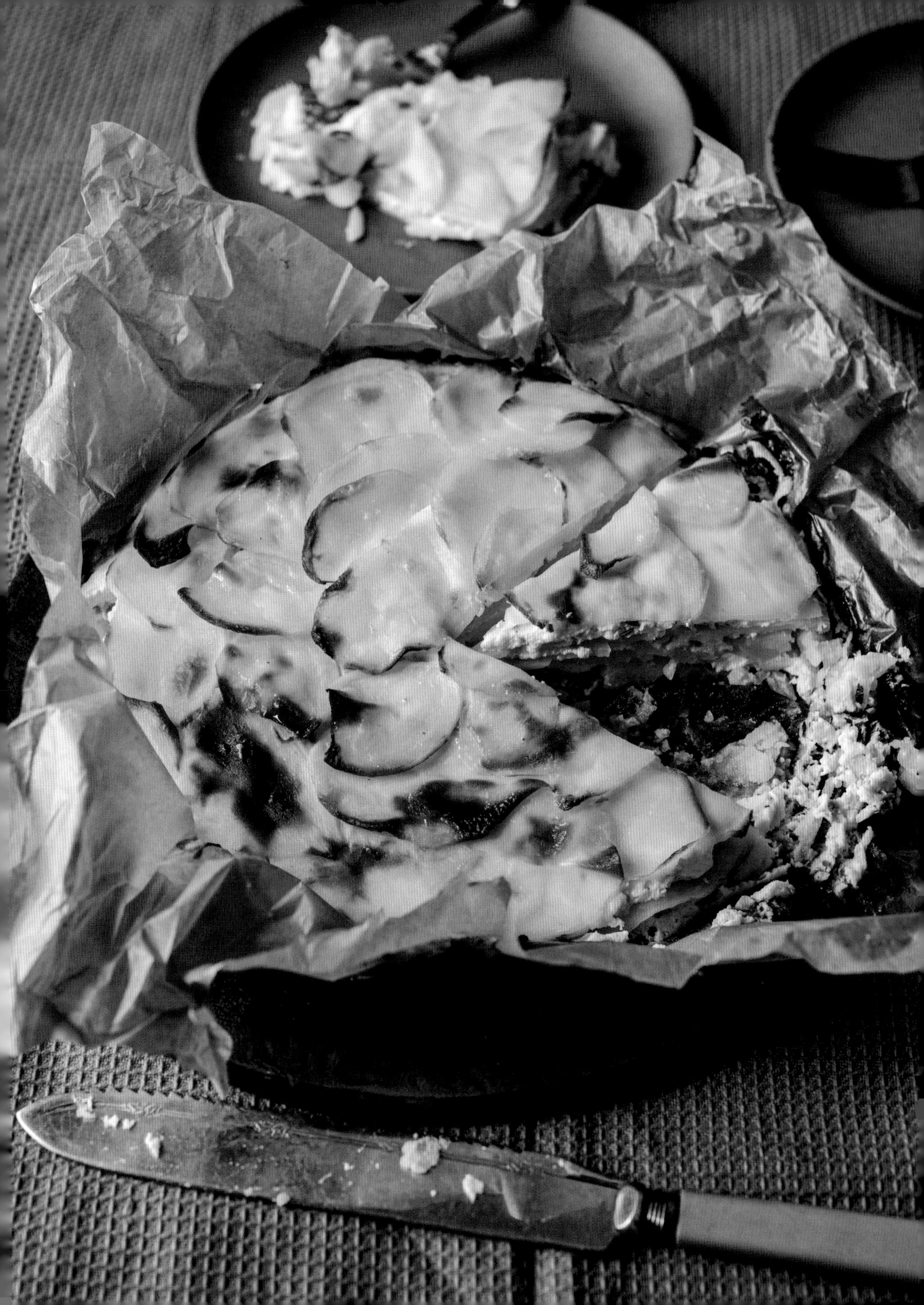

PUDS

SERVES: 4
PREP: 10 MINS
COOK: 15 MINS
CALORIES: 303

CHOCOLATE LAVA CAKES

A little memory of school, these cakes, though Paul has gussied them up somewhat with the addition of apple sauce (you'll note the same replacement in the confetti cake recipe) instead of a flurry of sugar. Trust him, for he knows what he does. You know, school dinners (and their matching puddings) get a lot of stick, but I have nothing but wonderful memories. Admittedly, I went to a fairly posh school (though be under no illusion, that was purely happenstance because it was the only high school for miles around; I still took my PE kit into school in a Netto bag) and we were served cheese and coffee after lunch, but even so. Even in little trousers I was a smooth talker and so it was that all the dinner-ladies would give me extra. My little heart soared (and likely spluttered) on Friday, which was always sausage and chips, and it was always something like the wonderful lava cakes below for dessert. I have no doubt that Connie (Queen of the Queue) will have long since cashed in her chips, but I'll remain forever grateful for the fact she kept me pleasingly spherical for a solid four years.

- 120g (4oz) apple sauce
- 120g (4oz) fat-free yoghurt
- 3 tablespoons honey
- 2 eggs
- 1 teaspoon vanilla extract
- 60g (2¼oz) self-raising flour
- 40g (1½oz) cocoa powder
- ¼ teaspoon salt
- 4 squares of dark chocolate
- 2 teaspoons icing sugar

Preheat the oven to 170°C fan/375°F/gas mark 5.

In a bowl, whisk together the apple sauce, yoghurt, honey, eggs and vanilla, then add the flour, cocoa powder and salt and mix until smooth.

Spray four ramekins with a little oil and place on a baking sheet. Fill them about a quarter of the way up with the mix, pressing a square of chocolate into the centre of each one.

Top up with the rest of the batter and bake for 12–15 minutes, until the edges are set and the centre is still a little jiggly.

Remove from the oven and cool for 5 minutes, then gently run a knife around the edge to loosen the cakes and tip them out on to plates.

Dust with the icing sugar and serve.

Note: Connie taught me the importance of a finely-kept 'tache, too.

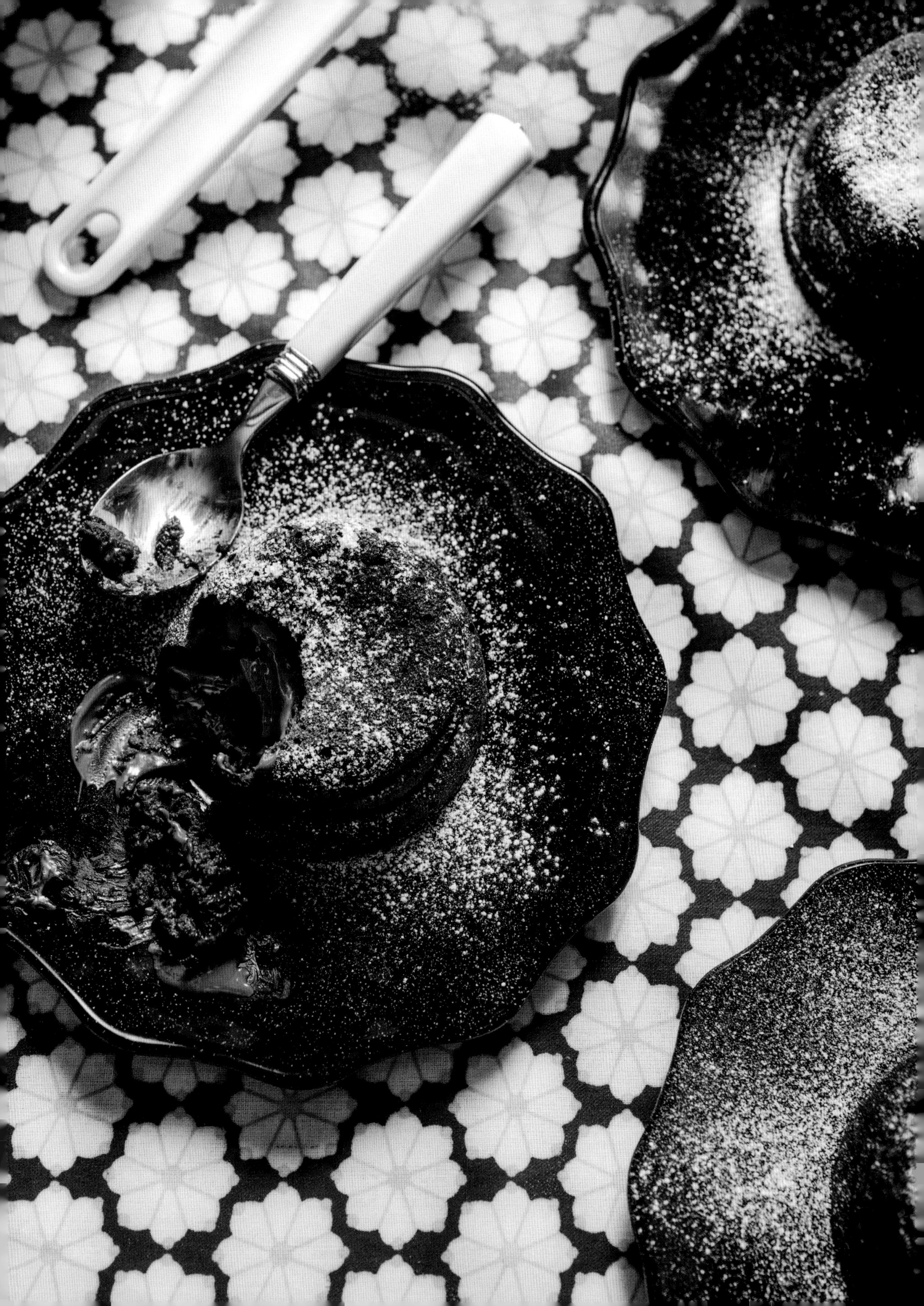

SERVES: 4
PREP: 15 MINS
COOK: 30 MINS
CALORIES: 495

STRAWBERRIES 'N' CREAM DUTCH BABY

Essentially a sweet Yorkshire pudding or a giant thickened pancake, this is a dessert for the ages – and if the idea of sweet Yorkshire pudding fills you with dread, just give it a go regardless. You don't need to fill them with the strawberries and cream that we suggest here, either: I've been witness to all sorts of unusual toppings in my time, some served with spoons in a way you might not expect, and can recommend banana, peanut butter and whipped cream as a personal favourite. Yes, high in calories, and no, perhaps not ideal if you're on a very restricted diet, but let me reiterate the twochubbycubs mantra one more time: a little of what you fancy does you good.

- 70g (2½oz) strawberries
- 2 tablespoons caster sugar
- 120ml (4fl oz) whipping cream
- ¼ teaspoon + ⅛ teaspoon vanilla extract
- 3 large eggs
- 120g (4oz) plain flour
- 120ml (4fl oz) semi-skimmed milk
- 3 tablespoons brown sugar
- 3 tablespoons butter
- 1 teaspoon icing sugar
- ½ teaspoon ground cinnamon

Preheat the oven to 220°C fan/475°F/gas mark 9.

In a blender or a food processor, blitz most of the strawberries (keep 2 or 3 aside for later) with the caster sugar until syrupy.

Whisk the cream in a bowl with ⅛ teaspoon of vanilla extract until you reach soft peaks, add the strawberry mix and whisk until you reach stiff peaks, then pop into the fridge.

In another bowl, whisk together the eggs, flour, milk, brown sugar and the remaining vanilla extract until smooth.

Put the butter into a 25cm (10 inch) baking tin (or oven-safe frying pan) and pop it into the oven to heat for 5 minutes. Remove the tin from the oven and carefully pour in the batter, then return it to the oven and bake for 18–20 minutes.

Remove from the oven and allow to cool for 5 minutes.

Top with the cream and the reserved strawberries, and dust with the icing sugar and cinnamon. Cut into quarters, and serve.

Notes: Don't be put off by the 'heavier' ingredients in this – it's all completely worth it!

A stand mixer is your friend here – but if you don't have one, a whisk and a strong arm will do the job just fine.

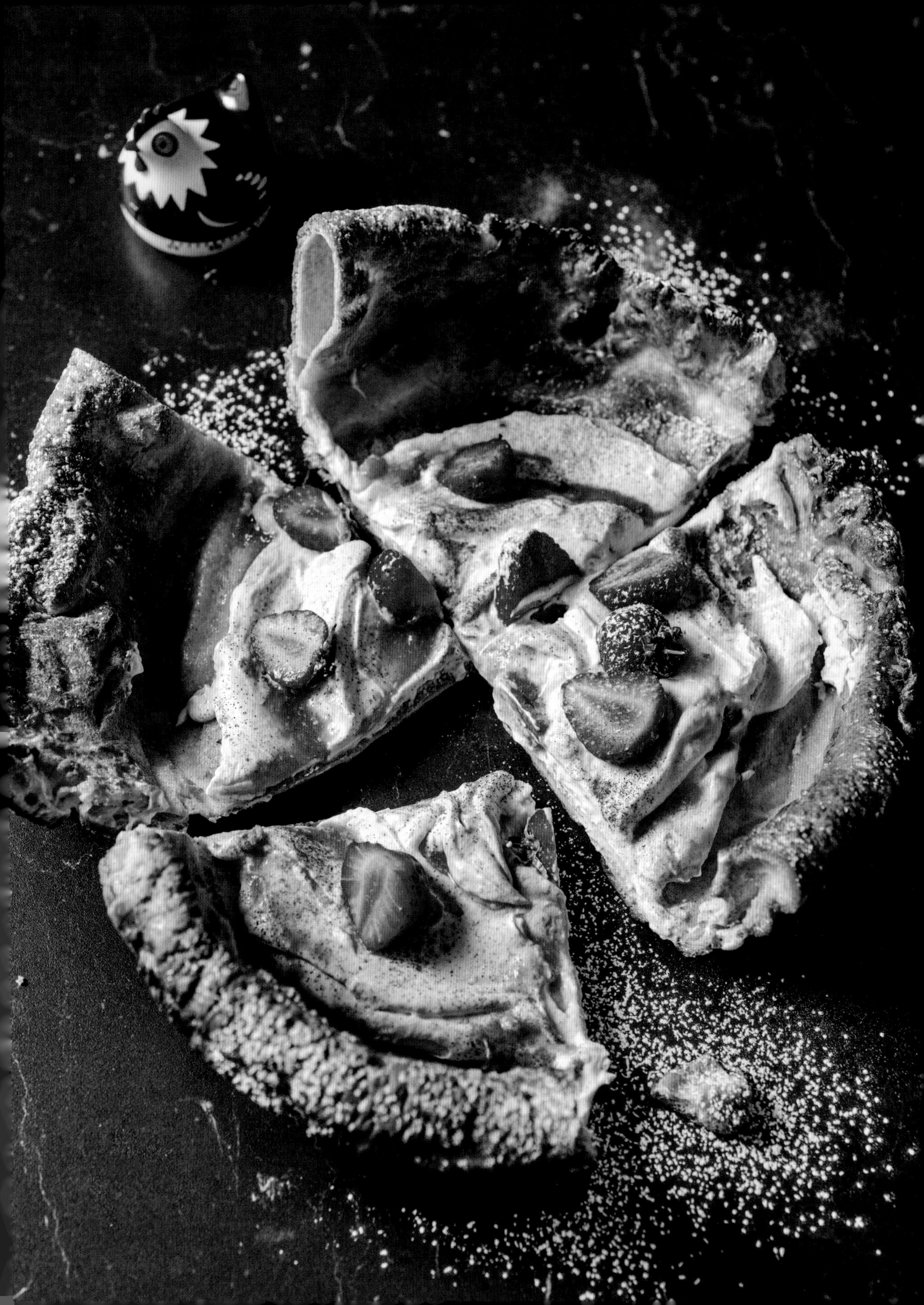

SERVES: 4
PREP: 10 MINS
COOK: 30 MINS
CALORIES: 156

↑30 mins · serves · 10 · V · GF

(CHOCOLATE ORANGE) MILK PUD

Although you would traditionally use whole milk for this pudding – and if you're not fussed about calories then we absolutely encourage you to do so – it works just fine with semi-skimmed. Paul and I are lucky enough to have a dairy farm within walking distance of our house which has recently branched out into providing, among other things, fresh milk that you bottle yourself via a very clever bottling machine. We did a post about it on our Facebook page on our first visit, accompanied by a picture of me pretending to grimace as I swallowed a mouthful of milk, and, by a quirk of the photo tagging process, inadvertently ended up as their business page cover photo for seven months. We like to imagine that tourists turned up in their droves to see the two fat cows dressed in knock-off Fred Perry and Asda slacks, we truly do. The pudding, then . . .

- 2 large eggs
- 2 tablespoons granulated sugar
- 2 tablespoons cornflour
- 300ml (10fl oz) semi-skimmed milk
- 1 teaspoon vanilla extract
- 2 teaspoons cocoa powder
- 1 orange

Beat the eggs in a large bowl, then gradually add the sugar and cornflour, whisking until the sugar has dissolved.

Gradually pour in the milk, whisking continuously. Pour the mixture into a saucepan and place over a medium heat, then gradually, while still continuing to stir, bring the mixture to the boil.

Reduce the heat to low and continue to cook for 2–3 minutes, stirring! – until thickened. Remove the pan from the heat and stir in the vanilla, then set aside to cool for 15 minutes.

Scoop the mixture into bowls (or glasses) and place in the fridge to set.

Before serving, sprinkle over the cocoa powder and add a slice of orange on the rim.

Note: They also offer 'raw milk', which we can't bring ourselves to try: that's a little too rustic, even for our rough-hewn tastes.

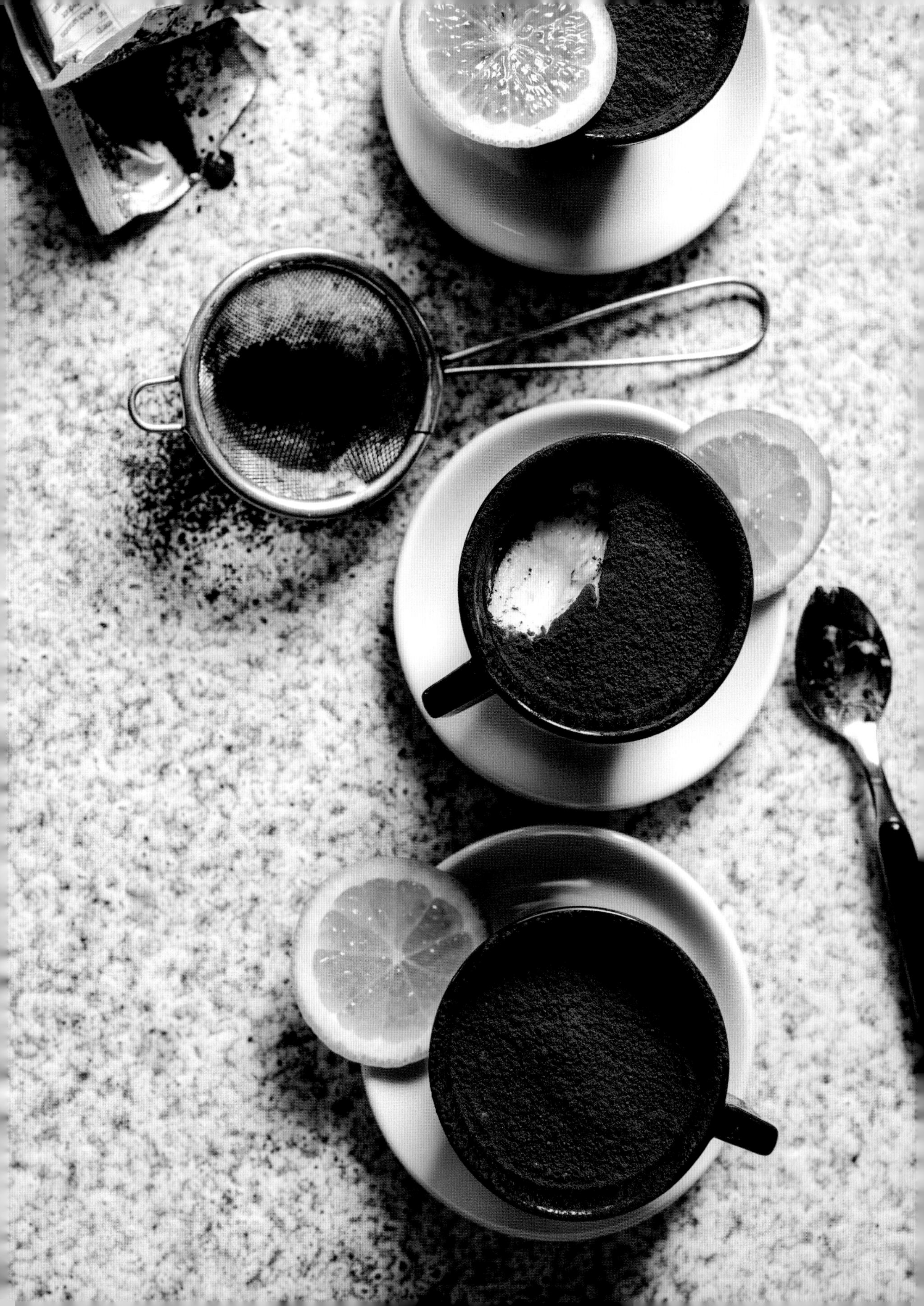

SERVES: 4
PREP: 5 MINS
COOK: 50 MINS
CALORIES: 260

- 4 medium apples
- 45g (1½oz) porridge oats
- 35g (1¼oz) plain flour
- 35g (1¼oz) brown sugar
- 50g (1¾oz) butter
- 1 teaspoon ground cinnamon
- ¼ teaspoon ground nutmeg
- ¼ teaspoon salt

EASY APPLE CRUMBLE

Everybody's good at cooking something, and I'm good at cooking crumble . . . wait, what year is this? Good heavens. Two reasons for including this in the book: one is the simple fact that this crumble is a decent, low-fat, high-taste dessert, and second, we have a steady access to apples now thanks to the allotment my parents now spend twenty-three hours of their day toiling at. Of course, I'm minded to exclude this recipe as a big screw-you to Mother Nature, no matter the malus-marvels or blossomiest blossom she throws our way. See, at the time of writing, I'm a few weeks into hay fever season, and it never gets any easier. One night I'll go to sleep happy and content, the next morning I wake with a swollen face and a nose dripping like I'm one intervention away from a rehab stint. Crueller still, the hay fever this year seemed to bypass me and I spent spring airily telling Paul that my new healthier diet must have been the key to success. But of course not. Yet, despite my itchy eyes and sternutation fits, we can't ignore sweet, delicious apples. So here's the apple crumble recipe, and I hope it was worth it.

Preheat the oven to 180°C fan/400°F/gas mark 6.

Peel and core the apples, chop them into small pieces, and place them in the bottom of a medium baking dish.

In a bowl, mix together the oats, flour, sugar, butter, cinnamon, nutmeg and salt until crumbly.

Sprinkle the crumble mixture over the apples and bake for 45–50 minutes, until golden brown.

Notes: My nana used to make the most amazing apple crumble using her classic 'eight times as much topping as needed' – a mantra I've adhered to in all things – and we've never quite been able to replicate it. This is nothing but a compromise.

Yes, I've tried the 'eat local honey' technique to combat my hay fever. My sister's partner is an apiarist: I get the good stuff. But no joy.

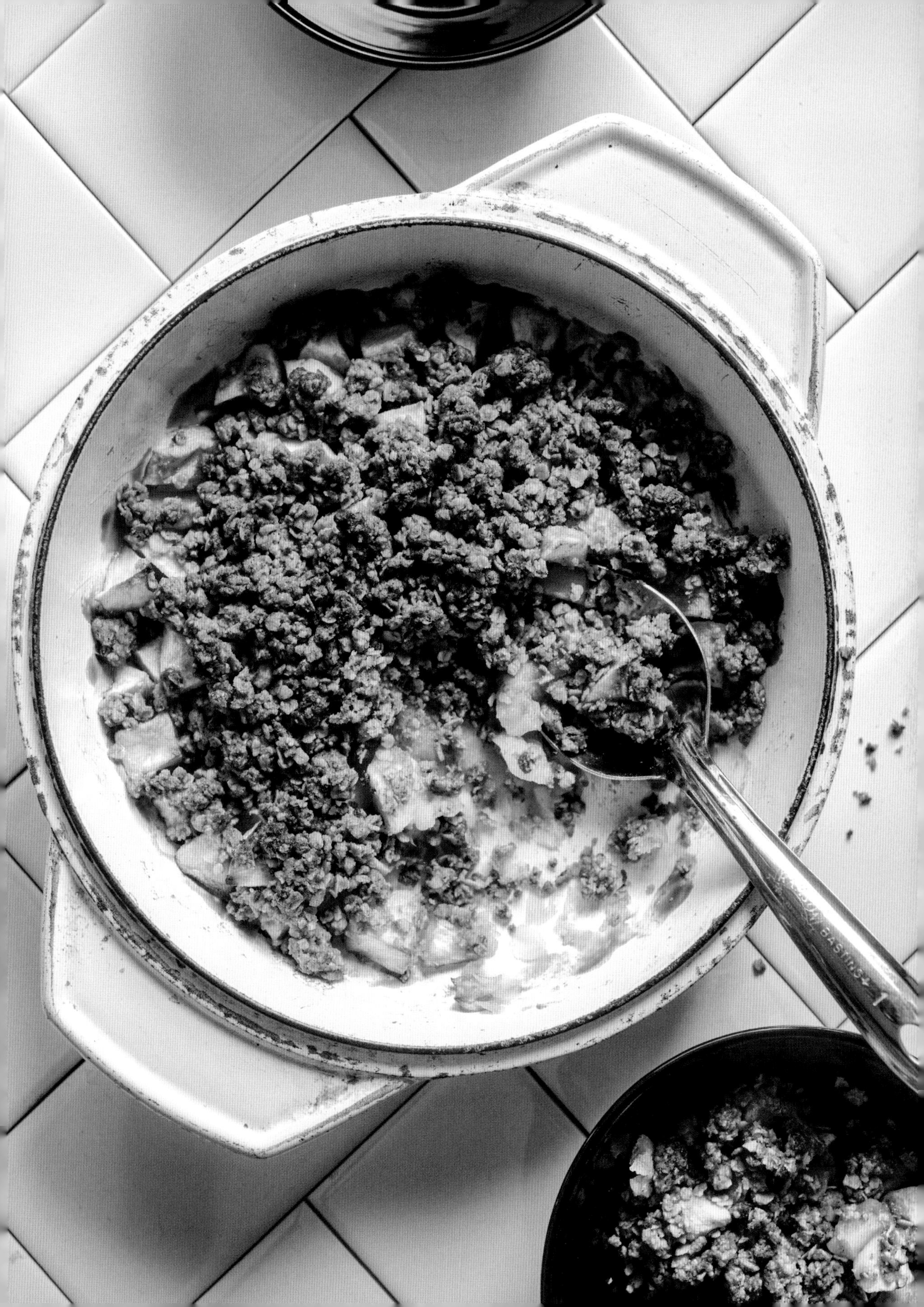

SERVES: 4
PREP: 2 HRS 10 MINS
CALORIES: 105

EASY CHOCOLATE MOUSSE

A chocolate mousse recipe which only came about after some experimentation with tofu, a block of which we received entirely accidentally in a good subscription service. We've used tofu plenty of times before, but turning it into such a sweet, easy and delicious dessert is a new one on us. Of course, me being here at all to provide you with such a delicious recipe is a miracle in and of itself. See, a couple of months ago, and without so much as a hint of hyperbole, I almost died. I had taken it upon myself to actually be proactive about some DIY (when my normal level of effort is to scrawl through those 'hire a builder' websites and choose the one I'd most like to bundle me around on the carpet) and set about clearing our vegetable patch. I hired a skip – one of the most exciting things you can do as an adult, frankly – and spent a full day shuttling wheelbarrows full of soil and wood and lost dreams back and forth. I didn't so much work up a sweat as I did marinate in it: I was glowing. Not as glowing as I nearly was, though. See, once I'd cleared the patch of the spare soil, I started trying to fork over the soil that was there. Everything was going great until I hit what I assumed was an old roof-tile and started trying to prise it out with a spade. Turns out what I was attempting to lift out with my very metal spade was the protective cover for a very thick, very exciting armoured cable carrying electricity under the garden. Honestly, the things I'll do for a ride in an air ambulance. That'll teach me for trying to be all butch, it really will.

- 250g (9oz) silken tofu
- 60ml (2fl oz) almond milk
- 30g (1oz) cocoa powder
- 60g (2oz) maple syrup
- 1 teaspoon vanilla extract
- ¼ teaspoon salt

Using a stand or a hand mixer, mix the tofu until it's smooth.

Add the rest of the ingredients and mix until smooth and well combined, then keep going for another 5 minutes or so until it becomes light and fluffy.

Transfer to serving dishes and chill in the fridge for 2 hours.

Note: No maple syrup? Golden syrup or honey are just fine.

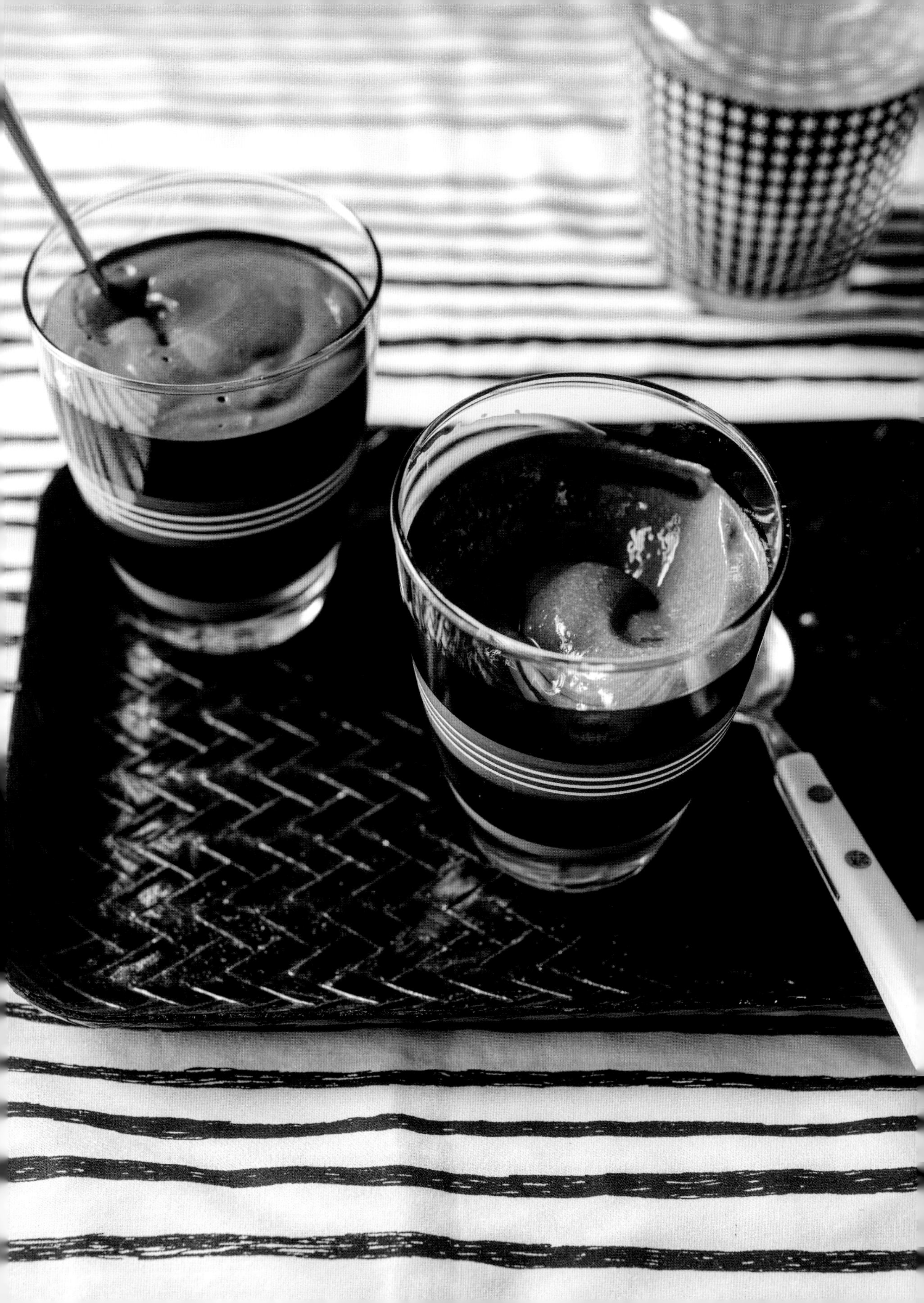

CONFETTI CAKE

MAKES: 8 SLICES
PREP: 10 MINS
COOK: 40 MINS
CALORIES: 128

We ummed and aahed about including this in our recipe book, because lord knows we've made such a song and dance about 'proper' cooking being the only way forward when it comes to cakes and biscuits and the like. But we've got more faces than the town hall clock, and so in it goes. Anyway, this recipe is different to most of the other 'slimming' treats out there as it contains that oft-missing ingredient: flavour. We do caveat this recipe by saying it isn't a light, fluffy wonder, but rather quite a dense, squidgy affair, but then so am I and I rarely get any complaints. As a result it is unlikely to win any beauty awards at the village fête, though it could come in useful as an unlikely murder weapon when *Midsomer Murders* starts running out of ideas. I wrote the above reference to village fêtes without considering whether they are still a thing – I do hope so. Growing up in the countryside with little else to do, I spent many a happy afternoon playing ring toss and smacking a rat. And some days, we went to a village fête! Oh shush, you know the score by now.

- 1 egg
- 2 tablespoons honey
- 120g (4oz) apple sauce
- ½ teaspoon vanilla extract
- 120g (4oz) self-raising flour
- 5 tablespoons hundreds and thousands
- 30g (1oz) reduced-fat soft cheese
- 20g (¾oz) icing sugar

Preheat the oven to 180°C fan/400°F/gas mark 6.

In a bowl, whisk together the egg, honey, apple sauce and vanilla, then gently fold into the flour, being careful not to overmix.

Fold in around 3 tablespoons of the hundreds and thousands and transfer the mixture to a small loaf tin.

Bake in the oven for 35–40 minutes, then remove from the oven and allow to cool.

In a small bowl, mix together the soft cheese and icing sugar. Spread this on top of the cake, and sprinkle over the remaining hundreds and thousands.

Notes: You can also cook these in muffin cases if you prefer.

Freeze without the icing.

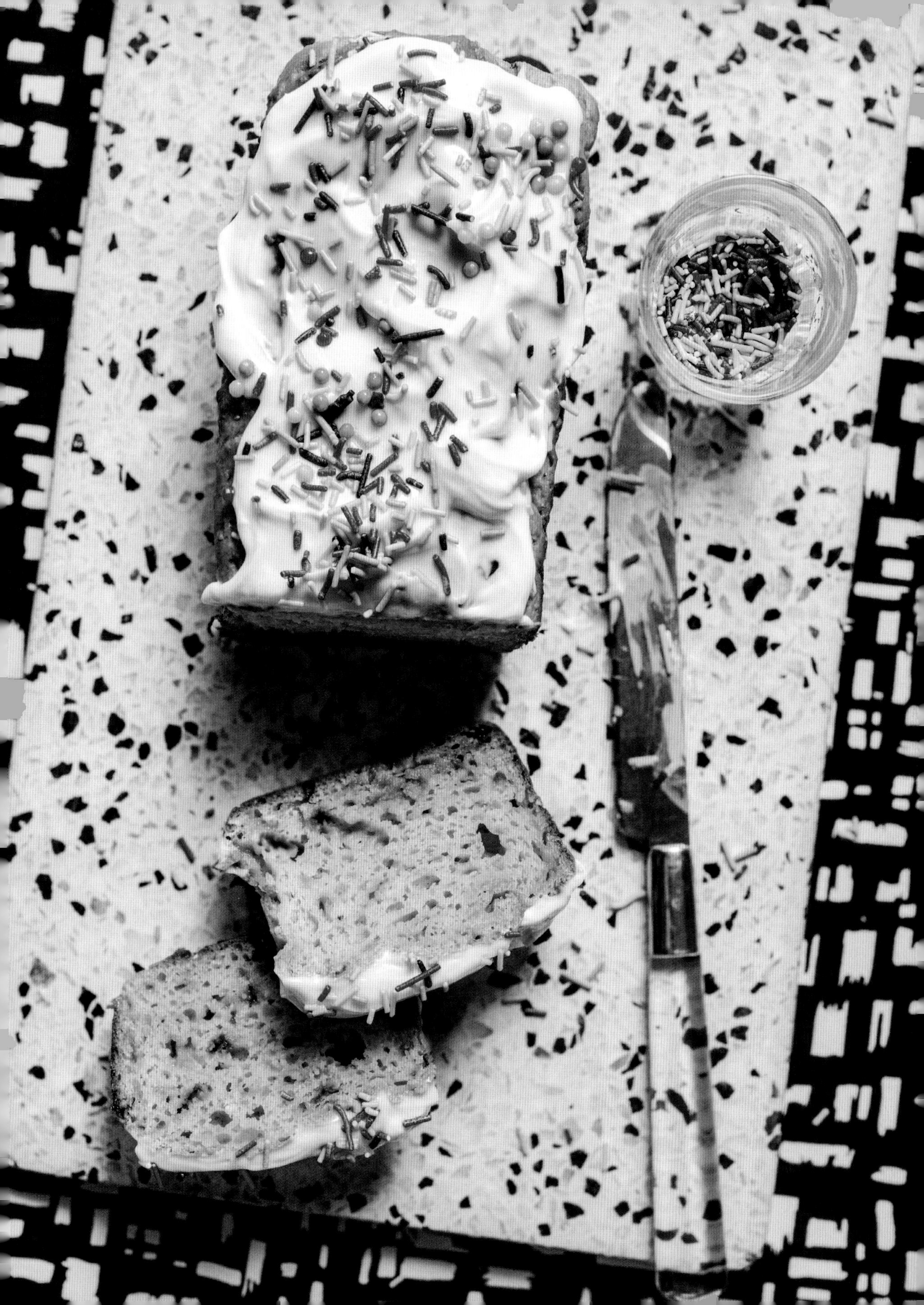

SERVES: 4
PREP: 5 MINS
COOK: 40 MINS
CALORIES: 303

GOOD OLD-FASHIONED BREAD & BUTTER PUDDING

We're finishing the book with an old classic dessert from days of yore which seems to have fallen out of fashion: well, not on our watch. And surprisingly, we can squeak it under 500 calories, although we like to think if you've made it this far, you'll indulge yourself regardless. Unusually, this is the last intro I have left to do – normally when preparing the book we write 'out of sequence', so one morning I'll be adding the gloss to a recipe in chapter two, the next I'll be whipping out an intro – it's never consistent. I always have the romantic notion that I'll finish the book with some sort of ritual, like Paul Sheldon's champagne and cigarette from *Misery*, but let me let you in on the reality: I'll click the 'Save' button, tell myself I must start earlier next time, and then spend the next four months agonising over whether I've managed to make you smile. I hope you do, readers, because it's always a pleasure.

- 2 tablespoons butter
- 3 slices of bread
- 75g (2¾oz) mixed dried fruit
- 425ml (15fl oz) semi-skimmed milk
- 2 eggs
- 40g (1½oz) granulated sugar

Preheat the oven to 180°C fan/400°F/gas mark 6.

Butter the bread and cut it into triangles. Place the triangles in a dish and toss over the dried fruit.

Pour the milk into a jug and microwave for 30–45 seconds, until warm.

Beat the eggs with the sugar and gradually pour in the milk, while whisking. Pour the eggs and milk over the bread.

Bake in the oven for 35–40 minutes, until set.

Notes: Please, don't be tempted to use wholemeal bread here. It has a place in polite society, absolutely, but no place at all in a bread and butter pudding.

You can make wee versions of this using the hundred or so ramekins that you've been keeping in the cupboard for best. Come on, we all do it.

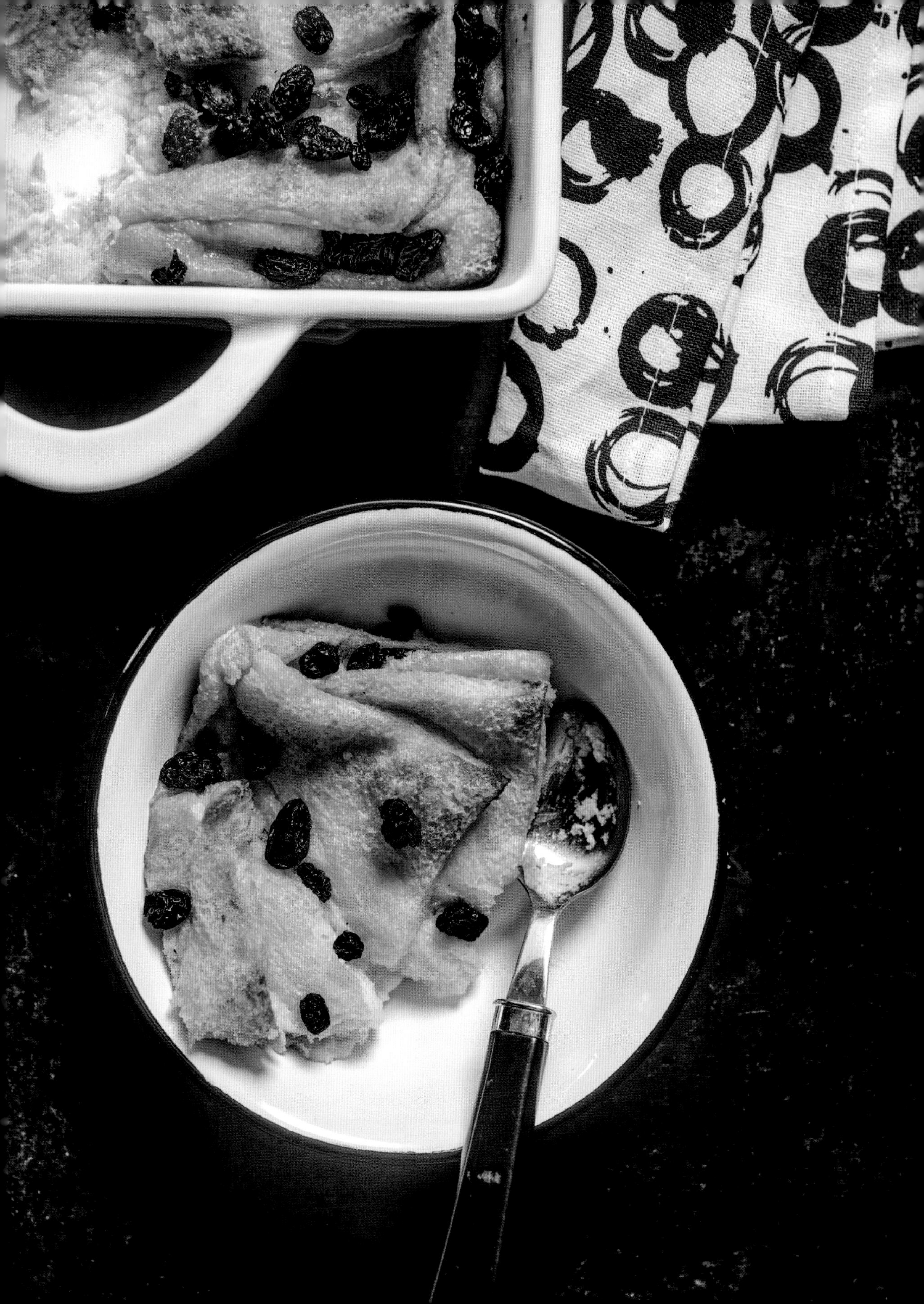

INDEX

T

V

W

Y

Z

ACKNOWLEDGEMENTS

Here's an unusual thank you to start these parting words with: Sarah Doick, a friend we made back in the heady days when I used to work for a living. Sarah had been a fan of the blog since day one and forwarded to me, perhaps cognisant of the fact my belly used to drag along the photocopier controls when I was making coffee at work, a flier for *This Time Next Year*. That was the programme which kicked off our weight loss and brought us a book offer, and we've never looked back. I don't believe in fate or the cosmos but it really makes me think – such a small random act that caused two lives to change so dramatically. A great Doctor said once that '. . . every great decision creates ripples, like a huge boulder dropped in a lake – the ripples merge and rebound off the banks in unforeseeable ways', and boy howdy is that true. Without Sarah deciding to send that flier to me, you wouldn't be reading this. Plus she knitted us an amazing Bob-omb! Thank you, Sarah :)

Speaking of friends, turning up next to collect their medals (no cash value, no refunds) are those who we can grandly call our collective muses: Paul and Martin Hawkins for me, Emma and Danielle for Paul. Paul and Martin have provided many things over the years: receipts, accusations, sheer volume, surprising mass, but almost always laughter and wise (if certainly exhaustive) counsel. This year Paul suggested his nan's corned beef hash as a recipe and it's a banger. The recipe, not Ann, though we've certainly heard rumours. For Paul, Emma and Danielle bring coarse chat and more gynaecological illumination than is decent to talk about in a cookery book. Let me tell you, readers – as someone who hears the voice notes that get played as Paul chokes his breakfast down, well, you wouldn't get that sort of discussion in *The Archers*.

Paul would also like to thank everyone at Project:U Fitness for keeping his moobs under some control and pushing him to better himself. Andrew Hodge, his co-sweaty-sausage at Project:U, deserves some praise too: I've been downwind of a sweaty Paul, so mate, you're a brave lad. Paul also wants to thank everyone he works with for being accommodating of the sometimes short-notice changes needed when you're a writer's strumpet. He singles out Cyndi, his long-suffering work wife, for special praise indeed – and I've met her and can sign off on what a lovely sort she is.

Finally, a mutual appreciation from the two of us for all the members of the Newcastle Ravens: for continuing to give me a reason to admire Paul in his rugby kit *and* for making me feel very welcome on my much-delayed arrival. That said, they can take singular blame for the reeking of our airing cupboard now we throw our soiled rugby boots in there on a Wednesday evening and leave them there to fester until they're next needed. Seriously, I spent almost a fortnight this summer trying to find what had died behind a radiator in our house, only to fish them out, gagging.

If Paul gets to single out some special mentions, then so must I, and although she was mentioned earlier in the book, first goes to Emma Lebovitch, my ex-work-wife. Our fortnightly strolls where I bounce ideas off you, listen to your stories and patiently explain how clouds are made or work through your seven-times-table are such a highlight. Next: Iain and

Darren – the latter for being an equal to my bitchery and the former for being a catalyst to my self-improvement and together for being such wonderful friends. Gary Main and Shaun Dicks merit a special mention because they're so damn cute together it makes my teeth itch, and together they're Main Dicks and if that's not a power-couple name, what is?

Because I'm not entirely sure they've locked their wills and powers of attorney down yet, my family earn some recognition too – partly because they keep us in catering-levels of allotment goodies, but mainly because they've always made Paul so welcome at the table.

While we were down supervising the food photography for this book (for supervising, read eating everything we could get our hands on and guiltily stealing spoons from the cupboard), we were struck by how utterly tireless and magnificent our team really is. Don't get us wrong: we've known they're amazing from day one, but watching a group of people – all experts in their craft – work on making your scribbled notes and clumsy ideas into something as beautiful as this book: it's incredible to witness.

Just by happenstance, the daughter of our food photographers wanted to show off her superior photography skills and asked to take a photo of all of us in the kitchen. We think it is a cracking photo (and, don't fret, the Magic Circle legal team she keeps on retainer have cleared us for copyright), and showing it here lets us put a face to the names of just some of the golden stars of our team.

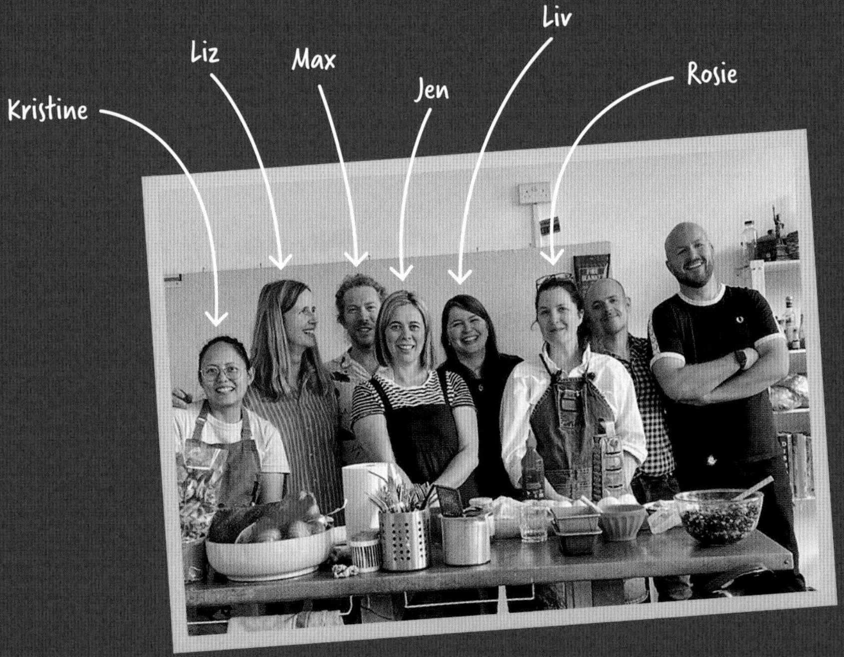

Our photographers, the hilarious and talented Liz and Max Haarala Hamilton, who not only made the food photography sparkle but also managed to take pictures of us both that didn't leave us dry-heaving into our elbows.

Liv Nightingall, our wonderful new project editor, whose ability to be patient, kind and polite in the face of our looming deadlines is second-to-none.

Rosie Reynolds and Troy Willis were tasked with taking our recipes and making them look presentable and, once again, have gone above and beyond anything we could hope for. If you were to look at those photos you'd almost believe we were cultured sorts.

Our prop stylist Jen Kay, who not only has the **best** job in the world but also does it perfectly – every dish, plate, spoon or errant budgerigar you see in this book is a result of her tireless attention to wonderful detail.

There was one very important team member missing here: the spectacular Lauren, our long-suffering Cub Wrangler, who is in charge of keeping us on the relatively straight and narrow and never fails to be a cheery presence!

There's so many others, of course: there's Abi at Hart Design, who – as you might guess – designed how the book looks. There's also our copyeditor Annie Lee, who has perfectly edited every word of our last four books and learned some exciting and terrifying terminology as she goes. Honestly, you should see the stuff that has to be cut out! There's our long-suffering publicist Becca, who tries to wrangle us into doing media despite us having faces for radio, and even then only switched off and thrown in a river. It is the terrific Kerry Torrens you have to thank for her careful wrangling of our calorie counts and sensible, welcome suggestions for tinkering. To name everyone else would take forever, but know this: every single soul we have spent time with when we travel to our publishers has been just a treasure.

It really is a joy unbound to be among such dedicated professionals and it goes without saying, we love them all. Without them and our wider team, we'd still be two coarse Northern scruffs forgetting to update their blog.

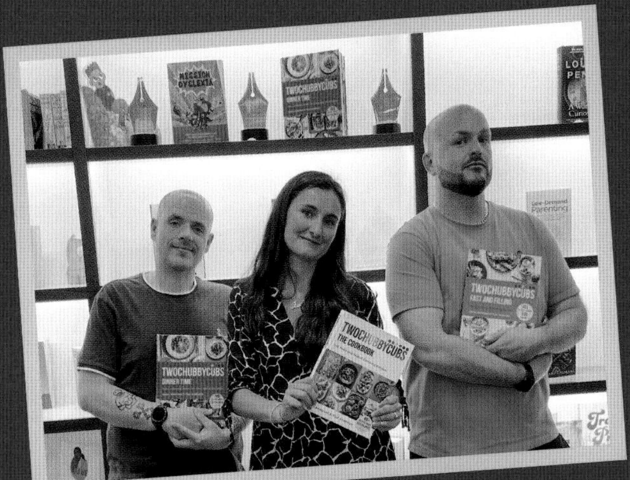

A catch-up meeting with our wonderful Lauren always makes us smile, although someone tell our faces that

Finally, as ever, the biggest thank you is saved for you. Yes, you, sitting there acting like butter wouldn't melt. Without you, what would we be? That you enjoy our content so much you've bought, borrowed or shoplifted our book never ceases to amaze us. You'd think at four books in we might become complacent, but good heavens no – you're the most important cog in our machine. We can only hope that the meals we suggest bring you comfort and that the endless nattering creates a smile. It's what we do it for. Well, that and keeping Goomba in expensive daycare.

Until we meet again, with love and endless pride in a time where both feel more vital than ever,

James and Paul

x

DOROTHY "LEGEND" BARRON

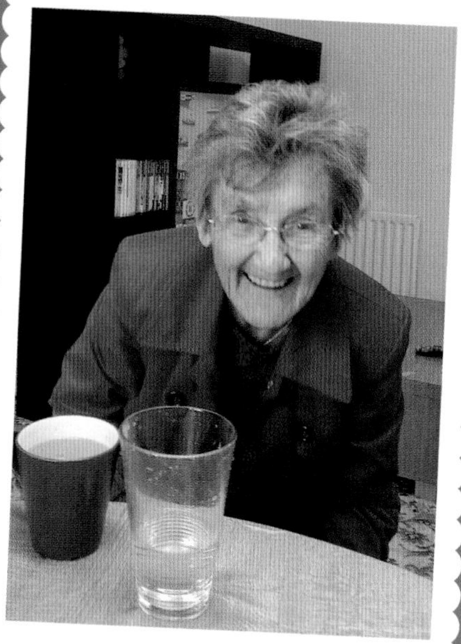

THE ABSOLUTE BEST NANA ANYONE COULD EVER HOPE FOR
ALWAYS IN OUR HEARTS, THANKS TO ALL THE BUTTER AND SALT YOU USED TO FEED US
JAMES & PAUL X

Oh, missing the lovely sickly-sweet dedications Paul and I usually leave for each other? Listen, there's only so many superlatives we can use in these books to illustrate our love for one another, so we came up with a limerick each:

There once was a munchkin called Paul,
Whose height barely mattered at all,
He stood up on one leg,
And out shot an egg,
Laying waste to his stolen food haul.

(That's one for those who have been with us since the beginning.)

There exists a young wonder named Jamie
Whose appendage is especially gamey
But luckily I'm accustomed
To him as my husband
Which works because I am a gay, me.

Yeah, see, you judge us, but this is why we write cookery books!

First published in Great Britain in 2023 by Yellow Kite
An imprint of Hodder & Stoughton
An Hachette UK Company

1

Copyright © James and Paul Anderson 2023
Photography by Liz and Max Haarala Hamilton © Hodder and Stoughton 2023, except pages 12, 13, 17 (top and middle) © James and Paul Anderson 2023, page 17 (bottom) © Darren Etherington 2023, page 18 (top and bottom) © Chris Welch 2023, page 18 (middle) © Andrew Sims 2023, page 253 © Coco Haarala Hamilton and page 254 © Lauren Whelan 2023

The right of James and Paul Anderson to be identified as the Author of the Work has been asserted by them in accordance with the Copyright, Designs and Patents Act 1988. They've got a pretty mean dog too, so consider yourself warned...

All rights reserved. No part of this publication may be reproduced, stored in a retrieval system, or transmitted, in any form or by any means without the prior written permission of the publisher, nor be otherwise circulated in any form of binding or cover other than that in which it is published and without a similar condition being imposed on the subsequent purchaser.

A CIP catalogue record for this title is available from the British Library

Hardback ISBN 978 1 399 70197 6
eBook ISBN 978 1 399 70198 3

Publisher: Lauren Whelan
Senior Project Editor: Liv Nightingall
Copyeditor: Annie Lee
Nutritionist: Kerry Torrens
Designer: Hart Studio
Photography: Liz and Max Haarala Hamilton
Food Stylists: Rosie Reynolds and Troy Willis
Prop Stylist: Jen Kay
Senior Production Controller: Matt Everett

Colour origination by Alta Image London
Printed and bound in Italy by Lego SpA

Hodder & Stoughton policy is to use papers that are natural, renewable and recyclable products and made from wood grown in sustainable forests. The logging and manufacturing processes are expected to conform to the environmental regulations of the country of origin.

Yellow Kite
Hodder & Stoughton Ltd
Carmelite House
50 Victoria Embankment
London
EC4Y 0DZ

www.yellowkitebooks.co.uk
www.hodder.co.uk

Not Milquetoast Milky Toast: *whisk 100g (3½oz) of sugar into 600ml (20fl oz) of milk together with a pinch of cinnamon and a drop or two of vanilla, and warm through. Toast some white bread, tear into chunks, and pour the milk on top. Not good for the diet, but a victory breakfast none the less.*

<u>*Notes*</u>

The information and references contained herein are for informational purposes only. They are designed to support, not replace, any ongoing medical advice given by a healthcare professional and should not be construed as the giving of medical advice nor relied upon as a basis for any decision or action.

Readers should consult their doctor before altering their diet, particularly if they are on a set diet prescribed by their doctor or dietician.

The calorie count for each recipe is an estimate only and may vary depending on the brand of ingredients used, and due to the natural biological variations in the composition of foods such as meat, fish, fruit and vegetables. It does not include the nutritional content of garnishes or any optional accompaniments recommended for taste/serving in the ingredients list.

Where not specified, ingredients are analysed as average or medium, not small or large. Eggs are medium, butter is unsalted and milk is semi-skimmed unless otherwise stated. All vegetables are washed.